AF731817

Concise Medical Dictionary

Gurjeet Ahuja

PEEPEE
PUBLISHERS AND DISTRIBUTORS (P) Ltd.

Concise Medical Dictionary

Published by:
Pawaninder P. Vij & Anupam Vij
Peepee Publishers and Distributors (P) Ltd.
Head Office: 160, Shakti Vihar, Pitam Pura, Delhi-110 034
Correspondence Address:
7/31, Ansari Road, Darya Ganj, New Delhi - 110002 (India)
Ph: 41512412, 9811156083
e-mail: peepee160@yahoo.co.in
peepee160@gmail.com
www.peepeepub.com

© 2023 Peepee Publishers and Distributors (P) Ltd.

All rights reserved

No part of this publication may be reproduced or transmitted in any form or by any means, electronic, mechanical, photocopy, recording, translated, or any information storage and retrieval system, without permission in writing from the publisher.

This book has been published in good faith that the material provided by authors/contributors is original. Every effort is made to ensure accuracy of material, but publisher and printer will not be held responsible for any inadvertent errors. In case of any dispute, all legal matters to be settled under Delhi jurisdiction only.

ISBN 978-81-8445-299-0

Preface

It can be challenging for students to navigate the various medical dictionaries available in the market and find one that meets their needs. The size of a medical dictionary does not necessarily reflect its usefulness or accuracy. It is essential to consider the credibility and authority of the source and the intended audience for the dictionary.

A good medical dictionary should provide concise and accurate definitions of medical terms and concepts, along with relevant examples and references. It should be easy to use, with clear organization and cross-referencing. Additionally, it should be updated regularly to reflect new advances in medicine and changes in terminology. This will help ensure that the information provided remains accurate and up-to-date, which is essential in the fast-paced field of healthcare.

Students can also consider using online resources such as medical databases, online medical dictionaries, and medical search engines to supplement their learning. These resources can provide more information and can often be searched using keywords, making them more efficient to use than traditional print dictionaries.

That sounds like a great initiative to bridge the gap and provide a useful resource for students and professionals in the medical field. It's important to provide concise and accurate information in a user-friendly format that is easy to navigate and understand. Including commonly used medical terms and pharmaceutical products will make the dictionary relevant and useful for its intended audience.

Gurjeet Ahuja

Contents

A

A symbol for accommodation. ***First*** item to denote in any medical enumeration; Human blood type containing A antigen; Adult motion picture certificate – A movie

A. An age of achievement

A_2 symbol for heart sound produced in **aortic** area, *heard by auscultating by stethoscope*

Å symbol for **angstrom**. *a unit of a physical measure.*

a *an indefinitive* article such as a liver, a spleen, a bone, a muscle and so on; Medical prefixing to denote **opposite of normal** such as apraxia meaning mind blindness or object blindness, a condition in which there is a lack of apprehension of the trueness of a thing; atony meaning absence of normal tone etc.,

a. abbreviation for L. ***an'num*** meaning year, *a'qua meaning* water, and *arteria meaning* artery. Total acidity is denoted by **a.**

a- a prefix denoting separation, or away from. Common word a'peks means away from the base i.e., the top of a conical part

a symbol for **acceleration** and activity . It denotes intensification, denotes intensified pulse, denotes intensified respiration

α alpha, the first letter of the Greek alphabet; shown to represent the heavy chain of IgA and the alpha chain of hemoglobin.

α- a prefix designating part of a chemical name ; the carbon atom adjacent to the principal functional group, e.g., α-amino acids (first of a series of isomeric compound), succeeding letters, β, γ, δ, etc., being used to designate succeeding carbon atoms in the chain; the specific rotation of an optically active substance, e.g., α-D-glucose; the orientation of an exocyclic atom or group, e.g., 3α-hydroxy-5α-androstan-17-one (androsterone); a plasma protein migrating with the α band (subdivided into α_1 and α_2 bands) in protein electrophoresis, e.g., α-fetoprotein; one in a series of related chemical compounds, particularly a series of stereoisomeric, isomeric, polymeric or allotropic forms, e.g., α-carotene; and one in a group of related entities, e.g., α-ray. For compounds prefixed with the symbol α—such as alphanaphthol, alphatocopherol, alpha-leucocyte, alphadinitrophenol are common in organic chemistry.

AA Denotes achievement age; Alcoholics Anonymous; amino acid. Meant '**of each**' in doctor's prescription writing.

aa. Abbreviation for **arteries**. Denote the vessels that carry blood away from the heart except coronary arteries

AAA Abbreviation for American Association of Anatomists. Amateur Athletic Association

AAAS Abbreviation for American Association for the Advancement of Science.

AABB Abbreviation for American Association of Blood Banks.

AACP Abbreviation for American Academy of Child Psychiatry.

AAE Abbreviation for American Association of Endocrinologists

AAFP Abbreviation for American Academy of Family Physicians.

AAMD Abbreviation for American Association on Mental Deficiency.

AAP Abbreviation for American Academy of Pediatrics.

Aaron's sign In appendicitis pressure over McBurney's point produces pain in precordial region or in epigastric region

AAV Abbreviation for Adeno Associated Virus

AB abbreviation for L. *Artium Baccalaureus,* **B**achelor of Arts. Human **blood type** under Landsteiner's ABO blood grouping which contains both A antigen and B antigen

Ab abbreviation for **Antibody**. Globulin portion of the serum is modified which reacts specifically both in vivo and in vitro. Common antibodies known are – agglutinins, antitoxins, haemolysins, opsonins and precipitins

ab Latin preposition meaning ***from.*** In Medicine under etymologies usage is in 'departing from a rule' as in ab-normal psychology, ab-normal behaviour, ab-normal position of organs

ab- prefix meaning ***away from,*** very common adjective form in medicine is aberrant, It adds to meaning such as eccentric, irregular, anomalous and insane,

abacterial Free from bacteria. No contamination in case of non living items in the universe; No infection in case of animate and human beings; Very specific for material used in surgical intervention which are sterilised and autoclaved and made free from bacteria ; Medical field is engaged in a bacterial procedures through a) Hospital disinfection procedures b) Operation Theatre disinfection procedures and c) Ship disinfection procedures

Abadie's sign In case of locomotor ataxia insensibility of the Achilles tendon to pressure is seen. Spasm of levator palpebrae superioris muscle occurs in case of Exophthalmic goiter

abaptiston An instrument which is designed to remove a small circular disc of skull bone in case of sub dural haematoma, extra dural haematoma which occur in concussion injury; depth of entry of this instrument is designed in such a way that it will not produce injury to brain tissue during surgical intervention.

abarognosis One who cannot perceive the weight sense; Lesions of posterior roots are known to cause loss of weight sense which is due to loss of Proprioceptive sensation from muscles, joints and toes

abarthrosis Denotes abnormal movements of joints; as in case of syphilitic joints free pivot like mobility of knee joint is seen; It is freely movable articulation of a joint; Usually the meaning is abnormal movement; Movement of a joint which cannot occur in a normal physiological condition of a person.

abarticular That which is not connected with a joint, Lesion not in the joint but is in other sites away from a joint, On examination it is found that the joint is free and not affected by pathology

abarticulation End of the bone within the synovial capsule is separated from natural attachment with other bones. Freely movable joint in which articular surface of bones are covered with cartilage, are connected with ligaments and are lined with synovial membranes

abasia Not able to walk owing to defective coordination in muscles that are Neurogenic in nature.

abasic Related with inability to stand without support.

abate lessen as in the case of pain after palliative treatment, decrease in intensity or in number as in the case of mosquito control with residual insecticide; also a proprietary name for an insecticide

abatement decrease in the severity of a pain or a symptom.

abbau 1. Breakdown of chemical substances. 2. products of catabolism

Abbe's condenser Lens attachment beneath the microscope for good illumination.

Abbe's operation Side to side or lateral anastomosis of intestine with the help of rings of cat gut.

Abbocillin-DC Commercial trademark for preparations of procaine penicillin G.

Abbott's method Treatment method adopted for scoliosis by pulling and counters puling on the spinal column.

Abbott-Miller tube A soluble channel intestinal tube used in the diagnosis and treatment of intestinal obstruction.

Abbott-Rawson tube Double barrel Gastro Enterostomy tube.

ABCD therapy In cancer therapy four drugs used in sequential manner are **A**driamycin, **B**leomycin, **C**CNU (lomustine) and **D**acarbazine.

abciximab It is an antithrombotic used in percutaneous transluminal coronary angioplasty; by I V infusion.

Abdomen It is that portion of the body which lies between the thorax and the pelvis; it contains a cavity separated by the diaphragm from the thoracic cavity above, and by the plane of the pelvic inlet from the pelvic cavity below, and lined with a serous membrane, the peritoneum which contains the abdominal viscera. Colloquially it is called belly. Anatomically there are 9 regions of abdomen. They are: right hypochondriac, epigastric, left hypochondriac, right lateral, umbilical, left lateral, right inguinal, pubic, and left inguinal..

Abdominal That which is related to abdomen.

Abdomino Combining form which denotes **relationship to the abdomen**.

abdominocentesis Paracentesis of the abdominal cavity..

abdominocystic Related to abdomen and gall bladder .

abdominogenital Related to abdomen and genital organs

abdominohysterectomy Surgical removal of uterus with its appendages through abdominal route.

abdominohysterotomy Surgical incision made on uterus through abdominal route.

Abdominoscopy Visualisation of abdominal organs through laparoscopy

Abdominoscrotal Pertaining to the abdomen and scrotum.

Abdominovaginal Related to the abdomen and the vagina.

abdominovesical Related to abdomen and urinary bladder.

abducens Latin adjective used in names of structures such as a nerve which serves to abduct a part.

abduct to draw away from the median plane, abduction

abduction It is the state of being abducted.

ABE Abbreviation for **A**cute **B**acterial **E**ndocarditis.

Abelcet Commercial trademark for amphotericin B antibiotics

abembryonic denotes away from the embryo.

Abernethy's fascia Fascia lying over the external iliac artery.

aberrant deviating from the normal course.

aberration deviation from the normal course, unequal refraction in case of eye, aberrant electrical impulse in the heart.

abetalipoproteinemia It is an autosomal recessive disorder of lipoprotein metabolism. It is characterized by hypocholesterolemia, progressive ataxic neuropathy, pigmentary retinal degeneration and deficiency of fat-soluble vitamins.

ABG Abbreviation for **A**rterial **B**lood **G**ases.

abiatrophy loss of vitality or tissue substance very early in young age.

abient That which respond to a stimulus.

Abies Belong to firs group of plants which yield Canada Balsam.

abietic acid This is an acid resin that is used in the production of soaps and varnishes.

abiogenesis spontaneous generation of life from the non living.

abiogenetic That which is related to spontaneous generation.

abiosis No sign of life or absence of life.

abiotic Not capable of living; That which is an antagonistic to life.

abiotrophy Referrable to degenerative disease Huntington's chorea.

abirritant A soothing agent. An agent that relieves irritation.

abirritation No response to stimulation.

abirritative soothing.
ablactation Slow and over a period cessation of breast milk giving by the mother to the young one.
ablate remove by cutting; extirpation
ablatio detachment or separation.
ablation detachment, separation
ablepharous pertaining to eye without eyelid.
abluent A cleansing agent.
abluminal directed away from the lumen of a tubular structure.
ablution the act of cleansing by the application of water by the hand.
ablutomania A symptom of Obsessive compulsive neurosis. A compulsion to clean unnecessarily rather that necessarilily.
abmortal Medical instruments with electric gadgets are kept away from injured tissue to overcome further trauma.
ABMT Abbreviation for **A**utologous **B**one **M**arrow **T**ransplantation.
abnormal That which is not normal as far as their structure, position, condition or behaviour con-cerned.
abnormality That which is abnormal Refers to birth defects.
abnormity Defects or abnormalities in an individual.
abomasotomy Surgical removal of 4th stomach or a ruminant
abomasum the fourth stomach of a ruminant animal which contain gastric glands for digestion.
aboral away from other than oral route
aboriginal people who are native to the place inhabited.
abort miscarriage before the fetus is viable or abortion, Not allowed to develop.
abortifacient That which causes abortion.
abortion Premature expulsion from the uterus of the products of conception embryo or a nonviable fetus. Uterine contractions leads to uterine hemorrhage, dilatation of the cervix, and expulsion of the products of conception.
abortionist The person usually qualified who performs abortions.
abortive Effecting an abortion; abortifacient. In case of illness, cutting short the course of a disease.
abortus This refers to a fetus weighing less than 500 gm. (17 oz.) or which is less than 20 completed weeks' gestational age at the time of expulsion.
abouchement The process of getting into a big vessel by a small tributary.
ABP Abbreviation for **A**rterial **B**lood **P**resure.
abrachia A birth defect where arms are not developed.
abrachius A person without arms.
abrade to peel away the external covering of a part
Abrams' heart reflex When chest wall is stimulated, there is reflex contraction of the lung.
abrasion the structural changes of skin or teeth over the age or through mechanical processes. Denuded of skin or mucous membrane by abnormal mechanical process.
abrasive That which causes abrasion.
abrasor Any instrument that is used for abrasion.
abreaction Reliving of an experience or the repressed emotions which usually is by resulting in an insight.
Abrikosov's tumor Name given to Myoblastoma
abrism a plant poisoning caused by consumption of local bean which is the jequirity bean found in subtropical Asia and the Americas.
abruptio status of detachment
abs- a prefix used in words like **abs**ence, **abs**cissa, **abs**orb, **abs**cess etc.,
abscess collection of pus in tissues, organs, or spaces.
abscise to remove by cutting as in case of tissue, bone or an organ in surgical excision.
abscissa In two dimentional structure or diagram, abscissa constitute the horizontal data entered in the diagram.
abscission originally from the root word scindere which means removal by cutting.
abscopal When Cobalt therapy is done on a tissue as a part of treatment of cancer, effect of Cobalt irradiation can burn adjacent tissues. This phenomenon is called abscopal which pertains to the effect on nonirradiated tissue
absence One of the stage of fits which is manifested in temporary loss of consciousness, absence can also occur in hysteria patients.
abs. feb. Abbreviation for L. ***absen'te feb're,*** to denote 'Fever is absent'.
absinthe Crude alcohol or toddy from plant which when consumed is known to cause loss of vision due to optic neuritis or/and death due to neurotoxin.
absinthium Name of the plant which yield toddy containing crude alcohol. Particularly it refers to leaves and flowering top of the plant.
absolute Not relative. Not combined but full in it's content such as absolute alcohol,
absorb When a substance gets entry into the skin or tissue through semipermeable membrane. When radiation ion gets entered into tissue and gets deposited within it without any clinical manifestations
absorbefacient An agent that causes or that promotes absorption. It can be an adjuvant in medicine, which helps in absorption of indented medication.
absorbent Agent which can get incorporated in another. Any tissue, which is involved in the process of absorption,
absorption It is used in case of absorption through the skin, through intestine or through kidney tubules where a substance is absorbed across tissues. Getting into head through attention.

absorptive That which is related with absorption

abstergent Substance used for surface cleaning, Iodine paint in surgery.

abstinence Total control in refraining from food, drug or sex.

abstract To write the summary of an article, of a book or of a research. Consolidated view of clinical findings.

abstraction To take away one ingredient from a chemical compound.

abterminal This is the expression for the current flowing periphery to the centre. Electrical current in muscle is an abterminal in nature.

abulia A state of mind where will power is absent and the person cannot take decision.

abulic Condition of a person when he or she cannot take decision.

abuse wrong use or misuse, particularly excessive use of anything.

abut to touch or border upon.

abutment When abutting occurs; When a structure sustains pressure; Abutment in case of a denture is a common expression.

ABVD It is an abbreviation for the drug regimen in Hodgkin's disease. This consists of the following:

- **A**driamycin
- **B**leomycin
- **V**inblastine
- **D**acarbazine

a.c. Abbreviation for Before Meals in Pharmacy prescription. [L]. *ante cibum,* before meals.

ACA Abbreviation for **A**merican **C**ollege of **A**ngiology

Acacia Common term for African tree, which yield gum. They belong to family Leguminosae in plant kingdom. Acacia trees in India and Burma yield catechu. South African plants yield cape gum. Acacia leaves world over has been known to cause to poisoning in livestock.

acalculia When a person is unable to do simple arithmetical calculation.

acampsia When a person cannot move or bend a joint.

acantha It refers to thorn like projection of vertebra.

acanthamebiasis Parasitic infection and infestation by Acanthamoeba species of amoeba which causes brain infection (encephalitis) and infection and inflammation of retina (keratitis)

acanthesthesia Feeling of a sharp point pressure on the body or on the part of the body which actually is not so. It is a false sensory perception.

acanthion Small thorny projection at anterior nasal spine.

acantho That which is related to spine or thorn like projection.

Acanthocephala They come under Phylum Nemathelminthes which have hooks in their head end for the purpose of attachment to the host.

acanthocephaliasis Intestinal parasitism with Nemathelminthes worms causing symptoms of infestation.

Acanthocheilonema They belong to group of filaria worm under nematodes.

acanthocyte Erythrocytes with irregular projections a common manifestation in malnutrition.

acanthocytosis When there are plenty of acanthocytes in the blood.

acantholysis This is seen in case of cellular degeneration process where there is disruption of intercellular connections.

acantholytic That which is related with acanthlysis.

acanthoma This is the term used for squamous cell carcinoma.

acanthopelvis a pelvis with a very sharp and prominent pubic crest

Acanthophis They are snakes found in Australia and New Guinea, which are poisonous snakes.

acanthosis hyperplasia of the skin.

acanthotic That which is marked by acanthosis.

acarbia It is a clinical condition where bicarbonate level in the blood is lowered.

acarbose This is used in the treatment of NIDD (Non Insulin Dependent Diabetes) as antihypoglycaemic agent. Chemically it is an α-glucosidase inhibitor

acardia congenital absence of the heart in a person.

acardiac Colloquially 'a cruel person'; Anatomically it refers to a person without a developed heart.

acardius It is birth defect state where heart is not formed during embryogenesis. This defect is common in one of the twin in twin pregnancy. Acardia is invariably is associated with other birth defects also.

acari It refers to many mites.

acarian That which is related to mites

acariasis Infested with mites

acaricide A chemotherapeutic agent used to kill or destroy mites. In Pharmacology it is called Scabicidal drug.

Acaridae Acarina group of mites that cause skin manifestations causing known clinicians such as grocers' itch, copra itch and vanillism.

Acarina This refers to class Arachnida including ticks and mites.

acaro That which is related with mites.

acarodermatitis Skin lesion in the form of inflammation of the skin due to mites.

acaroid That which resembles a mite.

acarologist An Entomology consultant who is specialised in the study of mites.

acarology The scientific study of mites and ticks.

acarophobia Fear for mites under the skin which is a common psychological disturbances in women.

acarotoxic Chemicals that destroys mites and are used as scabicides.

Acartomyia This refers to the group of mosquitoes that belong to Culex, Aedes and monsonoides. They are responsible for the spread of known communicable diseases.

Acarus They are ectoparacytes causing itch and colloquially called itch mite.

ACAT Abbreviation for **A**cyl **C**oA Cholesterol **A**cyl **T**ransferase.

acatalasia This is a genetic disease which is an autosomal recessive in nature. Geographical distribution is Japan and Switzerland. Clinically it is called Takahara's disease. Main clinical manifes-tations are oral gangrene and oral ulcers.

acathectic That which is related to or pertaining to or characterized by acathexia.

acathexia When the body cannot retain bodily secretions.

acathexis No attachment with social feelings. No emotion on any objects,

acaudate Animal that do not have tail or lacking a tail.

ACC Abbreviation for **A**merican **C**ollege of **C**ardiology

Acc Abbreviation for accommodation.

accelerant A substance which acts as a catalyst. A chemical, which stimulates and hastens the action of another in a chemical reaction.

acceleration When a thing gets intensified, anything that quickens from its normal dictum such as pulse rate, respiratory rate or velocity in the movement of a substance.

accelerator an agent which helps to increase the rate at which a substance acts or at which some reaction occurs. When a nerve or a muscle bring about hastening of a function,

accelerin This is a blood coagulation factor and is called factor VI in the description of haematology.

accentuation This refers to raised loudness of extra sounds like murmur in the heart. Heart sound and lung sound intensification are described as accentuation.

access a means of approaching something.

accessiflexor It refers to any supplementary or access-ory flexor muscle.

accessorius In naming anatomical structures which serve or perform supplementary functions in the body.

accessory Any anatomical structure which help in performing more important function in the body such as accessory nerve.

accident This refers, usually to a traffic accident where an unforeseen event can occur which are described as injury. This also can mean rare complications of a disease or of an operation.

accidentalism This is a theory in medical science which states the illness is by accidental situations and the changes are accidental changes from physiological status that can be cured by euthenics i.e., by changing external conditions. Accidentalism leads to symptomatic treatment of illness rather than going on to eitiological pathological basis.

accident prone One who is vulnerable to accidents owing to many psychological factors that lead to accident.

acclimatation Physiological adjustment to varied physical environment. Synonym acclimation, acclimatisation.

accommodation Latin word meaning to get adjusted to as in the case of lens of the eye accommodation for vision either for near vision or for distant vision.

accommodative That which is related to the condition called accommodation.

accomplice It is a French word denoting to a pathogen which is found accompanied with the true infective agent and cause severe infection.

accouchement This is French word which denotes the process of child-birth which is colloquially called delivery.

accoucheur One who conducts the delivery who is she or he. In allopathy he/she is called Obstetrician.

accoucheuse a lady who is trained in midwifery and who helps in conducting delivery

ACCP Abbreviation for **A**merican College of **C**hest Physicians.

accretio Latin root word meaning adhesion which is not normal, Anatomical parts which are separate anatomically gets fused.

accretion The process of adhesion of two parts which are anatomically different.

accuracy This refers to precision in health science where we describe the closeness of an expecte value to the true value. The value which is free of bias in research work.

ACD It is the abbreviation for **A**cid **C**itrate **D**extrose.

ACE It is the abbreviation for **A**ngiotensin **C**onverting **E**nzyme.

acebutolol This is a Beta adrenergic blocking agent which shows sympathomimetic activity in the body. Pharmacological effect is similar to the common drug Propranolol.

aceclidine Pharmacologically it is similar to Pilocarpine. Common use is in the treatment of Glaucoma to reduce intraocular tension.

acedapsone It is Dapsone derivative containing two acetyl groups. Chemically it is Diacetyl Diamino Diphenyl Sulphone used in the treatment of Leprosy.

acellular That which do not contain cells or that which is not made of cells.

acelomate Organisms which do not have body cavity.

acenesthesia The sense is lost with regard to physical existence and/or to the physiological function of an organ.

acenocoumarol It is a synthetic anticoagulant orally given that show rapid onset of action.

acentric A Greek word which denotes that a thing is not located in the center. Very common term used in genetics with respect to the chromosomes.

ACEP **A**merican **C**ollege of **E**mergency **P**hysicians.

acephalia Condition in the newborn where head is not developed, congenital absence of the head.

acephalobrachia Birth defect showing the congenital absence of the head and arms.

acephalobrachius a fetus showing the birth defect of congenital absence of the head and the arms.

acephalochiria Head and hands are absent since birth

acephalochirus Condition of a fetus which exhibits absence of head and hands.

acephalogastria When head, thorax and upper abdomen are absent in a fetus which is due to failure of embryogenesis. Such fetus is called acephalogaster.

acephalopodia congenital absence of the head and feet in a fetus. Such fetus is called acephalopodius.

acephalostomia No head in a fetus but possess a sort of mouth on superior aspect of body part. Such fetus is called acephalostomus.

acephalothoracia congenital absence of the head and thorax in a fetus which is called acephalothorus.

acephalous headless fetus

acepromazine maleate It is a tranquilliser used in veterinary science for immobilisation of elephants, hippos, tigers and lions.

acerola It is popularly called Barbados cherry and is rich in vitamin C. Nutritional value of vitamin C is about 1700 mg per 100 grams of fruits. It has value in therapeutic diet for cases of allergy to citrous fruits.

acetabula Two cup shaped cavity on either side of pelvis, lateral to the os coxae to which head of the thigh bone joins.

acetabular That which is related with acetabulum

acetabulectomy Surgical excision of the acetabulum.

acetabuloplasty Re constructive surgery done on the acetabulum

acetabulum Singular form of Acetabula From Latin word meaning vinegar holding cup like structure.

acetaldehyde It is a chemical liquid which has flammable characterstics and has pungent odour. This acetaldehyde is used in the preparation of acetic acid, some of the known flavours and some of the known perfumes. It is irritant to mucous membrane.

acetamide It is crystal in nature and has no colour that are used in chemistry as solvent.

acetaminophen It is very common preparation in the market in the pharmacological preparation as Para Acetyl Amino Phenol or PARACETAMOL that is used as antipyretic. It has very weak anti inflammatory effect on the body. Oral preparation is very common in clinical practice.

acetanilid Used to be common ingredient in APC. But is not commonly used due to its toxicity. Acetaminophen and phenacetin are para aminophenol derivatives.

acetarsone It is an Arsenical preparation used in amoebiasis, Ulcerative gingivitis, TV infection. This is commonly given to dogs as anthelmintic.

acetate It is the salt of acetic acid.

acetate–CoA ligase This is responsible in the formation of Acetyl Co enzyme in the body. This enzyme is present in Mitochondria of the cell which help the formation of acetyl coenzyme A from Acetate and coenzyme A.

acetazolamide This is a carbonic anhydrase inhibitor. Acetazolamide has many clinical used such as:

- Urinary alkaliser
- Glaucoma
- Epilepsy
- Acute mountain sickness

Preparations for oral, intra muscular and intra venous administration are available.

Acetest This is qualitative test for the detection of acetone in urine by putting a drop of urine on the tablet. Appearance of purple tint is indicative of presence of acetone in urine.

The tablet contains a) Sodium nitroprusside, b) Aminoacetic acid, c) Disodium phosphate and d) lactose.

Deep purple indicates heavy concentration of acetone in urine.

acetic That which is related to vinegar or acid vinegar which is sour.

acetic acid Chemically it is CH_3COOH which is the component of vinegar. It is used as solvent in the preparation of topical solution that contains nearly 35 to 40 percent of acetic acid.

acetin It is a glyceryl acetate which is commonly used in tanning, as food additive and as dye solvent.

aceto- This word is used when an acetyl radical or acetic acid molecule is present in a chemical. Always it is seen as a prefix to denot the presence of the acetyl radical

acetoacetate This is a salt acetoacetic acid.

acetoacetic acid This is a ketone body that is produced in liver. It's presence in blood or urine in excess indicate KETOSIS.

acetoacetyl-CoA reductase This an enzyme of the oxidoreductase class that catalyzes the reduction of 3-ketoacyl coenzyme A

acetoacetyl coenzyme A This is a thioester of acetoacetic acid and coenzyme A. It is an important metabolic intermediate in the oxidation of fatty acids. This is commonly referred to as Acetoacetyl Co A in the citric acid cycle in nervous tissue metabolism. This is also is a precursor of Cholesterol.

Acetobacter A gram-negative, aerobic, rod-shaped bacteria of the family Acetobacteraceae that produce acid and are present in fruits and beverages.

Acetobacteraceae This a family of gram-negative, aerobic, ellipsoidal to rod-shaped bacteria.

acetohexamide This belongs to Sulfonylurea compound which has the chemotherapeutic effect as Hypoglycaemic agent in Type 2 Diabetes mellitus. It is an effective oral hypoglycaemic agent.

acetohydroxamic acid This is used as drug in the treatment of urinary tract infection caused by urease producing bacteria. It is effective as oral drug in UTI.

acetolysis It is the decomposition of an organic compound using acetic acid

acetonaphthone This is a Naphthalene derivative with acetyl compound. This has the effect of Bactricide particularly as antitubercular agent. One of the isomer of acetonaphthone is used as mosquito repellent.

acetonation This is the chemical process of combination with acetone.

acetone Acetone is produced as ketone body in ketoacedosis. This is used in pharmacy as solvent. In a concentration of 80 percent it acts as an antiseptic

acetonemia This is a clinical condition where high level of acetone and acetic acid gets accumulates in blood producing pathological conditions.

acetonuria This is clinical condition where acetone is high in urine and clinically it is called ketonuria.

acetophenazine maleate It is a phenothiazine compound orally administered as an antipsychotic

acetosulfone sodium A derivative of dapsone having actions similar to Dapsone as leprostatic in the treatment of lepsory.

acetous That which produces acetic acid.

acetpyrogall This is used as a topical keratolytic.

acetrizoate A radiographic contrast medium, used in hysterosalpingography.

acetyl Depicts the monovalent radical, CH_3CO—.

acetylase This refers to Acetyltransferase an enzyme that catalyzes the addition or removal of an acetyl group

acetylation It is the chemical process where an acetyl group is introduced to an organic compound.

acetylcholine Being cholinergic agonist it is helpful in the neurotransmission at myoneural junction of striated nuscles. It gets rapidly hydrolysed and has diffuse action and thus has few therapeutic action.

acetylcholinesterase This is present in gray matter of nervous tissue, in RBC and in motor endplate of skeletal muscle. It is popularly called as Choline esterase I. It is abbreviated as AChE.

acetyl-CoA *C*-acetyltransferase Acetyl Co A C-acetyltransferase catalyzes the synthesis of acetoacetyl coenzyme A

acetyl-CoA carboxylase This is a biotin-containing enzyme that catalyzes the carboxylation of acetyl coenzyme A

acetyl coenzyme A This is a precursor of steroids. Acetyl coenzyme A is a thioester of coenzyme A and acetic acid. The coenzyme A derives the acetyl group from fatty acids and amino acids.

acetyldigitoxin This is obtained from degitoxin compound and has the same effect as digitalis. It is administered orally.

acetylene This is an explosive volatile and colourless gas belongs to unsaturated hydrocarbon alkyne group.

acetyleugenol This is one of the constituent of clove oil comes under essential oil.

α-*N*-acetylgalactosaminidase This is hexosaminidase enzyme present in lysosome. In case of it's deficienency, it produces Infantile Neuroaxonal Dystrophy which is an autosomal recessive trait.

***N*-acetylglucosamine-6-sulfatase** This is the enzyme of lysosome that has the catalytic action on cleavage group sulphate groups as a chemical degradation process. The deficiency of this enzyme is associated with the Sanfilippo Syndrome which is an autosomal recessive trait.

β-*N*-acetylhexosaminidase This is responsible for degradation of gangliosides and is found to be related with gangliosidosis and Tay-Sachs disease. In short form it is called Hexosaminidase

acetylization This refers to the chain of reaction called acetylation.

***N*-acetylmuramic acid** This is the constituent of bacterial cell wall and is polysaccharide in nature.

***N*-acetylneuraminic acid** Neuraminic acid is amino sugar acid that is found in glycoproteins and polysaccharides.

acetylsalicylic acid Acetyl salicylic acid is chemically ASPIRIN. It is commonly abbreviated as ASA i.e., **A**cetyl **S**alicylic **A**cid.

acetylsulfadiazine When sulfadiazine is excreted in urine that is identified by dark green crystalline the form and they are acetylsulphadiazine.

acetylsulfaguanidine This is urinary excretory form that is identified by their appearance of oblong crystalline plates; Sulfaguanidine is excreted in urine in the form of acetyl sulfonyl chloride.

acetylsulfathiazole Urinary excretion of thiazole is in the form of n-acetyl sulfathiazole that is identified by its sheaves of wheat crystals form.

acetyltributyl citrate This is produced by acetylation of citric acid. The main use of this is as a plasticizer.

ACG Abbreviation for **A**merican **C**ollege of **G**astroenterology

ACHA Abbreviation for **A**merican **C**ollege of **H**ospital **A**dministrators.

achalasia When Gastro Oesophageal sphincter fails to relax with swallowing, there may not be proper peristaltic activity of oesophagus that can produce CARDIOSPASM, a common clinical manifestation.

Achard's syndrome Described by Achard and Thiers which is described as DIABETES IN BEARDED WOMEN

ache This refers to fixed and continuous pain which is different from twinges.

acheilia Absence of lip which is always a birth defect.

acheilous One who is not having lips.

acheiria Hands are not developed in a person which is birth defect. It also refers to the feeling of absence of hands which occurs in certain clinical disorders.

acheiropodia congenital absence of hands and feet.

achillobursitis inflammation and thickening of the bursae of the Achilles tendon

achillorrhaphy Reconstructive surgery of Achilles tendon

achillotenotomy surgical division of the Achilles tendon.

achiria Touch sensation is lost where a person is unable to perceive which side of his body is touched.

achlorhydria Because of atrophy of gastric mucosa, there will not new HCl secretion even with stimulation. Clinically it is called gastric anacidity.

achlorhydric Person who is having achlorhydria.

acholia absence of secretion of bile.

acholic That which is free from bile.

acholuria Condition where bile pigment is absent in the urine.

acholuric That which is related with acholuria such as acholuric jaundice.

achondrogenesis This is clinical condition with bone Hypoplasia and short limbs and normal head and trunk. This is a hereditary disorder

achondroplasia Clinically the condition that results is achondroplastic draft where epiphyseal growth is retarted giving raise to inadequate bone formation. Children have lordosis and trident hand in additional to above defects.

achondroplastic That which is related to Achondroplasia

achordate This refers to animals which do not have notochord.

achromasia No normal pigmentation on the skin of a person. This also refers to tissue staining where there is no usual staining.

achromatic That which do not produce discolouration, Tissue that cannot stain properly,

achromatin This refers to tissue staining process where certain portion of cell like karyolymph, linin and nuclear membrane do not take up staining normally.

achromatinic pertaining to or containing achromatin.

achromatolysis Destruction or lysis of achromatin of a cell, Histological appearance of disorganisation of cell

achromatophil Opposite of chromatophil where cell do not take up the stain in staining process: If the tissue is not staining properly,

achromatophilia the property of resisting the coloring action of stains.

achromatosis There is no skin pigmentation. There is no iris pigmentation. There is no good staining of tissues in a staining process.

achromatous That which does not have color or colorless.

achromaturia The excretion of colorless urine in a person.

achromia Lack of normal color or pigmentation in the skin.

achromic That which is related to Achromia.

Achromobacter They are rod shaped flagellated bacteria found in water and in human intestine. They are associated with certain infections which are found as significant association

achromophilous Refers to tissue staining where cells do not show any affinity for stains.

Achromycin Pharmacological ingredient is tetracycline, a trade name.

achroodextrin Dextrin which is not coloured by iodine and is of low molecular weight in nature.

achylia When gastric juice do not contain HCl and pepsinogens.

achymia When the chime formation is absent

acicular Any structure which is needle shaped.

acid Acid is a chemical substance which lowers the pH by increasing the Hydrogen Ion Concentration, when a chemical substance is sour to taste, when a chemical substance turns litmus to red and when a chemical reacts with alkalis to form salts.

Other two definitions are:

a) When a substance acts as a proton donor in solution.

b) When a substance accepts a pair of electrons to form a covalent bond.

acidalbumin Allbumin that show acid in its reaction and which gets dissolved in acids.

acidemia Low pH in terms of increased Hydrogen Ion Concentration of the blood.

acid-fast This is denoted by the abbreviation AFB (**A**cid **F**ast **B**acilli) where bacteria is not readily decolorised by acid after staining (say after Z.N.Staining). Common examples are:

- Mycobacterium tuberculosis
- Mycobacterium leprae
- Nocardia species

acidic That which is related with acid or acid forming

acidifiable Substance which can be readily made acidic

acidifier Any chemical substance which can cause acidity or any substance that can increase gastric acidity.

acidify To make a substance or a chemical acid by the addition of another strong acid.

acidity This is the quality of a chemical substance which is measured by the Hydrogen Ion concentration. That which is acid or sour in nature.

acidogenic In clinical practice this refers to urine acidity if no specification is made. A substance that produce acid.

acidophil A cell or a tissue that readily stains with acid dyes. It also refers to a bacteria that can grow well in acid media.

acidophilic This refers to microorganisms that stains readily with acid dyes.

acidosis When there is increase in Hydrogen Ion Concentration or decrease in Bicarbonate content in the blood or in the body fluids pH decreases

acidotic That which is related with acidosis.

acid phosphatase It is an enzyme which is found in the liver, in bone marrow, in prostate gland and in the spleen. In laboratory practice determination of serum acid phosphatase activity is an important diagnostic test.

acidulated That which produces acid in a chemical reaction, rendered acid in reaction.

acidulous That which is acid in nature. Or that which is somewhat acid.

aciduria Any acid excess in urine such as increased glutaric acid in urine

aciduric It refers to bacteria which can withstand acid in vivo or in vitro which other bacteria cannot tolerate to thrive.

acidyl It refers to any acid radical.

Acinetobacter Neisseriaceae group of bacteria which are Gram negative paired coccobacilli that cause severe infections in man. Otherwise they are seen as normal flora in mammals including man

aciniform That which is grape like in structure and arrangement.

acinitis Infection and inflammation of the acini of a gland.

acinotubular Glands which are composed of tubular ending in the gland structure.

acinus It is singular form of acini meaning grape like or sac like anatomical structure such as that of lung, salivary gland etc.

acitretin This is Etretinate substance used in the treatment of Psoriasis as oral preparation.

acladiosis This is fungal infection of the skin which show ulceration and complications. The causative organism is Acladium. Geographical distribution is South East Asia region.

Acladium A group of fungus which cause tropical fungal infection in South East Asia.

aclasia Denotes the invasion to neibouring structure or continuity of pathology such as Multiple Exostoses.

aclasis Pathological continuity in organs.

aclastic That which is related to continuity of pathology in neibouring organs.

aclusion absence of occlusion in case of opposing tooth surfaces.

acme When patient reaches to critical stage or seen in the stage of emergency

acne Common in adult who sweat a lot and is indicated by the inflammatory changes of pilosebaceous unit. Colloquially it is called acne vulgaris.

acnegen This refers to a substance that causes acne.

acnegenic A substance which is causing or capable of producing acne.

acnemia Clinical condition where calf muscle gets atrophied.

acnitis Infection and inflammation of pilosebaceous unit on the face.

acoelomate It refers to platyhelminths which do not have body cavity.

ACOG Abbreviation for **A**merican **C**ollege of **O**bstetricians and **G**ynecologists.

aconative Lack of desire in a person who cannot act.

***cis*-aconitate** an intermediate product in Tricarboxylic acid cycle when interconversion of citrate and isocitrate occurs by dehydration process

aconitate hydratase This enzyme otherwise called Aconitase is responsible for the catalysis of citrate and isocitrate in Tricarboxylic acid cycle.

aconite Aconitic acid and related alkaloids which are poisonous substances are obtained from the root of Aconitum plant. This is known to produce Ventricular Fibrillation and Respiratory paralysis.

aconitine This is the active principle of Aconite plant which is dangerously poisonous.

aconuresis One who is not willing to urinate or clinical condition of urinary incontinence.

acoprosis There is no stool formation and intestine is free of fecal matter.

acorea absence of the pupil in the eye.

acoria Person concerned does not have sensation of satisfaction of eaten well. Appetite will not be there but dissatisfaction will be there as far as eating is concerned.

Acorus This plant belongs to family Araceae. It's rhizome is used as insect repellent and also as flavouring agent.

Acosta's disease This refers to Acute Mountain Disease.

acousma When a patient hears buzzing or ringing sounds which are fake. This is called auditory hallucination.

acousmatamnesia When a patient is unable to recall the sound or the nature of sound. Forgetfulness to sound or noice.

acoustic That which is related to sound.

acousticophobia Unwanted and uncalled for fear to external sound which is irrational in nature.

acoustics The Scientific study of the nature, occurrence and effects of sounds.

acoustogram Sound tracing through recording in the graph which is done with respect to knee joint movement to trace the sound produced while movement of the joint. Accoustogram can record the following through sound produced:

- Movement of semilunar cartilage
- Contact sound by the rubbing of articular surfaces
- Blood flow in synovia

ACP Abbreviation for **A**merican **C**ollege of **P**hysicians

acquired That which is obtained by the person from environment. That which is not genetic in origin, such as acquired immunity from getting infection.

acquisition Progressive achievement in learning which can be measured through psychological tests.

ACR Abbreviation for **A**merican **C**ollege of **R**adiology.

acral That which is related with legs or extremities. Anything that affects limbs.

acrania Birth defect involving absence of skull.

acranial Relates to the person who does not have cranium or skull.

acranius It is abnormal foetus without skull.

Acrel's ganglion Ganglion on the extensor tendons of the wrist.

Acremoniella This is a fungus belonging to class Hyphomycetes that cause lung infection

acrid pungent and that produces irritation on exposure

Acremonium This fungus is common to produce opportunistic infections among immunocompres-mised patients.

acridine Dibenzopyridine used in the synthesis of acridine dyes and antiseptics.

acriflavine It is a topical antiseptic for external application on skin and mucous membrane.

acr(o)- a combining form denoting relation to an extremity, top, or summit, or to an extreme.

acroagnosis When sensation of limb is lost to the extreme end. This is also referred to as acroanaestesia.

acroarthritis arthritis of the extremities.

acrobrachycephaly When the anteroposterior diameter of the skull is very short and abnormal.

acrocentric When chromosome having the centromere near one end of the replicating chromosome that results in one arm longer that the other

acrochordon Brownish skin lesions on neck, chest and axilla due to light exposure which is common in elderly lady.

acrocontracture contracture of limbs which involve muscles.

acrocyanosis Bluish discolouration of limbs which is characterstics of Raynaud's disease.

acrodermatitis When skin of legs and hands get highly inflamed.

acrodynia This is common in childhood when a child is sensitive to chemicals, when mercury poisoning occurs. The illness is characterised painful fingers, painful toes, photophobia, perspiration. This refrs to toxic effect of chemicals particularly due to mercury

acrolein This is obtained when glycerine gets decomposed. This is associated with the occurrence of bleeding and neoplasms in man.

acromastitis inflammation of the tip of the breast (nipple)

acromegaly This is a clinical condition characterised by enlarged skeletal system, osteoarthritis changes in joints, due to hypersecretion of growth hormone. Acromegaly is associated with diabetes, high blood pressure and abnormal calcium metabolism.

acromial That which is related with acromion.

acromio When a structure is related with acromion.

acromioclavicular That which is related to acromion and clavicle such acromioclavicular joint.

acromiocoracoid That which is related to acromion and coracoid process

acromiohumeral pertaining to the acromion and humerus.

acromion the lateral extension of the spine of the scapula, projecting over the shoulder joint and forming the highest point of the shoulder

acromionectomy Surgical resection of the distal end of the acromion, done in the treatment of acromioclavicular arthritis.

acromioplasty surgical removal of hook of the acromion to relieve mechanical compression

acromioscapular pertaining to the acromion and scapula.

acronym Nickname derived from first letters of a word

acroparalysis paralysis of the lower limb or upper limb or both

acroparesthesia By nerve compression tingling and numbness occurs in fingers and hand which is usually associated with pain.

acrophobia Fear for heights which is uncalled for.

acrosclerosis This systemic scleroderma in combination with Raynaud's disease

acrosome This is derived from Golgi apparatus of the nucleus of spermatozoon that facilitate spermatozoal entry for conception.

acrosyndactyly Terminal fingers get fused with a small cleft in-between

acrotic pertaining to weakness of the pulse.

acrotism Unable to feel the pulse in a person absence or imperceptibility of the pulse.

acrylamide a vinyl monomer used in the production of polymers with many industrial uses.

acrylate a salt acrylic acid.

acrylic This is polymers of acrylic acid used in dental prostheses, intraocular lenses, age resins, and as adsorbents in chromatography.

act an act of doing, or a thing done; a performance involving motor activity.
ACTH Abbreviation for **A**dreno **C**orticotropic **H**ormone.
actin This is a protein of the myofibril that is responsible for muscle contraction and muscle relaxation that acts through myosin particles.
actiniform formed like a ray;
α-actinin This is a muscle protein which help in binding actin molecules in the muscle actions.
actiono That which is related with some form of radiation.
Actinobacillus A gram-negative, fermentative nonmotile, coccoid or rod-shaped bacteria of the family Pasteurellaceae which are pathogenic to man.
actinodermatitis skin inflammation due to excessive exposure to sunlight or to X-rays.
Actinomadura A bacteria of the family Nocardiaceae, order Actinomycetales, consisting of branched filaments.
actinomycelial Related to the mycelium of an actinomyces.
Actinomyces A bacteria of the family Actinomycetaceae, consisting of gram-positive, with branched filaments. They are non–acid-fast and nonmotile.
Actinomycetaceae a family of bacteria containing five major genera consisting of gram-positive, nonsporulating irregularly shaped rods, which tend to form branched filaments.
actinomycetin a substance derived from cultures of the actinomycete
actinomycin Antibiotics obtained from cultures of various species of Streptomyces which has antifungal, antibacterial and cytotoxic effects.
actinomycoma Reactive lesion which looks like a tumour in actinomycetes infection.
actinomycosis An infectious disease caused by Actinomyces in man which prodeuce lumpy jaw by lymph node enlargement in the neck and mouth. Other clinical manifestations are Liver abscess, Lung abscess.
actinomycotic pertaining to with actinomycosis.
actinomycotin An antibiotic prepared from the culture for the use in the infection of actinomyces.
actinotherapy Treatment with light rays which is called phototherapy.
action Performance of a function or a movement either of any part or organ or of the whole body such as Capillary action, Reflex action etc.
activate to render active.
activation This is the biological process of rendering active such as Proenzyme transformation, activated sludge purification of seweage, induction of brain activity in EEG.
activator Any substance which possesses catalytic action.
active characterized by action and is not passive
activin This is produced in Pituitary gland and in Gonads and has the stimulatory action of FSH in the body.
activity The ability to produce some action such as Muscular activity, Nervous activity, Radioactivity, etc.
actomyosin This is present in Muscle as a complex protein containing actin and Myosin.
acu- a combining form denoting relationship to a needle such as acupuncture.
acuity This refers to the clarity or clear vision.
acuminate Refers to a structure which is sharp and pointed.
acupoint a specific point for needle insertion along a body meridian in acupuncture.
acupressure Adjacent tissues are pressed for the relief of pain which is not that scientifically proved for itsefficacy.
acupuncture It is a traditional Medical practice from China. This is practiced through the insertion of fine needles into specific exterior body locations to relieve pain.
acute having a short and relatively severe course.
acyanotic characterized by absence of cyanosis.
acyclic This refers to open chain structure in chemistry. When a symptom or illness occur independently of menstrual cycle.
acyclovir This is an antiviral synthetic preparation which is chemically acyclic purine nucleoside. It is found useful in the treatment of herpes, Epstein-Barr and cytomegalovirus. Dermatological preparation for genital and mucocutaneous herpes are available.
acylation An acyl raldical is introduced into a compound which is a chemical reaction.
acyl coenzyme A A thiol ester of a carboxylic acid whose formation is the first step in fatty acid oxidation.
acylglycerol lipase This enzyme is present in small intestine which is responsible for digestion of lipids
acystia A birth defect with absence of urinary bladder.
acystinervia defective nervous tone in the bladder.
ad It indicates that a substance be added
adactylous No fingers or toes in the hand or feed . Related to adactyly.
adactyly It is a developmental anomaly characterized by the absence of digits on the hand or foot.
Adair Dighton's syndrome This is the clinical condition of osteogenesis imperfecta Type I.
adamantine Related to enamel of teeth
Adams' operation Sub cutaneous division of the palmar fascia at various points for Dupuytren's contracture.
Adams-Stokes syndrome A clinical condition which is characterised by sudden attacks of unconscious-ness which may or may not be associated with convulsions. This is always associated with heart block.
adaptation The adjustment of an organism to its environment, adjustment of eye to light, adaptation of denture
adaxial located alongside of the axis.

add. Abbreviation used in prescription which means to add.

addict Because of physiological and psychological dependency a person who resist his habit of consuming drug or alcohol. Status of drug or alcohol dependence which is associated with strong compulsion is called substance abuse.

Addison's disease This is due to hypofunction of adrenal gland and colloquially called bronzed skin. Condition is associated with prostration, anaemia, hypotension diarrhoea and gastrointestinal disturbances.

additive This normally refers to food additive where addition of a flavouring agent, a preservative or a vitamin are added to a food item to normalise the required nutrients.

adducent Performing the movement of adduction.

adduct Movement of limb made towards the median plane. Movement of digit made towards the axial line of the limb.

adduction the act of adducting a limb or a digit.

adductor That which performs or functions as adduction which, refer to the muscle which bring about adduction.

adenalgia This refers to the pain in a gland

adenectomy Surgical removal of a gland.

adenine This is the component of Nucleic acids and Nucleotides which is a major purine base

adenitis Infection and inflammation of a gland.

Adenium African plant which contain substance called somalin which is similar to action of Digitalis on heart

adeno That which is related with a gland or with many glands.

adenoacanthoma Cancerous tissue of gland in which majority of cells show squamous cell changes.

adenoblast This is an embryonic cell that gives rise to glandular tissue.

adenocyte Secretory cell of a gland which is matured.

adenoepithelioma This is a tumor composed of glandular and epithelial elements.

adenofibroma This is a tumor composed of connective tissue and glandular structures.

adenofibrosis When we notice fibroid changes in a gland.

adenogenous That which orginates from glandular tissue.

adenography Radiography of a gland

adenohypophysis The anterior lobe of the Pituitary Gland which secretes Growth Hormone, ACTH, FSH, LH and prolactin. It regulates Thyroid gland, Gonads and Adrenal Cortex.

adenoid That which resembles a gland.

adenoidectomy Excision of the adenoids.

adenoiditis Infection and inflammation of the adenoid tissue of the nasopharynx.

adenoids Common name for enlarged tonsil which usually occurs among adolescents.

adenolipoma This is a tumor which is composed of glandular and fatty tissue elements

adenolymphoma This is tumour of parotid gland which is benign in nature

adenoma Tumour which contain recognisable glandular structure; but is an epithelial tumour in the true sense

adenomalacia Very soft gland which is pathological in nature.

adenomatoid That which resembles adenoma.

adenomyofibroma Adenomatous and myomatous tissue containing tumour which is a fibroma

adenomyometritis Inflammatory lesion of the endometrium, which leads to adenomyosis.

adenomyosarcoma This is a mesodermal tumour which contains striated muscle.

adenomyosis A benign condition of Myometrial stroma and endometrial glands. This is always associated with hypertrophy of myometrium.

adenopathy Always refers to Lymphadenopathy meaning Enlargement of lymph node.

adenopharyngitis Infection and inflammation of Tonsils, Pharynx and Adenoids.

adenophthalmia Infection and inflammation of the meibomian glands.

adenosarcoma A Tumour containing Glandular elements and Sarcomatous elements. Typical example is Wilms' Tumour.

adenosclerosis This refers to the hardening of a gland.

adenosine This is the component of RNA which belongs to a purine nucleoside Adenosine is a regulator of body metabolism.

adenosinetriphosphatase This enzyme is represented as ATP that works as catalyser in the biological process of Hydrolysis of ATP to Adenonine Diphosphatase. The said catalytic process brings about the biological action of muscle contraction, chemical transport in the cell membrane

adenotome This is a surgical instrument used in ENT for the excision of the adenoids.

adenovirus They belong to adenovirus species of viruses.

adenylic acid This is chemically Adenosine Mono Phosphate which is the phosphorylated adenosine

adeps Adeps is the common and usual ingredient of skin ointment which contain purified mental fat.

adequacy When a substance is enough or sufficient for a specific purpose in biological use or in chemical use

adermia This refers to no dermis or no skin which is a birth defect and is associated with many complications.

ADH An abbreviation for **A**nti **D**iuretic **H**ormone.

adherence When a substance adheres to another substance which can be chemical in nature or biological in nature.

adhesin In the external wall of bacteria adhesion is stipulated as molecule which is responsible for the process of adhesion

adhesion The anatomical expression of abnormal adhesion of the omentus and intestine in certain pathological conditions.

adhesive A chemical or a biological substance which cause close adhesion of two surfaces.

adhesiveness The quality of remaining adhesive of a substance.

adiadochokinesia This is the inability to perform rapid alternative movement of a part of a body or of an extremity.

adiaphoria This refers to refractory period to a biological stimuli which has resulted by earlier exposure of such stimuli.

adicillin This is the other name for Cephalosporin N antibiotic which is used in the treatment of Gonorrhoea and Typhoid.

Adie's syndrome This is a pathological pupillary reaction called Pupillotonic. The pupil on the affected side contracts on near vision more slowly than of the pupil of opposide side. The same slowness is observed in dilatation also.

adipo That which is related with fat.

adipocele This refers to a hernia which contains fat tissue.

adipocyte Refers to a fat cell.

adipokinin This is the other name for Beta Lipotropin.

adipolysis The breaking down of fat in tissue metabolism, which is also called as lipolysis.

adiponecrosis Necrosis of fatty tissue.

adipose Fat in excess quantity is present in the given tissue.

adiposity This refers to Obesity.

adiposuria The presence of fat in the urine

adjunct Any thing that is an accessory

adjustment This refers to modification of a structure or of an organ to adapt to new circumstances. Hormony of a person with other in case of social or phychological conditions. This can be denture fixation adjustment in dentistry. This can be adjustment of a microscope in microscopic examination of slides.

adjuvant This is usual in vaccine preparation to add a substance which assist in producing immunity in an individual. In case of treatment it can be a substance which aids other substance in producing remedy.

Adler Theory Austrian psychiatrist who was a student of Freud during 1870–1937. He developed a psychoanalytic theory which states 'the neuroses are developed as compensations for a social or physical inferiority.'

adnexa This refers to appendage or for an adjunct part.

adolescence This is the period of 11 years to 19 years in a boy or a girl who starts the period of life beginning with the appearance of secondary sex characters.

adolescent That which is related with adolescence.

ADP This is the abbreviation for Adenosine Di Phosphate.

adrenal This relates to 2 glands located above the kidneys. They are also called Supra Renal Glands.

adrenalectomy excision of one or both adrenal glands;

Adrenalin It is the hormone secreted by adrenal gland which is otherwise called epinephrine.

adrenalinemia Presence of epinephrine in the blood.

adrenalinuria Presence of epinephrine in the urine.

adrenalism Adrenal gland disorder in the form of Hyper or Hypo function.

adrenalitis Infection and inflammation of adrenal gland.

adrenergic This refers to Symphathetic nerve fibres that produce norepinephrine at synapse. That which secretes adrenaline.

adreno That which is related with adrenal gland or a combining form denoting relationship to the adrenal gland.

adrenocortical That which is related with adrenal cortex.

adrenocorticoid This refers to corticosteroid hormone.

adrenocorticotrophic Which has the stimulating effect on adrenal cortex.

adrenogram X-ray or Imaging of adrenal glands.

adrenomegaly enlargement of the adrenal glands.

adrenostatic Agent that inhibits the activity of the adrenal glands.

adrenotropic having specific affinity for hormonal influence on adrenal gland.

Adrian English physiologist 1889–1977 who won Nobel Prize for Medicine and Physiology for Medicine for his work on Neuron function.

adsorbent Refers to chemical agent which attracts particles to its surface by the process of adsorption.

adsorption The process of attachment of particles on the surface of another which yield high concentration of a liquid or of a gas.

adult Person male or female having attained full growth

adulterant When a substance is added in the interest of commercialisation and that can be harmful to the body which is also called as sophistication. Common adulteration is by adding adulterant to food.

adulteration It concludes mixing, substitution, concealing the quality, unsafe food sold, misbranding and addition of toxicants.

advance Performing the operation of advancement in a given situation.

advancement It is furthering process in surgery or in orthopaedics where reattachment at an advanced point is done or a part is moved forward.

adventitia Connective tissue which covers the outermost covering of an anatomical structure such as vewssel or organ.

adventitious Not natural, structure found other than its usual place.

adynamic Not dynamic

Aeby's muscle One of the compressor muscles of the lips.

Aeby's plane One passing through the nasion and basion perpendicular to the median plane of the cranium.

Aedes One of the genus of mosquitoes which are vectors in the transmission of diseases like Dengue, yellow fever, which annoying because of their bites. Common species are – A. aegypti, A sympsoni, A. africanus, A. albopictus.

aerated Charged with either air or with carbon dioxide such as aerated water.

aeration Gaseous exchange in the lung during respiration by taking oxygen and leaving carbon dioxide.

aero The root word which is combined to described to denote its relation to air or to gas.

Aerobacter The group of bacteria belonging to family enterobacteriaceae which are Gram negative and facultative anaerobic.

aerobe a microorganism that can live and grow in the presence of free oxygen.

aerobic Organism that grows in the presence of oxygen or that requires oxygen for tissue respiration.

aerobiology It is that branch of biology which deals with the distribution of living organisms in outdoor air.

aerocolpos It is the clinical condition with the distention of vagina with gas.

aerodontics The branch of dentistry which is concerned with effects on the teeth at high altitude

aerogen Gas-producing, bacteria.

aerogenesis Gas production.

aerogenic Bacteria that produce free gases.

aeromedicine This refers to Aviation Medicine.

aeropathy Illness that occurs in either low or high altitude such as air sickness or decompression sickness.

aerophagia This is a physical disorder associated with anxiety which result in abdominal distension and belching.

aerophobia Fear for air with the conceptual idea of getting air borne infections.

aerosis This is the process of production of gas in the tissues

aerosol Medication in the form of liquid which can be atomised into a fine mist for inhalation therapy.

aerotaxis Presence of molecular oxygen makes an organism to move towards it.

aesculapian That which is related to or pertaining to Aesculapius, the God of medicine, or to the art of medicine.

Aesculapius He is the Mythological God of healing.

AF Abbreviation for **A**trial **F**ibrillation.

AFCR Abbreviation for **A**merican **F**ederation for **C**linical **R**esearch.

afebrile Clinical description to express that person is not having fever.

affection This is common state of human being showing emotional attachment with other beings. It also mean that a person is affected with an illness.

afferent The arrangement is or the distribution is centripetal in nature which means that given items are conveying toward a center

affiliation This show an interdependent relationship of one on another, which is a social drive in nature in the society.

affinity A special attraction for a specific element, organ, or structure which is common occurrence in chemical reactions or in electron charging.

afflux a flow of something, especially water or air.

afibrinogenemia The clinical condition in which there will be lack of fibrinogen or coagulation foctor I in the blood.

aflatoxicosis This is due to contamination of Aspergillus flavus fungus in groundnut or peanut causing mycotoxic effect. The toxin is aflatoxin which produces liver necrosis.

aflatoxin a toxic factor produced by Aspergillus flavus molds in ground nut or in peanut .

AFP Abbreviation for **Alpha Feto Protein**.

afterbirth This refers to the III stage of labour where the placenta and membranes are delivered from the uterus after the birth of the child.

aftercare the care and treatment of a recovering patient especially one who has undergone surgery

afterload This is the force against which cardiac muscle shortens that is described in cardiac physiology. This depends on peripheral vascular resistance and blood volume.

aftermovement This is called Kohnstamm phenomenon where the arm is elevated spontaneously when the body part is stuck with a rigid object .

afterpains This is due to contraction of the uterus after the birth of the child that produce the cramplike pains

afterperception the perception of a sensation after the stimulus producing it has ceased.

AG Abbreviation for Atrial Gallop.

Ag This is the symbol for **Antigen**

agalactia Failure of the secretion of milk called also galactosis.

agamete the product of asexual multiple fission in protozoa.

agammaglobulinemia Actual meaning is the absence of Immunoglobulins in the blood. In clinical practice situations are very often hypogammaglobulinemia.

agamo This is the combining form meaning asexual.

agamous Having no recognizable sexual organs.

aganglionic That which is related with the absence of ganglion cells.

agar This is a mucilaginous complex sulfonated polymer of galactose units, extracted from *Gelidium cartilagineum, Gracilaria confervoides,* and related red algae. This is used in culture media for microorganisms.

agastria Clinical condition with the absence of the stomach.

age The duration of individual existence measured in years. Other usages are Anatomical age, Mental age, Gestational age, chronological age etc.

agenesis Absence of organ due to developmental defect.

agenitalism 1. absence of the genitalia. 2. a condition caused by failure to secrete gonadal hormones.

agenosomia congenital absence or rudimentary development of the genitals

agent Any substance capable of producing an effect, whether physical, chemical, or biological.

agerasia A person is unusually youthful in his/her advanced years.

ageusia Absence of the sense of taste

agglomerated That which is crowded into a mass.

agglutinable That which is capable of agglutination.

Agglutination This is the immunological action of an agglutinant substance. It is an antigen antibody reaction.

agglutinin This is an antibody that aggregates a particulate antigen such as bacteria

agglutinogen This refers to any substance which, acting as an antigen, stimulates the production of agglutinin.

aggregate This refers to crowding or clustering together.

aggregation This refers to massing of materials or clumping of material

aggression This is a form of behaviour which leads to self-assertion or is an innate drive due to frustration.

aging At the passage of time with man, we observe gradual general changes called senescence .

agitation Restlessness or excess motor activity due to tension or anxiety.

aglossia Condition with the congenital absence of the tongue.

aglycemia Virtually total absence of sugar from the blood;

agnathia A birth defect where lower jaw is absent.

agnosia When a person cannot perceive any of the sensory stimuli such as auditory, visual, olfactory, gustatory or tactile.

agonadism Clinical condition without gonads or sex glands which are called anarchism in males and Turner's syndrome in females.

agony severe pain or extreme suffering usual reference to extreme pain at the time of death.

agoraphobia Marked fear of being alone or being in public place where escape is difficult is felt.

agranulocytosis Decreased number of granulocytes called leukopenia.

Agrobacterium It is a soil bacteria found in roots or stems of plants. They are known to produce galls on plant stems.

AGS This is the abbreviation for **A**merican **G**eriatrics **S**ociety.

ague In ancient times Malaria was called as ague since it used to produce sharp chill in illness.

agyria This refers to smooth surfaced brain and convolutions of the cerebral cortex is not formed.

AHA This is the abbreviation for **A**merican **H**eart **A**ssociation

AHF This is the abbreviation for **A**nti **H**aemophilic **F**actor VIII which is responsible for coagulation of blood.

AHG This is the abbreviation for **A**nti **H**aemophilic **G**lobulin which again is factor VIII.

aichmophobia Irrational fear of sharp-pointed objects

AID This is abbreviation for **A**rtificial **I**nsemination **D**onor.

aid Assistance by extending help through helping device. examples are visual aids, hearing aids etc.,

AIDS Abbreviation for **A**cquired **I**mmuno **D**eficiency **S**yndrome.

AIH Abbreviation for **A**rtificial **I**nsemination **H**usband.

ailment Illness of the body which is usually milk in nature.

ainhum This is manifestation in African black adult males wherein toes or fingers have a linear constriction leading to spontaneous amputation .

air It is the gaseous mixture which makes up the earth's atmosphere is an odorless, colorless gas consisting of 1 part of oxygen and 4 parts of nitrogen and small amount of carbon dioxide.

airborne This refers to spread of infectious disease through air which is one of the common mode of transmission of diseases.

airway This is the passage for the air to enter and get exit during inspiration and expiration. Airway clearance is the first mode of reviving a person in First Aid.

Åkerlund deformity This is radiographic appearance of duodenal ulcer where indentation and niche are present as a deformity of the duodenal cap.

akinesia Lack of control of voluntary muscle movements which can be by disease or by a local anaesthetics.

Akureyri disease *Akureyri is a* town in Iceland where an apidemic of neuro myasthenia was occurred among thousands of patients during the year 1948.

alacrima Deficiency of secretion of tears can be acquired or congenital in origin.

Alangium a genus of shrubs and trees of the family Alangiaceae of Indian species is used as an emetic in place of Ipecac.

alanine This is a nonessential amino acid,

β-alanine an ω-amino acid, β-aminopropionic acid; it is not found in This is the precursor of Acetyl Co A and is an intermediate product in the metabolism of cytosine.

alanine transaminase Abbreviated as ALT this is present in serum and body tissues mainly in liver. In case of liver disease and in Infectious Mononucleosis Serum enzyme activity in terms of SGPT is increased.

Alanson's amputation Alanson's amputation is described as a circular amputation where the stump is shaped like a hollow cone.

alastrim This the viral infection Variola Minor.

alba used as an adjective for anatomical structures such as substantia alba and pityriasis alba.

Albee's operation This is Hip surgery for Ankylosis which consists of cutting upper surface of head of femur and freshening a corresponding point on the acetabulum to allow two new surface be in contact.

albendazole Broad-spectrum anthelmintic used against helminths and in hydatid cyst disease including neurocysticercosis

Albers-Schönberg disease *Albers-Schönberg,* German radiologist. This refers to Osteopetrosis.

Albert's diphtheria stain Stain is used to demonstrate Diphtheria bacilli in throat swab. The stain contains Toluidine blue and Malachite green. When the slide is treated with Iodine solution metachromatic granules appear black, Bars look dark green and the bacilli look light green.

Albert's operation, suture In case of Flail joint of the Knee, surgical escision of the knee is undertaken for the relief of symptoms.

albicans This word denotes the colour of whiteness.

albinism This clinical condition is associated with Aminoacidopathy affecting melanocytes of eye and skin which cause hypopigmentation .

albino This refers to an individual affected with albinism.

Albright's hereditary osteodystrophy This is the clinical condition of Pseudohypoparathyroidism.

albumin This is one of the major plasma protein which constitutes 60 percent of total plasma protein which help in maintaining plasma colloidal osmotic pressure and help in the transport of organic anions.

albuminoid That which resembles albumin

albuminuria This is clinically referred to as Proteinuria where albumin is excreted in the urine which is pathological.

Alcock's canal This is the original name of Pudendal Canal after its inventor.

alcohol Methyl alcohol, Ethyl alcohol, Butyl alcohol etc., are series of organic compounds from Hydrocarbons with the substitution of hydroxyl groups of H atoms. Official preparation of Ethyl Alcohol contains 92 to 93 percent of ethanol by weight.

alcohol dehydrogenase This an enzyme of the oxidoreductase class that catalyzes the reversible oxidation of alcohols to aldehydes which is the first step in the alcohl metabolism in Liver.

alcoholism This is the outcome of alcohol dependence which is a disorder characterized by a pathological pattern of alcohol use that causes a serious impairment in social or occupational functioning.

aldehyde Acetaldehyde, Formaldehyde, Glyceraldehyde etc are organic compounds containing the group — CHO i.e., carbonyl group,

aldehyde dehydrogenase This is an enzyme of the oxidoreductase that catalyzes the oxidation of aldehydes

Aldomet tradename for preparations of Methyldopa

aldose This is the group of Monosaccharides containing Glucose, Galactose and Mannose.

aldosterone This is the Mineralocorticoid hormone secreted by the Adrenal Cortex which promotes the retension of sodium, excretion of potassium and secondary retention of water in the body.

aldosteronism A clinical pathological condition because of Hyperaldosteronism which causes electrolyte imbalance in the body. Primary and Secondary Aldosteronism are known clinical entities.

aldrin An insecticide which come under the chlorinated hydrocarbon insecticide similar to dieldrin. Aldrin toxicity are tremors ataxia and convulsions.

Alexander's operation Gynaecological correction of displaced uterus by shortening of round ligament s of the uterus.

alexia Ability to understand written language is lost due to cerebral lesion

algae Chlorophyll containing algae which belongs to a group of cryptogamous plants, in which the body is unicellular

algesia Excessive sensitivity to pain which is a type of hyperesthesia.

algesio That which is related with pain or a combining form denoting relationship to pain.

algesiogenic That which produce pain

algid chill or very cold

algorithm This is step by step planning and solving medical problems through decision.

alicyclic Chemical which has the properties of both aliphatic and cyclic substances.

alignment This refers to that things are put in a straight line such as alignment of teeth.

alimentary Related with the organ of digestion.

alimentation To give food for nourishment where nutrient is given to an individual.

aliphatic They are organic compound which contain straight chain or branched chain in its structure.

alkali Chemical compounds that go to form soluble soaps with fatty acids. They turn red litmus to blue. They have pH value of above 7.

alkaline Chemicals that have the reactions of an alkali and have the pH of above 7.0

alkaline phosphatase It is an enzyme present in normal tissues and also in malignant tissues. Serum Alkaline Activity can help in the diagnosis of certain diseases.

alkalinity This gives the degree of alkalinity of a chemical or of a biological agent.

alkalizer A chemical agent which neutralizes acids

alkaloid Alkaloids may be plant origin such as atropine, cocaine, caffeine, morphine, nicotine, strychnine etc., or may be synthetic such as procaine. They are nitrogenous substances in plant and are found pharmacologically active.

alkalosis Too much accumulation of base leads to alkalosis which can be demonstrated by the decrease in H ikon concentration.

alkane They are saturated Hydrocarbons with general formula C_nH_{2n+2}.

alkaptonuria This is an autosomal recessive disorder which is characterized by accumulation of homogentisic acid (HGA). This is always associated with arthritis.

alkyl When an Aliphatic Hydrocarbon loos one H atom radical alkyl is produced.

alkylation If one active H atom is introduced to alkyl group the process is called alkylation.

allanto That which is related with sausage .

allantochorion A Membrane is formed by the fusion of the allantois and chorion.

allantoin This is present in Allantoic fluid and foetal urine. History of medicine has described that allantoin was used for Ulcer healing, for Osteomyelitis and for the formation of epithelial cells.

allantoinuria This denotes that allantoin is present in the urine.

allantois This is vestigial in man which becomes vessels of the umbilical cord.

allele Gene that occupy the chromosomal locus. In humans they diploid and have two alleles one on each chromosome of a homologous pair.

Allen's paradoxical law This law states that when sugar is given more and more to a normal person it is utilised more and more, but in case of diabetes it is quite reverse in nature.

Allen's test This is a qualitative test done to find out dextrose in urine. The urine is added to the boiling Fehling's solution and later is allowed to cool. If dextrose is present, it is seen by the appearance of turbidity.

Allen-Doisy test This test is done to find out oestrogenic substance in vaginal secretion. Presence of cornified epithelial cells is positive and presence of only leucocytes is negative.

allergen Antigen which produce the hypersensitivity or allergy in a person.

allergic That which is allergic or that which is related with allergy.

allergy Usually refers to harmful reactions in immunology. Due to exposure to an allergen which is an antigen, a state of hypersensitivity induced

alliance Members unite together for furthering their interests or with an agreement to cooperate for each other with a specific purpose

allicin This is present in Garlic and is extracted in the form of an oil which seems to have anti bacterial activity.

Allis' sign This is sign of the fracture of neck of femur wherein, on examination the fascia between the crest of the ilium and the greater trochanter is observed to be relaxed.

allo The condition other than normal.

allodynia This is the result of a stimulus which is non-noxious in nature on the normal skin.

alloeroticism Sexual feeling directed to another person.

allograft Graft of tissue between individuals of the same species but of disparate genotype from cadaver or from relatives who may be related or not related.

allomorphism This refers to the change of crystalline form without change in its chemical constitution.

allopath This word is applied to a practitioner of Allopathic medicine.

allopathic That which is related or is pertaining to allopathy.

allopathy This is the system of Modern Medicine where treatment of disease is done on scientific basis on the ground of established diagnosis.

allopurinol Allopurinol is an isomer of hypoxanthine which is used in the treatment of hyperuricemia of gout

all or none This is the principle which postulate that the heart muscle under whatever stimulus will contract to the fullest extent or not at all. Similarly in case of nerve conduction stimulation of an individual fiber causes an action potention to travel over the entire fiber or not travels at all

allotoxin It refers to a chemical or biological substance which is formed by local tissue that serves as defence force.

allotrophic When the metabolic action of digestion renders the substance as non-nutritious

allotropic Individual who is preoccupied with others that on oneself.

allotropism When a given substance is available in more than one form it is called allotropism such as diamond and graphite are forms of carbon.

allowance When we allow or permit something such as RDA

alloxan This is a product of uric acid which has the capacity of destroying Islet of pancreas and thus can produce induced diabetes.

alloy Alloy is a mixture of more than one metal or metalloid that are mutually soluble with each other.

allyl This is the chemical which is an univalent organic group, —CH2[dbond]CHCH2.

allylamine Very commonly used chemical in the manufacture of pharmaceuticals, which is a caustic liquid with an ammoniacal odor

alochia This connotes Absence of the lochia.

alopecia This is colloquially called Baldness due to loss of hair from skin where normally hair are present.

alpha fetoprotein It is a plasma protein produced by the fetal liver. It declines by one year. It is seen elevated in liver associated disorders. Hence it is an indicator for treatment and for prognosis.

alpha-tocopherol This is Vitamin E.

ALS Abbreviation for **A**myotrophic **L**ateral **S**clerosis

alter This refers to castrate a house pet or livestock.

alternans This refers to alternate features such as pulsus alternans.

alternating An event occurring in regular succession

altrose This chemical sugar is an aldohexose isomeric with glucose at carbons 2 and 3.

altruism Responding with concern for other's need without any self interest.

alum This is from Hydrated Aluminum Oxide and Sulphuric acid with the addition of potassium. In public health it is used as an adjuvant in vaccines.

aluminum This a light white element from Bauxite and has use in the manufacture of prosthetic devices.

alveobronchiolitis Infection and inflammation of the bronchioles and alveoli of the lungs.

alveolus It is small sac like structure such as Alveolus of Lung or alveolus of Jaw.

Alzheimer's disease This is a clinical condition which is called Primary Degenerative Dementia with total forgetfulness of the individual leading to total disability.

AMA Abbreviation for **A**merican **M**edical **A**ssociation

amalgam This is an alloy in which mercury is one of the components.

amalgamate This is chemical process of union of a metal in an alloy with mercury to form an amalgam.

amalgamation This is the formation of an amalgam.

amantadine hydrochloride Basically this is an antiviral preparation used in Influenza- A infection. This acts as antidyskinetic in Parkinsonism and hence found useful in Parkinsonism.

amaranth A Dye from plant origin used in Food Cosmetics and Drugs as Colouring agent.

amasesis When a patient is unable to chew the food.

amastia Condition with congenital absence of the Breast in females.

amathophobia Unwanted and uncalled for fear for Dust in an Individual.

amaurosis This refers to clinical condition of the eye producing blindness from the cause arising from Optic nerve or brain.

amaurotic That which is related with Amaurosis.

ambenonium chloride A cholinergic Drug used in the treatment of myasthenia gravis

ambi- A prefix meaning 'on both sides'.

ambidexterity Manual skill is performed by both hands in equal status and in equal speed.

ambient surrounding or encompassing

ambilateral Related to both left and right side of an organ or part or the body.

ambiopia Refers to Double Vision or Diplopia.

ambiversion This denotes the balance of introversion and extroversion in man.

ambly- The word denotes the dullness in a cell, in a tissue, in an organ, in a part or the body of man.

amblyaphia Dim vision in a person in whom no detectable cause can be found out.

amblyopia Clinical ophthalmic condition showing impairment of vision without detectable organic lesion of the eye.

amboceptor This is Anti Sheep Red Blood Cell Antibody that is used in Complement Fixation Test which is an Immunological test first Described by Dr.Ehrlich.

Ambrosia This is well known Annual Plant in Tropical Countries which produce large quantity of pollen which are known to cause Hay Fever in Man.

ambulance A transportation vehicle which is equipped with emergency medicamentations and treatment used to transport the sick and invalid for emergency unit of a hospital. One of the Physiological conditions of Pregnancy is advanced labour when the ambulance is used to transport the woman.

ambulatory Patient who is not bed ridden but is able to walk and attend to his routine.

amcinonide This is a synthetic corticosteroid for topical use.

amdinocillin This is a semisynthetic penicillin used against Gram negative Bacteria as Chemotherapeutic agent.

ameba This refers to Protozoa which is unicellular organism and has pseudopodia for its motility. It is spelled as 'Amoeba'

amebiasis It is the infection with the parasite Entamoeba histolytica organism which produce Intestinal Amoebiasis. Rarely also it produces Liver infections.

amebicide An agent which is destructive to amoebae.

ameboid Movement that resembles the movement of Amoeba.

ameboma This is a tumor-like mass produced by localized inflammation from Amoebic infection in man.

amelanosis When the tissue is totally lacking with melanin which is called depigmentation of Hypo-pigmentation.

amelia When a limb or limbs are not developed which is due to congenital defect and defective embryo-genesis.

amelioration This denotes the clinical improvement of patient at retreatment.

amelo The word means 'enamel'

ameloblast Innermost layer of enamel which cover the dental papilla.

ameloblastoma Epithelial neoplasm of enamel organ which can be follicular or cystic in nature.

amenorrhea Absence of the menses.

amentia The term means Profound Mental Retardation in man.

amethocaine hydrochloride An anaesthetic containing Tetracaine Hydrochloride.

ametria No Uterus is found in a woman which is invariably due to congenital absence of the uterus.

ametropia Image is not focused on the retina and the clinical conditions are termed as Myopia, Hypermetropia and Astigmatism.

amidobenzene This is chemical name for Aniline.

aminacrine hydrochloride This is used in the treatment of wound as an antiseptic which is effective against many gram-negative and gram-positive bacteria

amination Chemical production of amine by the addition of an amino group to an organic acceptor compound. This is also done by the reduction of a Nitro Compound.

amine This is an organic compound containing nitrogen which can be primary amine, Secondary amine or Tertiary amine depending upon Hydrogen atom present in it. In organic chemistry the group are Methyl amine, Ethyl amine, Propylamine etc., are common amines in use.

amine oxidase This enzyme catalyzes the primary amines to form Aldehydes and Hydrogen Peroxide.

amino This is the monovalent chemical group —NH_2.

amino acid The organic compound containing an amino (—NH_2) and a carboxyl (—COOH) group is Amino Acid.

aminoacidemia If excess quantity of amino acid is present in the blood.

aminoacidopathy Diseases occurring due to aminoacid metabolism in the body.

aminoaciduria This is the excess of amino acids in the urine biochemically called hyperaminoacidemia.

aminobenzoate This is the salt of Para Amino Benzoic Acid.

***p*-aminobenzoic acid** Though it is not a nutrient, it is included in B vitamin complex which is required for the synthesis of Folic Acid by organisms.

aminoglycoside This biochemical agent inhibit protein synthesis by the process of binding with 30S Ribosomal Sub unit. Thus has antibiotic property. The common in use like amikacin, gentamicin and streptomycin are derived from Streptomyces.

***p*-aminohippurate** This is the salt *p*-aminohippuric acid.

6-aminopenicillanic acid The main source of 6 amino penicillanic acid is Penicillium which is the active nucleus to all penicillins. This has an established anti bacterial activity.

***p*-aminophenol** This is from Acetaminophen which likes an allergen that causes asthma and methemoglobinemia in man.

aminophylline This is prepared from Ethylenediamine and Theophylline and has good bronchodilator property. The preparation is available for oral, IM and IV administration. It's additional properties are cardiac stimulation Diuresis and Antispasmodic.

aminopurine Aminopurine contains Adenine and Guanine and is the component of Nucleic Acid.

aminoquinoline With the addition of one amino group we get Heterocyclic compound. Commercially we have two major groups a) 4 amino quinolines and b) 8 Amino quinolines. It is powerful weapon as Anti Malaria Treatment.

aminosalicylic acid Amino salicylate has Anti TB activity. PAS (**Para Amino Salicylic acid**) is used in TB treatment. By inhibiting Folic acid synthesis PAS inhibits the growth and multiplication of Myco-bacterium tuberculosis.

amitosis This is direct cell division without the formation of spireme spindle figure or chromosomes.

amitriptyline This is an antidepressant which has sedative effects in enuresis, chronic pain and peptic ulcer

Ammon's horn It is the name for Hippocampus.

ammonia An alkaline Gas NH_3 which has penetrating odor

ammoniacal Treated with excess ammonia.

amnesia Unable to remember past experiences.

amnio Denoting relationship to the amnion.

amniocentesis To obtain amniotic fluid percutaneous transabdominal puncture of the uterus is done.

amniography Radiography of the gravid uterus to outline fetus and amniotic cavity.

amnion This is derived from Trophoblast which envelops the fetus.

amniotic That which is related with amnion.

amniotomy Rupture of the fetal membranes to induce labor.

amodiaquine This is a 4-aminoquinoline used in the treatment of malaria Giardiasis and Extra Intestinal amoebiasis.

Amoeba Human parasite belonging to the genus of amoeboid protozoa

amorphous If a chemical is not crystalline form, if an item is shapeless.

amorphus Fetus which is malformed and has no shape.

Amoss' sign Patient suffering from painful flexure of spine when asked to sit from lying position supports himself with hands to sit.

amoxicillin Antibiotic used against Haemophilus influenza, E. coli, Proteus and Neisseria organisms. This is synthetic derivative of Ampicillin.

amphetamine This is a Sympathomimetic drug used as stimulating drug. Abuse of Amphetamine leads to dependence.

Amphibia Vertebrates that breathe by gills in the larval state and later breathe by lungs

ampho Ampho is a prefix meaning both.

amphoteric This means to have two opposite characteristics such as acid and alkali .

amphotericin B A broad spectrum anti Fungal antibiotic.

ampicillin This is Penicillinase sensitive penicillin used as broad spectrum antibiotic in day to day clinical practice against both Gram +ve and Gram –ve bacteria.

amplexation Treatment of fractured clavicle by an apparatus

amplexus This is pseucopulation seen in Frogs.

amplification An increase in visual stimulus or in auditory stimulus which is recorded in the progress during treatment.

amplitude Large or Wide range in a given situation.

ampule Small glass container used to put and preserve sterile liquid or medication sealed.

ampulla An anatomical structure which is flask like dilatation and is tubular in structure.

amputation Surgical removal of limb for therapeutic purposes.

amputee a person who has limb or limbs amputated.

amuck It refers to Wild and uncontrollable1

Amussat's operation This surgery is Lumbar Colotomy where surgical incision is done across the outer border of the Quadratus Lumborum.

amyelencephalia Congenital absence of the brain and spinal cord in the newborn.

amyelia No spinal cord since birth which is referred to as congenital absence of the spinal cord.

amygdala An Anatomical structure which is shaped like an almond such as Corpus Amygdaloideum.

amygdalic acid This is Mandelic Acid.

amyl Radical, $-C_5H_{11}$. (Univalent) such as Amyl nitrite, Amyl acetate

amylase This is a catalytic agent in the Hydrolysis or metabolism of polysaccharides. There are two types one is α amylase and the other is γ amylase.

amylin This is the component of Islet of Langerhans of Pancreas. It inhibits insulin stimulated glycogen synthesis in muscles.

amyl That which is related with Starch.

amyloid Substance which has the property resembling starch. It gets deposited in Amyloidosis. The biochemical types are Light Chain Protein Amyloid and A Protein Amyloid

amyloidosis Accumulation of Amyloid protein in organs and tissues which produces pathology of that organ or that tissue.

amylose It is the water soluble Glucan which a lesser constituent of Starch.

amylum Meaning Starch.

amyotrophy Atrophy of muscle tissue.

ANA Abbreviation for **A**merican **N**urses' **A**ssociation

anabolic pertaining to promote anabolism.

anabolism Constructive metabolic process by which organisms convert substances for its growth.

anaclasis Refraction of light.

anacrotic In the recording or tracing of Pulse it is the ascending limb that is described.

anaerobe Microorganism that lives and grows in complete absence of Oxygen.

anaerobic Lacking molecular oxygen or that which is related with Anaerobe.

Anagnostakis' operation This is an Ophthalmic operation for Entropion and the operation for Trichiasis.

anakmesis Arrest of maturation

anal Pertaining to the anus.

analeptic It is a restorative Drug or medicamentation such as Caffeine, Amphetamine etc.

analgesia absence of Pain on stimulation.

analgesic Substance that relieves pain

analog Electrical Equipment in which the data is by electrical signals in terms varying magnitude.

analogous Similar in some respect.

analogy The quality of being analogous

analysis The process of determining the component parts of an item.

analyzer This is a Polarising apparatus with a Nicol Prism to analyse polarised light, According to Dr. Pavlov CNS control of an organism

anaphase The stage in meiosis and mitosis

anaphylaxis In a person who is highly sensitised clinical manifestations like Pruritus, Urticaria, Angioedema, Vascular collapse, Shock and even Respiratory arrest occur. Depending on the severity they are classified as Systemic anaphylaxis, Generalised anaphylaxis, Anaphylactic Shock and Hypersensitive Reaction.

anaplasia This refers to the a loss of differentiation of cells which invariably refers to Tumour cells.

anasarca Generalized massive edema.

anastomose This refers to the connection with one another by Anastomosis particularly in arteries and veins.

anastomosis Connection between two vessels.

anatomical Pertaining to anatomy or to the structure

anatomy The science that deals with the structure or of the structure of the body

anchor This is the means by which something is held securely.

ancillary Assisting in the performance of a service.

ANCOVA Abbreviation of Analysis of Co Variance.

Ancylostoma Nematode parasites of the family Ancylostomatidae, which is popularly known as hookworms.

ancylostomiasis This refers to the hookworm

Andersen's syndrome This include triad of Vitamin A deficiency, Cystic Fibrosis of Pancreas and Bronchiectasis.

Anderson splint This a combined form of fixation for internal and external fixation in case of fractures. First Wire and nail are inserted through tissue into bone above and below the fracture. Wires and nails are attached to plate and the plate are joined by adjustable screws.

Andes disease This is clinical condition of chronic mountain sickness.

André Thomas sign This is a sign of Cerebellar lesion where in finger to nose test if the patient is directed to raise his arm over his head and then suddenly ordered to let it fall to his head, the arm will rebound.

andro Relationship to the male.

androblastoma This is benign tumour of testis which is of 3 types according to histological classification 1) Epithelial 2) Stromal and 3) Mixed

androgen Substance that promotes masculinization, Testosterone.

androgynoid The person is pseudohermaphrodite.

android resembling a man

andrology scientific study of the masculine constitution of male sex, the study of diseases of the male organs of generation.

andropathy Disease peculiar to males.

androsterone This is an androgen with exertion of male hormone effect in man.

anemic pertaining to or characterized by anemia.

anencephaly Small cerebral hemispheres in the skull which is congenital defect.

aneroid Not containing liquid.

anesthesia loss of sensation, usually by damage to a nerve or due to the administration of anaesthetic agent.

anesthesiologist A Physician or Dentist specializing in anesthesiology.

anesthesiology Branch of medicine which studies anesthesia and anesthetics.

aneuploid A chromosome number that is not an exact multiple of the normal diploid number or an cell having an aneuploid number of chromosomes.

aneurysm Dilatation of the wall of an artery a vein or the heart which can form a pulsating tumour.

Angelucci's syndrome The clinical condition with excitement palpitation and spring conjunctivitis.

angiectasis Dilatation and often lengthening of a blood or lymphatic vessel

angina Spasmodic choking or suffocative pain.

anginal pertaining to angina.

angio a combining form denoting relationship to a vessel.

angioblast Mesenchymal tissue of the embryo from which the blood cells and blood vessels differentiate

angioedema a vascular reaction involving the deep dermis or subcutaneous tissues with localized edema caused by dilatation and increased permeability of capillaries

angiofibroma a lesion characterized by fibrous tissue and vascular proliferation on the face

angiogram A radiograph of blood vessels taken during angiography.

angiolipoma a lipoma containing clusters of blood vessels

angiology the study of the blood and lymph vessels of the body.

angiolymphangioma A mixed angioma in which lymph vessels and blood are present.

angioma a tumor whose cells tend to form blood vessels or Lymphatics and accordingly it can be Haemangioma or Lymphangioma.

angiomegaly enlargement of blood vessels Common site is eyelids.

angionecrosis Necrosis of the walls of blood vessels.

angioneuropathy Neuropathy of blood vessels such as angiospasm or angioparalysis.

angiopathy Disease of the blood vessels or lymphatics.

angioplasty an angiographic procedure to eliminate narrowing in blood vessels.

angiorrhaphy Suture of a vessel or vessels.

angiosarcoma Malignant neoplasm arising from vascular endothelial cells

angiosclerosis Hardening of walls of blood vessels

angiotensin A Vasopressor hormone from Renin.

angitis Infection and inflammation of blood vessels.

angina Spasmodic, choking, or suffocative pain. commonly referred to Angina Pectoris.

angioblast Mesenchymal tissue of the embryo from which the blood cells and blood vessels differentiate

angiocardiography By injecting contract material angiography of the heart and great vessels are taken and images are analysed for Ventricular functions.

angiodystrophia Disorder of blood vessels caused by a defective supply of nutrients.

angioedema Vascular reaction involving the deep dermis or subcutaneous tissues representing localized edema caused by dilatation and increased permeability of capillaries

angiofibroma a lesion characterized by fibrous tissue and vascular proliferation on the face.

angiogram Radiograph of blood vessels taken during angiography.

angiography A diagnostic investigation where in the radiographic visualization of blood vessels following introduction of contrast material is done.

angiolipoma A lipoma containing clusters of blood vessels which is painful.

angiology The study of the blood and lymph vessels of the body.

angioma a tumor whose cells tend to form blood vessels or Lymph vessels

angiomatosis Diseased state of the vessels with the formation of multiple angiomas.

angiomatous The nature of angioma.

angionecrosis Necrosis of the walls of blood vessels.

angioneuropathy Disorder of the Vasomotor system which produce angiospasm, angio paralysis.

angioplasty Procedure for elimination of areas of narrowing in blood vessels.

angiorrhaphy Suture of a vessel or vessels.

angiotensin Vasopresor hormone from Renin.

angle The point of junction of two intersecting borders or surfaces

Ångström's unit see under This is the unit of Wavelength which is $1/10^{th}$ of a millimicron

angstrom A unit of length used for atomic dimensions and light wavelengths

angular That which has corners or angles.

angulation Angulation that occurs in poorly set bone, Sharp angle formed in intestine or ureter which gives raise to obstruction.

anhidrosis Severe deficiency of sweating which may be due to obstruction of sweat glands or due to paralysis of sweat glands.

anhydrous deprived of water.

aniline Colorless oily liquid arylamine derived from coal tar

anima Soul or inner being of a person, as opposed to the personality the social role

animation The state of being alive.

anion an ion carrying a negative charge

aniso That which is unequal or not similar.

anisocytosis R B C of different sizes present in the blood. Depending small or big they are called Microcythemia or Macrocythemia respectively.

anisometropia The refractive power of the two eyes are found to be different.

anisopoikilocytosis RBCs are of different size and different shape in the blood of a patient.

anisotonic When two solutions are compared one is having high osmotic pressure than the other,

anisotropic Substance that has the unlike properties such as having a double polarising power.

ankle It is the region of ankle joint.

ankylo That which is bent or fused.

ankyloglossia Restricted movement of the tongue

ankylosed That which is fused.

ankylosis This refers to the immobility of a joint

Annelida They are Metazoan invertebrates with body segmentations such as leeches and earthworms.

annular Ring like or circular.

anococcygeal pertaining to the anus and coccyx.

anode Electrode at which oxidation occurs, i.e., the positive electrode in a storage battery.

anoderm The epithelial lining of the anal canal.

anodyne That which relieves pain such as Morphine, Aspirin, Opium etc.,

anomaloscope Instrument used in testing the anomalies of color vision through spectral lines.

anomaly Birth defect which is not normal or is abnormal in nature.

anonymous Nameless

Anopheles They are insects of public health importance which transmits Malaria fever. Common species in India are A. culicifacies, A. Fluviateles, A. Stephensi, A. sundaicus, A. subpictus, and A. minimus.

anophthalmia a developmental defect characterized by complete absence of the eyes.

anorectal Pertaining to the anus and rectum.

anorexia lack of the appetite

anorgasmy Unable to experience orgasm.

anosmia absence of the sense of smell

anosteoplasia Defective bone formation.

anovaginal That which is related with Anus and Vagina such as Anovaginal fistula.

anovesical That which is related to Anus and Urinary Bladder.

anovular Menstruation which is not accompanied with the discharge of an ovum.

anovulation Absence of ovulation.

anoxia Reduced Oxygen supply to tissue or a total lack of oxygen

ansa General term used in anatomical nomenclature to designate a loop

Antabuse This drug is Disulfiram which is used in De addition treatment among alcohols.

antacid Drug that neutralises the acidity and is used in gastric acidity.

ante- a prefix meaning prior to

antebrachium This refers to the Forearm.

antecardium This refers to Epigastrium.

antecedent This refers to Precursor.

ante cibum Abbreviation for Before Meals.

antecubital situated anterior to the elbow.

anteflexion Forward curvature of an organ or part such as Anteflexion of the Uterus.

ante mortem This means before death.

antenatal This period is called Prenatal period in pregnant woman.

antenna They are feelers in the mouth parts of Arthropoda.

Antepar Preparation of Piperazine Citrate which used as Antihelmenthic.

antepartum That which occurs childbirth, with reference to the mother.

anteposition Forward displacement of the uterus.

antepyretic Occurring before the stage of fever.

anteriad toward the anterior surface of the body.

anterior situated in front of or in the forward part of an organ.

antero Prefix signifying before.

anterolateral Structure or an organ is situated anteriorly and to one side

anteromedial Structure or an organ is situated anteriorly and to the medial side; preferred to.

anteversion the forward tilting of an organ specifically referred to uterus in pelvis.

anthelmintic Drug which is destructive to parasitic (Helminths) worms

anthracosilicosis Pneumoconiosis consisting of both anthracosis and silicosis, caused by coal with a high silica content

anthracosis Pneumoconiosis caused by deposition of coal dust in the lungs. When the dust accumulates in large amounts, it may result in coal workers' pneumoconiosis.

anthrax Bacterial zoonotic disease by Bacillus anthracis from infected carcasses. Common in animal handlers in agriculture. Types of anthrax are Cutaneous anthrax, Gastrointestinal anthrax and Inhalational anthrax.

anthropocentric Considering human beings as the center of the universe.

anthropoid Resembling that of a man

anthropometric Related with measuring the body by height, weight, chest circumference, head circumference or Mid upper arm circumference.

anthropometry The science which deals with the measurement of the size, weight, and proportions of the human body that is done in Nutritional assessment of the community.

anthropophilic preferring human beings to other animals for sucking blood by insects particularly mosquitoes.

anti A prefix signifying opposite

antiabortifacient An agent that promotes successful gestation.

antiarrhythmic Drug that prevents cardiac arrhythmia.

antibacterial Drug that suppresses the growth of bacteria.

antibiotic Chemotherapeutic agents or drugs that inhibit the growth of organism that are used in infections to cure the infectious diseases.

antibody This is Immunological molecule that interacts with antigen to produce Antigen Antibody reaction. that is required for body protection mechanism. Common antigens in immunology are:

- Agglutinins
- Bacteriolysins,
- Haemolysins
- Opsonins
- Precipitins

anticarcinogen Drug used in cancer treatment.

anticholelithogenic Agent or substance that serves to prevent the formation of gallstones.

anticholinergic Blocking the passage of impulses through the parasympathetic nerves.

anticoagulant Drug that prevent the blood clotting. Common drugs are Heparin, Warfarin, Dicumarol.

anticonvulsant Drug that prevents or relieves the event of convulsions.

anticurare an agent that counteracts the action of curare on skeletal muscle.

anti-D IMMUNO globulin or antibody against the "Rh_0" Rh blood group antigen

antidepressant Drugs that prevents or relieves depression in man.

antidiabetic Drug used in alleviating diabetes.

antidiarrheal Drugs that counteracts Diarrhoea.

antidiuretic Drug that suppresses the rate of urine formation

antidote A remedy for counteracting a poison.

antiemetic Drug that prevents or alleviates nausea and vomiting.

antifilarial Drug that is effective against filaria.

antiflatulent That which relieves or prevents flatulence.

antifungal Drug used in the treatment of fungal infections called antimicotic drugs.

antigen Substance which is capable of inducing a specific immune response with specific antibody.

antigenic Having the properties of an antigen.

antigenicity This is the property of being able to induce a specific immune response

anti-HBc Antibody to hepatitis B core antigen.

anti-HBs Antibody to hepatitis B surface antigen.

antihemorrhagic An agent that prevents Haemorrhage.

antihistamine The drug that counteracts the action of histamine.

antihypertensive Drug that brings down the blood pressure of patient.

anti-infective Drug capable of killing pathogens or capable of inhibiting the growth of pathogens

anti-inflammatory Drug that counteracts or suppresses the process of inflammation.

antilewisite Antidote to Dimercaprol o British Antilewisite which is warfare harmful chemical.

antimalarial Therapeutic agents that are effective against malaria.

antimicrobial That which kills microbes which are called antibiotics used in the treatment of infections.

antimycobacterial Drug which is effective against mycobacteria. or drug used in Tuberculosis.

antimycotic Drug used in the treatment of fungal infections.

antioxidant Substance that are added to food substance which prevent the deterioration by the action of oxygen in the air.
antiparkinsonian Effective in the treatment of parkinsonism.
antipruritic Drug used for relieving or preventing itching.
antipsychotic They are neuroleptic agents that are effective in the treatment of psychosis such as Phenothiazines, Dibenzoxazepine etc.
antipyretic Drug used in the relief of fever such as paracetamol or aspirin.
antiretroviral Drug used in HIV/AIDS that are effective against retroviruses.
antirheumatic Agent that relieves or prevents rheumatism.
antisepsis Chemicals that are used in the prevention of sepsis by antiseptic means.
antiseptic That which has the property of antisepsis.
antiserum Serum that contains antibody which is obtained from animal that has been immunized either by injection of antigen into the body or by infection with microorganisms containing the antigen. Both Monovalent or Polyvalent are available.
antisialagogue Drug to counteracting the formation of saliva.
antisocial Behavior that violates the rights of others societal mores and the law in society.
antispasmodic relieving spasm, usually of smooth muscle, bronchi, intestine, bile duct, ureters or sphincters
antithromboplastin Substance that prevents or interferes with the interaction of the blood coagulation factors
antithyrotoxic Drug counteracting the toxic effects of excessive amounts of Thyroid hormone.
antitoxin Antibody against a toxin.
antitussive Relieving cough.
antiulcerative Promoting the healing of ulcers.
antivenom Venom used in counteracting the poisonous effect of snake venom. Also called Antivenin.
antiviral Drug used in the treatment of Viral infections that suppresses their replication.
Anton's symptom Person who is blind fails to recognise that he is blind.
antrectomy Surgical excision of an antrum, such as Pyloric antrum.
antrum Anatomical nomenclature for a cavity or chamber especially within a bone.
ANTU Rodenticide which produce pulmonary oedema and pleural effusion that is chemically **A**lpha **N**aphthyl **T**hio **U**rea.
anuresis Retention of urine in the bladder.
anus Terminal orifice of the alimentary canal.
anusitis Infection and inflammation of the anus.
anxiety Emotional state consisting of psychophysiological responses to anticipation of unreal or imagined danger. This is manifested in the form of heart rate, altered respiration rate, sweating, trembling, weakness, and fatigue
anxiolytic Anti anxiety drug which reduces anxiety.
aorta This is main trunk from which the systemic arterial system proceeds.
aortic Pertaining to the aorta.
aortogram The radiography from aortography.
aortography radiography of the aorta After the I V injection of an opaque medium Radiograph of aorta is taken. Usual radiological procedures include a) Retrograde aortography and b) Translumbar aortography.
aortopathy Disease of the aorta.
aortopexy In the case of Tracheomalacia the compression caused by air obstruction is removed by suturing the anterior walls of aortic arch and right subclavian artery to the sternum to pull the attached trachea.
aortoplasty Surgical repair of the aorta
apathy Lack of feeling.
ape Term used to refer to monkeys of the larger old world.
aperture This refers to an opening or to an orifice. Microscope's objective lens. Diameter of the iris . Diameter of the camara lens.
apex Anatomical word to depict the superior aspect of the body or of a part or of the organ.
Apgar score This is a monitor done at 1 minute and at 5 minutes after birth. A score of 7 to 10 normal, 4 to 7 mild depression and 0 to 3 severe depression. Apgar score allows prompt action in severe depression.
APHA Abbreviation for **A**merican **P**ublic **H**ealth **A**ssociation.
aphakia absence of the lens of the eye either due to cataract surgery or due to congenital absence.
aphakic Pertaining to aphakia.
aphasia Loss of power to speak, Brain injury can cause loss of power of expression of speech, writing and comprehension.
aphonia loss of voice.
aphrodisiac Drug or chemical that arouses the sexual instinct.
aphtha a small ulcer which is a round lesion such as aphthous stomatitis.
apical Located at the apex.
apiphobia Unwanted fear of bees.
aplasia Undeveloped tissue or organ.
aplastic Undeveloped from the primordium or from the stem cell.
apnea cessation of breathing.
apoatropine An antispasmodic alkaloid derived from belladonna.
apocrine Gland secretion which contains apical portion of secreting cell is also cast off.
apoenzyme Protein component of an enzyme that is separable from the coenzyme but that requires the presence of the prosthetic group to form the functioning compound

apoferritin Colorless protein related to Transferrin.
apogamy Reproduction without conjugation of gametes and is called Parthenogenesis.
apolipoprotein Protein constituents of lipoproteins grouped under A B C and E.
apomorphine hydrochloride a derivative of morphine used as a central emetic in the treatment of drug overdose and accidental poisoning; administered subcutaneously.
aponeurosis Tendinous expansion, serving mainly to connect a muscle with the parts that it moves.
apophyseal Related with apophysis.
apophysis Bony outgrowth which is not separated from that bone science it is a part of that bone. This can be called a part, a tubercle or a tuberosity.
apoplexy Because of internal bleeding in the brain the existence of the clinical condition called Stroke. Because of its occurrence in other organs we have other clinical conditions like Adrenal apoplexy, Abdominal apoplexy, Ovarian apoplexy, Pancreatic apoplexy etc.
apoprotein This is the protein moiety of a conjugated protein
apostasis This suggests the end or crisis of an attack of disease.
aposthia Prepuce is not present since birth in man.
apothecary This refers to drug store or Pharmacist dispensing drugs.
apparatus In human body many parts act together to perform one specific function. In Instrumentation technology many items are assembled which can perform an assigned function. Sayer's apparatus for Plaster of paris jacket work, Biliary apparatus for biliary function etc.
appendage The part which is appended or added to main part.
appendicectomy Surgical removal of appendix after attending to it for its acute phase.
appendicitis Infection and inflammation of the vermiform appendix.
appendicular That which is related with vermiform appendix.
appendix Specifically referred to vermiform appendix of small intestine which is a vestibular origin without any function in man. Anatomically the term says a supplementary, accessory or an attached part of a main structure.
appetite Recurring and natural desire for food which may be or may not be associated with hunger contraction.
appliance Devices that are used in day to day Therapy such as Dental appliance, Surgical appliance, Orthopaedic appliance etc.,
applicator A device used to apply mendicamentation in day to day therapy such as loop applicator, drops applicator etc.
apposition Placing of things in proximity
apprehension Fear or anxiety.
approach Surgical approach meaning reaching the organ or tissue at surgery for operation or resection.
approximation Apposition or bringing close together.
apraxia Due to paralysis one is unable to carry out normal movements.
Apresoline This contains Hydralazine Hydrochloride.
aproctia congenital absence of the anus.
apterous This refers to insects which are wingless.
aptitude Ability and skill in certain lines of endeavour which is inborn in nature.
aptyalism When there ius no salivary secretion.
apyogenic That which is not caused by pus.
apyrexia There is no fever on clinical examination.
AQ Abbreviation for **A**chievement **Q**uotient.
Aq. Abbreviation to depict Water.
aqua water.
aquaphobia Irrational fear of water when a person approaches swimming pool, river, pond, sea
aquatic Inhabiting in water refers to animal.
aqueduct A channel or a passage or channel meant for passage another anatomical structure such as Cerebral aqueduct, Vestibular aqueduct.
aqueductus Channel in a body structure or organ, especially a channel for the conduction of fluid
aqueous Prepared with water.
arabin It is mainly Arabic acid which is an amorphous carbohydrate gum composed of residues of arabinose, rhamnose, galactose, and an aldobionic acid which is called as gum Arabic or Acacia.
arabinose This is an aldopentose present in plants in the form of glycosides, mucilages and polysacchar-ides; which is also found present in bacteria.
arachidic acid It is a fatty acid present in vegetables such as peanut.
arachidonic acid It is an essential fatty acid present in animal fat which is the precursor of prostaglandins.
Arachnida In Medical entomology they are in the class of the Arthropoda which include ticks, mites
arachnodactyly A clinical condition characterized by abnormal length and slenderness of the fingers and toes which is also seen Marfan's syndrome.
arachnoid That which resembles a spider web such as Arachnoid of brain or Arachnoid of Spinal cord.
arachnoide mater Membrane situated in between Dura mater and Pia mater; that is having subarachnoid space.
arachnoiditis Infection and inflammation of the arachnoide
Aran's law In injury to the vault of the skull, produce fracture of the base of the skull which is the extension of fracture through shsortest circle.
Aran-Duchenne muscular atrophy This Muscular atrophy which is by spinal pathology

arborescent That which looks like branches of a tree.

arbovirus The virus which is transmitted by the bite of insects which suck blood on man. This contains major group of viruses like Flaviviridae, Rhabdo-viridae, Rhabdoviridae and Togaviridae.

ARC Abbreviation for **A**IDS **R**elated **C**omplex

arc It is a projected structure which has the curve like a bow such as Visual Arc.

arcade Anatomical structure composed of a series of arches such as Arterial arcade, Dental arcade etc.,

arch Structure with a curved or bowlike outline.

archaic very ancient

archeo primitive.

arctation This refers to Stenosis or narrowing of vessels.

arcus Any structure having a curved or bowlike outline.

ARD Abbreviation for **A**cute **R**espiratory **D**isease

ARDS Abbreviation for **A**cute **R**espiratory **D**istress **S**yndrome.

area A demarcated surface which has definite function or unform structure such as Aortic area, Auditory area etc.

areata clinical manifestation in the form of patches such as alopecia areata.

Arenavirus This group of virus include Lassa Virus and other haemorrhagic producing viruses.

arenoid That which resembles sand.

areola Area surrounding nipple, Area surrounding pupil, area surrounding a pustule, Area surrounding a Vesicle.

Arey's rule This rule is relative calculation of gestational age in first five months of pregnancy. This requires thelength of the foetus and numbers of lunar months since conception.

Argas Ticks of the family Argasidae, some of which transmit diseases to humans

Argemone It is a prickly poppy that contains Argemone oil whose adulteration can cause Epidemic Dropsy.

arginase An enzyme that converts Arginine to Urea and Ornithine in Urea cycle within the Liver.

arginine This is from Protein digestion which is a nonessential amino acid. It helps in the synthesis of Creatine.

Argyll Robertson pupil In Myopia the pupil do not respond to light but responds to accommodation effort

Aristotle Aristotle was a Greek philosopher and student of Plato. He stressed the need for observation and induction and has described anatomy physiology and embryology. He postulated four theory of elements called Humoralism.

arm This refers to upper limb for mobility and independent function.

armadillo South American Ant Eater which has horny shield on the dorsal surface which was found successful in culturing leprosy bacilli.

armature A protective structure or a protective organ.

armpit Axilla which is the externally visible portion of upper limb.

Arneth count This is the ratio of different polymorphonuclear leukocytes by taking number of lobes as criteria.

- One Lobe .... 5 percent
- Two Lobes ...... 35 percent
- Three Lobes .... 41 percent
- Four Lobes ..... 17 percent
- Five Lobes ...... 2 percent

aroma Fragrance of medicine food drink or of spice.

aromatic Organic substance which has ring system of chemical structure with conjugated double bonds such as Benzene, Naphthalene

arousal When a person who is not responding is made to respond. When a person is made awakened from sleep, When a person is stimulated by sex stimuli

arrangement To arrange things, To arrange in position of items

arrector Structure that has raisen

arrest To stop such as cardiac arrest, Developmental arrest

arrested When the head of foetus is detained in pelvis, When bleeding is controlled by pressure or ligation

arrhythmia Normal rhythm of the heart is not present.

arsenic Brittle, lustrous, grayish solid which is toxic and carcinogenic. In ancient times arsenic preparations were used in medicine. Now used in some of the selected parasitic infections.

arsenic acid Arsenic pentoxide in hydrated form represented as $H3AsO_4$,

arsenite Salt of arsenous acid.

arsenous acid Arsenic trioxide in hydrated form represented as $H3AsO_3$

arsphenamine In olden days this was given as specific treatment for Syphilis yaws and other spirochetal infections. Nowadays it is replaced by newer drugs.

ART Abbreviation for **A**ssisted **R**eproductive **T**echnology.

arterial Pertaining to the arteries.

arteriogram Radiograph of an artery taken during arteriography.

arteriograph Film produced by arteriography.

arteriography angiography of coronary artery or by catheterisation angiography of arteries

arteriola Minute arterial branch proximal to a capillary.

arteriolith Concretion in an artery.

arteriolitis Infection and inflammation of the arterioles which can be necrotising or hyperplastic in nature.

arteriolonecrosis Necrosis of arterioles such as nephrosclerosis;

arteriolopathy Disease of the arterioles.

arteriolosclerosis Sclerosis and thickening of the walls of the smaller arteries

arteriolosclerotic pertaining to or characterized by arteriolosclerosis.

arteriomotor pertaining to or causing change in the caliber of an artery.

arterionecrosis necrosis of an artery or of arteries.

arteriopathy any arterial disease.

arterioplasty Surgical repair of an artery.

arteriorrhaphy Suture of an artery.

arteriorrhexis Rupture of an artery.

arteriosclerosis Thickening and loss of elasticity of arterial walls Which are of three types on histological basis. They are:

1) Arterial Sclerosis
2) Arteriolosclerosis
3) Atherosclerosis

arteriovenous Referred to both artery and vein.

arteritis Infection and inflammation of an artery.

artery This refers to a vessel or channel that carry blood to the heart from different parts of the body. The wall of artery is made of three layers. They are:

1. Tunica Externa the Outer layer
2. Tunica Media the Middle layer
3. Tunica Interna the Internal layer

arthral Pertaining to a joint.

arthralgia Pain in a joint

arthritis Infection and Inflammation of joints

arthro That which is related with joint.

arthrocele A joint swollen and there is fluid accumulation in that joint.

arthrocentesis Surgical puncture and aspiration of a joint.

arthrochondritis Infection and inflammation of the cartilage of a joint.

arthroclasia In case of fused or ankylosed joint, surgery is done to break the fusion to allow joint for normal physiological movement.

arthrodynia Pain in a joint due to pathology

arthrodysplasia Deformity of many joints which is hereditary in nature.

arthrogram Introduction of opaque contrast material into the joint and taking a radiographic recording for the purpose of diagnosis.

arthrokatadysis Bone softening and its absorption which results in limiting the movement. This is common in case of Hip joint surfaces.

arthrolithiasis The clinical condition is called Gout.

arthrology the scientific study of the joints and ligaments which is termed as Syndesmology.

arthropathology The scientific study of the structural and functional changes produced in the joints by disease.

arthropathy This refers to the disease of the joint.

arthrophyma Refers to the swelling of a joint.

arthrophyte Extra growth in a joint cavity which is called as joint mouse.

arthroplasty plastic surgery of a joint to allow free movement of that joint. Hip and Knee joint anthroplasty is common and well developed in terms of surgical technique and functional progress.

Arthropneumo radiography Radiography of a joint after injection into it of air, oxygen, or carbon dioxide.

arthropod They are jointed legged insects which are often responsible in the transmission of diseases.

Arthropoda Medically important insects which have jointed legs and come under Insects and under Arachnida. They are responsible in the spread of arbovirus infections and arthropod borne infections.

arthroscope Endoscopic examination of a joint for diagnosis and for therapy.

arthroscopy Examination and clinical observation of the interior of a joint with an arthroscope.

arthrosynovitis Infection and inflammation of the synovial membrane of a joint.

arthrotomy Surgical incision of a joint.

Arthus phenomenon This phenomenon is described by Arthurs when he noticed Local oedema and tissue necrosis after sub cutaneous injection of specific antigen in sensitised Rabbit.

articular Related with joints.

articulate Clear pronouncement, Clear speech made, A good and coherent verbal expression, To make a joint by dividing to small units, Proper relation for denture.

articulation To make speech sound, Occlusion surface contact in case teeth,

articulatory Related with making voice notice or utterance by a person.

artifact Artificial product. Additional structure introduced in histology or in microscopy. In X ray or Imaging any structure not normally present is found present.

artificial Artificaially made, Not natural, It is pathological

arytenoid shaped like a jug refers to arytenoid cartilage.

AS Abbreviation for **A**ortic **S**tenosis

As Symbol for Arsenic

asafetida Oleo-gum-resin obtained from the roots of *asafoetida* and other related species of Umbelliferae group of plants. The main odorous principle is isobutyl propyl disulfide. Used as a condiment and food flavouring,

asbestos It is Magnesium and Calcium Silicate which is incombustible and fibrous. There are two types in the land that are available. They are: a) Serpentine type and b) Amphibole type. Asbestos is associated with Mesothelioma of Pleura which is highly cancerous.

asbestosis A form of pneumoconiosis caused by inhaling asbestos which is a major occupational hazard.

ascariasis Roundworm infestation in man by Ascaris lumbricoides which is common nematode under Helminths.

ascaricide Drug used in the treatment of Roundworm infestation which destroys worms of Ascaris.

Ascaris Round Worm which comes under Nematode is common intestinal parasite in developing countries. This comes under family Ascarididae.

ascending That which has an upward course.

ascertainment This word is used in Genetic studies which signifies that traits are identified by the investigator. This can be single, multiple, complete or incomplete ascertainment.

Asch's operation This is an ENT operation for Deviated Nasal Septum or Nasal Deflection as a surgical correction procedure.

Aschheim-Zondek test This is a pregnancy test by injecting urine of pregnancy woman to immature female mice. The test is positive if there is swelling congestion and haemorrhage of ovaries and maturation of ovarian follicles.

Aschner's reflex By compressing eyes rhythm of the heart gets slowed down. Aschner's criteria for this oculocardiac reflex is as under;

- Diminished if heart rhythm is diminished by 1-5
- Normal if it is from 5 to 13
- Exaggerated if it is 13 to 50

Aschoff's bodies This is histological finding in Rheumatic myocarditis. Sub military collections of cells and leukocytes in interstitial tissues of heart is seen.

ascites Effusion and accumulation of serous fluid in the abdominal cavity.

ascitic Characterized by ascites.

Ascomycetes Fungus of the group Ascomycotina under Phylum Eumycota.

ascorbic acid This is vitamin C a water-soluble vitamin found in many fruits and vegetables that is required for some of the enzymatic action in the body. Deficiency causes Scurvy

ASCP Abbreviation for **A**merican **S**ociety of **C**linical **P**athologists.

ascus Spores of fungus is called ascus.

-ase Term used in forming the names of enzymes

asemia One who cannot talk, one who cannot understand speech, one who canno understand signs

asepsis Free from infection.

aseptic Free from infection or septic material called as Sterile.

asepticism This refers to the principles and practices of aseptic techniques.

asexual Refers to growth and development without sex in lower animals. That which is not related with sex.

asexuality Absence of sexual interests.

ASF a synthetic resin that contains **A**niline, **F**ormaldehyde and **S**ulphur which is used in mounting specimens in slides.

Asherman's syndrome a rare condition where scar tissue, also called adhesions or intrauterine adhesions, builds up inside your uterus.

ASI Abbreviation for **A**ddiction **S**everity **I**ndex.

Asklepios Aesculapius is Greek Mythological God of Medicine.

aspartame An artificial sweetener which is 200 times sweet as sucrose. It is used in therapeutic diet as low calorie sweetener.

aspartic acid Nonessential amino acid present in proteins and has the function of neurotransmission of CNS.

aspect It is the look or appearance of given item, Surface of orgain in a designed direction. such as dorsal aspect, posterior aspect etc.,

aspergillosis Fungal infection by Aspergillus fungus. Clinically lesions of skin, ear, orbit, nasal sinus lungs, bones an meninges are seen.

Aspergillus A genus of Fungi which are opportunistic pathogens in man.

aspermia Semen containing no sperms which causes infertility in man.

asphyxia Lack of oxygen causes pathological changes and choking.

asphyxiant Substance capable of producing asphyxia.

asphyxiation Causing of suffocation in a person

aspirate By suction taking out fluid or tissue as therapeutic procedure.

aspiration To take out fluid by needle suction, Process of inhalation, To crave for a thing in life.

aspirator Apparatus used for suction of fluids

aspirin Chemically it is acetylsalicylic acid which has anti-inflammatory analgesic, and antipyretic effects

assay Procedure to find out the quantity or quality of a substance, Determination of potency safty and clarity of a drug or vaccine.

assessment Evaluation, Appraisal, Testing, Examining. Usually referable to clinical assessment of a patient.

Assézat's triangle The Facial Triangle formed by lines joining the alveolar and basal pints and the nasion.

assident Not accompanied with a disease.

assimilable Capable of digesting or assimilation of food.

assimilation Food digestion to complete form there by one gets calories and nutrients. A process of anabolism. Getting new experience in life from psychological point of view.

Assmann's focus Exudative lesion of Tuberculosis in apex of the lung. Sometimes sub apical lesion of tuberculosis.

association Brain that links primary motor to sensory cortex, Attributers when tested show that their occurrence either by chance or not by chance - a statistical inference Association of genetic phenotype characteristics occurring, Connection of two or more ideas or feelings in the state of consciousness.

assortment a group of different things or of different types of the same thing; a mixture.

astasia Incoordination with inability to stand

aster The structure seen in a cell during the prophase of mitosis

asterion Star shaped suture produced by the joining of three sutures namely Lambdoid suture, Parietomastoid suture and Occipitomastoid suture.

asterixis The motor disturbance produced in hepatic coma where flapping tremor is produced.

asteroid Star-shaped

asthenia lack of strength and energy resulting in weakness.

asthenopia Fatigue of the visual organs with pain in the eyes, headache, dimness of vision

asthenospermia Reduction in the vitality of spermatozoa.

asthma Recurrent attacks of paroxysmal dyspnea which is associated with spasmodic contraction of the bronchi. Allergy and sensitiveness are found responsible for asthma.

asthmatic Person who is affected with asthma.

astigmatic That which is related with astigmatism.

astigmatism Here the refractive surface of the eye are having unequal curvature which do not allow light rays to focus at one point. The patient cannot see either horizontal lines or vertical lines at a given point of time.

astraphobia Irrational fear of thunder and lightning.

astringent Chemical or drug that causes cooling effect and vasoconstriction of area where it is applied.

astrocytoma It is also called as Astrocytic Glioma which is the primary tumour of the brain composed of astrocytes.

Astrovirus Under the family Astroviridae there are seven serotypes, which are known to cause G.E. in Man.

asylum A place of shelter for the support and care of helpless and deprived such as mentally sick individuals.

asymmetry Dissimilarity in corresponding parts or organs on opposite sides of the body which are normally alike.

asymptomatic Person who do not have any clinical manifestations. No symptoms.

asystole absence of a heartbeat which refers to missed heart contraction in cardiac cycle.

atactic The clinical condition which is characterized by ataxia.

ataraxia Calmness or peace of mind.

atavism Inherited characteristics of man has come from his great grandfathers rather than father. Gene recombination and Unusual environment are blamed for this condition.

ataxia condition characterised by muscular coordination and irregularity of muscular action..

atelectasis Collapse of the lung which was once normal. Incomplete expansion of lung which may be due congenital or acquired causes.

atenolol Beta adrenergic blocking agent prescribed in hypertension and in angina pectoris.

atherectomy Surgical removal of atherosclerotic plaque from an artery using a rotary cutter through a special catheter guided radiographically

atheroma Degeneration and thickening of plaque of atherosclerosis.

atherosclerosis Atheromas which are yellow plaques of cholesterol or lipoid material inside an artery.

atlanto Denoting relationship to the atlas.

atlas Name of First Cervical Vertebra which articulates with Axis bone below and with Occipital bone above. This also means in Medical sciences for Illustrated collection on a given topic.

atloaxoid Related with the atlas and the axis.

atloido-occipital Related with the atlas and the occiput.

atmosphere Gas envelope surrounding the earth and the pressure exerted at sea level is 760 mm Hg.

atmospheric That which is related with atmosphere.

atom An atom consists of a central nucleus that is surrounded by one or more negatively charged electrons. The nucleus is positively charged and contains one or more relatively heavy particles known as protons and neutrons.

atomic Pertaining to an atom.

atonia No tone or atony in a referred structure.

atony lack of normal tone as in a muscle deprived of its innervation.

atopen allergen involved in an atopic disorder.

atopy Person getting atopic allergy due to environmental antigen which is supposed to be genetic predisposition that is manifested in the form of Bronchial asthma or Allergic Rhinitis.

atoxic That which is not poisonous

ATP Abbreviation for **A**denosine **Tri** **P**hosphate

atraumatic Not causing damage or injury.

atresia congenital absence of a normal body orifice such as anal atresia, aural atresia etc.,

atrichosis No hair on the skin where there should be usually termed as alopecia.

atriomegaly Pathological dilatation of atrium of the heart.

atrioventricular That which is related with atrium and ventricle of the heart.

atrium Meaning a chamber the word always used and referred to the atrium of the heart.

Atropa Atropa belladonna plant that belongs to the Solanaceae which yield alkaloid Atropine, Hyoscyamine and Scopolamine which have high medicinal value.

atrophied Structure or an organ that is shrunken.

atrophy wasting of cell, tissue, organ or part of the body such Bone atrophy, disuse atrophy, nerve atrophy etc.,

atropine An alkaloid derived from species of belladonna that has anticholinergic and antispasmodic property.

Other properties are:
- o Dilatation of pupil
- o Antisecretory
- o Blocks vagus nerve which helps in chronic gastric ulcer
- o Anti tremor
- o Anti Parkinsonism
- o Relaxation of smooth muscles

atropinism Poisoning caused by ingestion of atropine which produce toxic effects such as dry mouth, dry throat, papillary dilation, fever, increased pulse rate, flushing of the face, mental confusion and hallucinations.

ATS Abbreviation of **A**nti **T**etanus **S**erum

attachment This refers to anatomical connection by which one thing is fixed to another. E.g., Epithelial attachment, Orthodontic attachment.

attack Sudden onset of disease such as Heart attack, Anxiety attack, transient ischemic attack etc.,

attar Volatile vegetable oil which is fragrant like Rose attar.

attention Awareness and response which is selective in nature to the environmental stimuli.

attenuation Reduced virulence of pathogens which cannot cause disease in man .

attitude Foetal position in the womb that one in the attitude of universal flexion. Positive or negative attitude of man in the society.

attraction In drawing of one part into another such as attraction of maxillary and mandibular structure giving raise to shortening of the face.

attrition The natural process of wearing away of parts of body such as teeth, hair, akin etc., as a part of senescence.

atypia Irregular and not conforming to normalcy.

atypical Common term used for unusual strains of bacteria or virus in microbiology. That which is not typical in nature and is unusual in appearance.

Aub-Dubois table This table gives the BMR (Basal Metabolic Rates) for given age in man

Auberger blood group is a type of human blood group in which the Aua antigen is expressed. It is found in 82% of caucasians. It may be related to the Lutheran antigen system. The blood group was named after patient Auberger, who was a 59-year-old French woman with oesophageal varices.

Aubert's phenomenon This is an optical illusion wherein vertical line appears to incline towards other side when the head is turned towards one side.

audio Related to hearing.

audiogram The record of the thresholds of hearing of an individual for various sound frequencies.

audiologist Specialist in audiology who helps in diagnostic testing and rehabilitation of impaired hearing.

audiology The scientific study of hearing for diagnostic purpose and for rehabilitation purpose.

audiometer A device to monitor and record stimuli of intensity and frequency for the measurement of hearing. This is used in testing hard of hearing or deafness.

audiometrician Technician specializing in the measurement of hearing ability (audiometry).

audiometry Measurement of hearing by an audiometer.

audioscope Instrument to detect hearing impairment with the help of otoscope and audiometer.

audition To listen to such as audition test in All India Radio.

auditory Related with the sense of hearing

Auenbrugger's sign In case of Pericardial effusion there will bulging of epigastrium.

Auer bodies (rods) In patient suffering from Leukaemia rod shaped bodies are seen in the cytoplasm of myeloblasts.

Auerbach's ganglion Small ganglia of Auerbach's plexus i.e., in nerve fibres situated in muscular coats of intestine

augmentation Addition of tissues in case of bladder or breast in plastic surgery. Surgical procedures are called Augmentation Cystoplasty and Augmentation Mammaplasty

Aujeszky's disease Bulbar paralysis by virus other than Ravie's virus causing Pseudo hydrophobia.

aura Term used in Fits or epilepsy where subjective sensation precedes and marks the onset of epilepsy.

aural That which is related with hearing or auditory or with aura of epilepsy.

Aureomycin An antibiotic with chlortetracycline hydrochloride.

auricle Refers to atrium of heart

auricula Portion of external ear.

auricular Related with ear

auriform Any structure which is ear-shaped.

auriscope Device to examine ear namely Otoscope.

auscultate Examination by listening to the sounds of the thoracic or abdominal viscera, with or without a stethoscope.

auscultation Listening for sounds within the body of lungs, heart, abdomen and other organs and also in pregnancy for foetal heart sounds.

Austin Flint murmur In case of Aortic Regurgitation a loud presystolic murmur is heart at the apex of the heart.

autemesia Functional or idiopathic vomiting.

autoagglutination Clumping of blood cell by one's own serum.

autoagglutinin A factor present in the serum which is called Autologous factor which helps in auto agglutination i.e., agglutination of one's own cellular elements.

autoallergy If the person is having autoimmunity.

autoamputation In case of an extra growth or of a polyp, sudden detachment occurs. In case of injury cutting of a finger, of a limb etc.,

autoantibody In response to one's own endogenous body element an antibody or immunoglobulin is formed which is called '*self antigen*'

autoanticomplement In a person self complement is formed for his own complement which is called '*self complement*'

autoantigen In a person self antigen is formed for his own antigen. This is a character of autoimmune disease.

autoclave In hospital disinfection procedure a bin which is fitted with device for regulation of pressure is used in sterilisation. Heat and pressure act on killing pathogens.

autodigestion This name is given for cellular tissue and organ lysis or digestion that occur after death called '*a post mortem change*'

autoerotism Self gratification by masturbation

autogamy fertilization within a single mother cell by union of chromatin which is called *self fertilisation.*

autograft For graft, tissue is taken from site and grafted in another site. Donor and recipient both are self or same individual.

autohemagglutination Clotting of blood cells which is called '*Haemagglutination of self*'

autoimmunity This is cell mediated immune response against ones own antigen that leads to '*Autoimmune disease*'

autoinfection infection or infestation in a person by pathogens present in him by mechanical means. Typical example of autoinfection is threadworm infection.

autokinetic One that has the power of voluntary motion.

autolysis Digestion of cellular components that is seen as a post-mortem change by endogenous hydrolases from lysosomes

automatic That which moves by self regulation. That which is self moving.

autonomic That which is functionally independent such as Autonomic Nervous System.

autonomous Pertaining to autonomy.

autonomy This is the state of functioning independently where outside force cannot act.

autoplasty Transplantation of one's own tissue.

autopsy The postmortem examination of dead body to find out the cause of death that is required for legal documentation

autoregulation In biological system body identifies and adjusts for the changes that have occurred. One of the example is maintenance of constant blood flow in hyper or hypo tension.

autosome In Human beings there are 22 pairs of autosomes that are paired chromosomes and are alike in both sexes.

autosuggestion Induction for acceptance of idea belief by self hypnosis.

autozygous Parental descent of a character in man.

auxiliary Helping hands, Afforded aids.

avascular A structure or an organ that is not supplied with blood supply.

Avellis' syndrome In this clinical condition there is paralysis of Nucleus ambiguous and paralysis of spinothalamic tract leading to the following conditions;-

- Loss of sensation for pain and temperature in contralateral leg trunk arm neck and in scalp skin
- Ipsilateral paralysis of vocal cord and soft palate

averaging Calculating mean of given data in a population. Considering a person to the average scale in terms of demographic or academic data.

avermectin This belong to Lactone group of chemicals that are used in the treatment of helminthic infestation and also as insecticides.

avian That which is related with birds.

Avicenna He is Persian Physician and Philosopher who wrote his famous medical book "Canon" during 17th century. This book is systematic compilation of speculative and practical medicine.

avirulence This refers to a pathogen which cannot produce disease.

Avogadro's law This law enunciated by Avogadro states 'Equal volumes of gases with the same pressure and temperature contain an equal number of molecules.'

avulsion Accidental tearing of a part especially refers to scalp skin.

axilla This is the 'Armpit' situated between arm and upper thorax wall. It is pyramidal in shape that contains anatomical structures like nerves, vessels and loose areolar tissue.

axis Revolving body turning line, Specific parts arranged line, Name of Second Cervical Vertebra. Designated X axis or Y axis in X and Y axis.

axolemma It is the plasma membrane of an axon

axon This is responsible for the impulse travel from nerve cell that are the processes of neurone cell.

Ayer's test For surgical spinal block anaesthesia the pressure monitored in L.P. should be equal to the pressure in the Cisterna Magna puncture. In normal subjects the pressures will be same.

Ayer-Tobey test In case of Lateral sinus thrombosis pressure on one jugular vein alone causes a rise in spinal fluid pressure that can be monitored in a manometer attached to L P needle.

azide Any chemical compound that contains the group —N_3.

azithromycin an antibiotic derived from Erythromycin that inhibits bacterial protein synthesis used against wide range of bacteriae.

azobenzene It is a nitrobenzene product used in azo dyes and pH indicators.

azoospermia Absence of spermatozoa in the semen a cause of infertility.

azotemia When high level of urea and nitrogenous compounds are found in the blood.

AZT Abbreviation for Zidovudine which is an antiretro viral drug used in HIV/AIDS

azygous Meaning unpaired.

B

β beta, Second letter of the Greek alphabet and symbol for Beta chain chemicals.

Babesia A protozoal parasite in R B C causing Babesiosis disease.

babesiosis Tick-borne diseases due to infection with protozoa of the genus Babesia attacking Red Blood Corpuscles.

Babinski's reflex On stimulating the sole of the foot dorsiflexion of big toe occurs which is due to Pyramidal tract lesion.

Baccelli's sign In patients suffering from Pleural effusion, clinician can hear the whisper over the chest.

bacciform Berry-shaped.

Bachmann's bundle This is a transverse band of muscle fibres that extends between the bases of right and left auricular appendages.

Bacillaceae This is a family of bacteria made up of endospore-forming rods and cocci.

Bacillary Related to rod like pathogens which cause illness in human beings.

bacilluria Presence of bacilli in the urine in urinary tract infections.

Bacillus This is a genus of bacteria of the family Bacillaceae that contain 48 species of pathogenic organisms.

bacitracin This is antibacterial preparation that contains polypeptide produced by Bacillus subtilis group of organisms.

backbone This is the column containing vertebral bones.

BACOP Abbreviated 5 drugs that are used in cancer treatment. They are **B**leomycin, **A**driamycin, **C**yclophosphamide, **O**ncovin and **P**rednisone.

bacteremia It is the presence of bacteria in the blood.

bacteria All pathogenic and non pathogenic organisms under Prokaryotae excluding Algae.

bacterial That which is related with bacteria

bactericidal Chemicals or drugs that kill bacteria.

bacteriofluorescin Dye produced by Pseudomonas organism which emits light (Fluorescent)

bacteriological pertaining to or related with bacteria

bacteriologist One who is expert in the study of morphology, life cycle, virulence, immunological aspect, culture , fermentation reaction and the study of sensitivity of known bacteria.

bacteriology The Scientific study of bacteria with respect of their morphology, culture, reaction and immunological aspect which is known as Microbiology.

bacteriolytic Agent or item which has to do with the destruction of bacteria.

bacteriophage One type of virus that eats away or destroys bacteria.

bacterioprotein Protein of bacterial origin.

bacteriopsonin Opsonic is an antibody that interacts with bacteria which makes bacteria more susceptible to phagocytosis.

bacteriostatic Chemical or drug which inhibits the growth or multiplication of bacteria.

bacteriotoxin Toxin produced by bacteria.

bacteriuria On laboratory examination we observe the presence of bacteria in the urine.

Bactrim Commercial trade name of drug that contains Trimethoprim and sulfamethoxazole.

badge This refers to Film badge or dosimeter used by radiologists and workers who work in radiology department.

Baelz's disease This is a clinical condition manifested by painless papules on mucous membrane of lips.

Baer's cavity In Embryology, associated with Blastoderm a cavity below the Blastoderm which is the cleavage cavity.

bagassosis This is an Occupational Pneumoconiosis produced by the inhalation of sugar cane dust called Bagasse. The clinical condition is by the hypersensitivity pneumonitis owing to dust and bagasse fungus.

Bainbridge reflex Heart rate is increased when there is raise in pressure in somatic veins.

Baker's cyst Swelling behind the knee produced by synovial cyst in popliteal bursa due to escape of synovial fluid into popliteal bursa.

balanic Related with Glans penis or Glans Clitoris (portion of genital organ)

balanoposthitis Infection and inflammation of the Glans penis (front of male sex organ under foreskin) and Prepuce (foreskin).

Balantidium This is a genus of ciliate protozoa which include parasites that cause intestinal paracytism.

baldness Loss of hair on the scalp which is called alopecia.

Baldy's operation This operation is a method adopted in surgical correction of Inguinal Hernia by obliterating the sac of that hernia.

Balkan splint Balkan came from the place name where the splint was first used in the treatment of fracture of femur. A metal ring and a overhead bar are provided which are supported with pulleys attached.

Ball's valve They are folds of rectal mucosa which are going to form sinuses of Morgagni at a later date.

ball Referred to spherical mass such as hair ball, fungus ball etc.

Ballance's sign This is sign of splenic rupture. When patient ies on the left side resonance of right flank is present.

Ballet's sign This is sign in Exophthalmic goiter and Hysteria. Pupil movement and automatic eye movement persist with loss of voluntary eye movements called ophthalmoplegia externa.

ballismus Movements caused by contractions of the proximal limb muscles due to destruction of the subthalamic nucleus

ballooning Done for therapeutic purpose by distending any cavity of the body with air or gas

ballottement This is the clinical technique to test pregnancy by pushing up the head of fetus by fingers inserted into vagina.

Balme's cough In case of obstruction of nasopharynx, cough is produced when patient lying down .

balneotherapy It is the treatment of disease by baths.

balsam Resinous liquid of vegetable origin composed of esters. Such as Canada balsam used in microscopic medium.

band The strip to hold two objects or two parts held together. Anatomical band that hold two parts are called Trabecula, Taenia or Frenulum.

bandage It is strip or gauze or cotton used to wrap round the part in case of fracture or injury. Bandages are used as dressings or strappings.

bandicoot Wild rat called wild rodent which acts as reservoir of Rat bite fever organism and Ictero haemorrhagica fever organisms.

Bandl's ring During labour ring shaped thickening of the uterus occurs just above the internal os which becomes the lower limit of the contractile portion of the uterus in labour.

Bang's bacillus This pertains to Brucella infection which cause abortion.

Bannister's disease This refers to Angiooedema.

Banthine Pharmacy trademark for the drug Methantheline Bromide

Banti's disease This refers to Congestive Splenomegaly.

Banting Sir Frederick Grant Banting Discovered Insulin in 1922

bar The unit of pressure, expressed in dyne/cm^2

Barber's psoriasis This refers to Localised Pustular Psorisis.

barbital The barbiturate that is a long-acting compound administered orally as a sedative and hypnotic.

barbiturate Sedative-hypnotic derived from barbituric acid or thiobarbituric acid and classified into long-, intermediate-, short-, and ultrashort-acting Barbiturates. Very common ones are:

- ✓ Phenobarbital as anticonvulsant
- ✓ Thiopental as I V anaesthetics

barbituric acid This is chemically 2,4,6-trioxo-hexahydropyrimidine. Addition of aryl or alkyl group form sedative and hypnotic.

Bard's sign This is the sign in Organic Nystagmus. Oscillations of the eye increase as the patient's attention follows the finger moved alternatively from one side to the other. The same Oscillations disappear in congenital Nystagmus.

Bardet-Biedl syndrome Syndrome consisting of Obesity, Hypogonadism, Mental deficiency, Skull defects and Retinitis Pigmentosa.

barium It is one of the earth material element which is yellow

Barkan's operation This is eye surgery Goniotomy for Glaucoma. This consists of opening of Schlemm's canal under direct vision secured by contact glass.

Barlow's disease This is clinical condition of scurvy among infants.

Barlow syndrome Many clinical entities by Mitral Valve Prolapse in an individual.

baroreceptor Receptors in blood vessels that get stimulated by the change in Pressure. They are pressure receptors.

Barr body This is Sex Chromatin described by Barr.

Barraquer's disease This is partial Lipo Dystrophy described by Barraquer.

Barraquer's operation This operation is done to remove lens in cataract by means of suction with the instrument called Erysiphale.

Barré's sign In mental retardation the contraction of the iris is also retarded .

Barré-Guillain syndrome Spastic paraplegia due to Acute Idiopathic Polyneuritis.

barren The word denote that a person is sterile.

Barth's hernia Hernia of loops of intestine between serosa of abdominal wall and persistent vitelline duct.

Bartholin's abscess Abscess of Bartholin gland.

Bartonella A genus of bacteria of the familia bartonellaceae order Rickettsiales present in RBCs and spread through arthropods.

basal Situated near a base.

basalis Related to the near of a base.

Basedow's disease This refers to Graves' disease described by Basedow.

baseline This is baseline or initial information in an experiment or survey which can be compared with information at a later date in Medical research.

basic Property as base which neutralizes acid. One which has the property of a base.

basilic Very important or prominent.

Basioccipital Related or pertaining to the basilar process of the occipital bone.

basis Opposite of Base or designated lowest part of a structure.

Basle Nomina Anatomica Recommendations of Anatomical structures in 1895 held in a meeting in Basle Switzerland. But the present Anatomical nomenclature are based on 1998 recommendations of Terminologia Anatomica.

basophil Referred to the cell which stains readily with basic dyes such as Granular Leukocytes.

Bassen-Kornzweig syndrome Referred to Familial Lipoproteinaemia described by Bassen and Kornzweig.

Basset's operation In surgical resection done for the surgical treatment of cancer of vulva, dissection of inguinal glands are done by a technique adopted by Basset.

Bassini's operation For radical cure of Inguinal hernia the surgical procedure is adopted as adopted by Bassini.

bassorin Gum extract which swell in water is used as a pharmaceutical adjuvant.

bastard Person born out of wedlock or a considered inferior.

Bastian-Bruns law In case of complete transverse lesion of spinal cord proximal to lumbar enlargement, the tendon reflexes of the lower extremities are absent.

Batten-Mayou disease This is Juvenile Amaurotic family idiocy with clinical manifestation of pigmentation of the maula and pallor of the optic disk.

Baudelocque's diameter He described the external diameter of the pelvis, which has the practical utility in obstetrics.

bauxite Name is derived from the place called Baux in France where first Bauxite mine was established. This contains Aluminum Hydroxides clay and some metal oxides, which form the source for Aluminum.

BCG Vaccine given for active immunization against Tuberculosis prevention is made up of strain of bacteria developed by Calmette and Guerin. Hence the Abbreviation **B**acilli **C**amette **G**uerin.

b.d. This is prescription abbreviation for twice a day.

beaded Anatomical structure having the appearance of a string of beads.

beaker A cup with a lip for pouring used in chemistry laboratory use and also in Pharmacy .

beam Electromagnetic radiation or particles.

beard Hair growing on the lower part of a man's face as a secondary sex characteristics.

bearing This refers to a supporting surface or point.

bearing down The labour effort or the expulsive effort of a woman in labor.

Bearn-Kunkel syndrome Refers to Lupoid Hepatitis described by Bearn and Kunkel.

beat Referred to pulse or throb of pulsation.

Beau's lines During the convalescence of wasting diseases, transverse lines on the finger nails appear.

beclomethasone dipropionate Synthetic glucocorticoid administered by inhalation for the chronic treatment of bronchial asthma

bedpan This is vessel given to patient who is bed ridden for receiving urine and stool in the bed itself.

bedsore Decubitus ulcer occurring in bed ridden and paralytic or unconscious patient.

Beevor's sign This is the sign of Functional Paralysis wherein patient is unable to inhibit the antagonistic muscles.

behavior Observable conduct of a person or it is how a person conducts in his society.

Behçet's syndrome Recurrent genital ulcers, aphthous lesion of mouth, uveitis, iridocyclitis with hypopyon.

Behring's law When the serum of a person which contains immune antibody is given to another person the other person also gets immunity against that illness.

bejel This is a Non sexually transmitted infection called endemic syphilis similar to Pinta and Yaws.

bel a unit of relative power intensity used for acoustic measurements are usually expressed in Decibels.

belching This is the other name for Eructation.

belemnoid Anatomical organ which is dart shaped.

Bell's muscle This is the musculi pylori of the ureters.

Bell's palsy Lesion of the facial nerve resulting in distortion of the face and the pathology is peripheral facial nerve paralysis.

belladonna A plant which yields alkaloids like atropine, hyoscyamine, scopolamine that are commonly used in medical treatment. These alkaloids are anticholinergic drugs.

belly Colloquially it is abdomen .

Benadryl Drug tradename for Diphenhydramine Hydrochloride.

Bence Jones protein This is one type of globulin present in urine and blood which has distinct character, present in multiple myeloma.

bend Flexed or curved part of an organ or of an anatomical structure.

bends Abdominal pain and pain in limbs by decompression or reduced air pressure. .

Benedict's test This test is done to detect dextrose (sugar) in urine. To 5 cc of Benedict's solution 10 drops of urine are added, boiled for 2 minutes and allowed to cool slowly. If sugar is present the precipitate will be red, yellow or green in colour depending on sugar content.

benign Harmless and that which is not cancerous growth.

Bennett's fracture This is longitudinal fracture of first metacarpal bone with subluxation.

bentonite Aluminum silicate, which on the addition of water swells to produce a slippery paste and is used as bulk laxative.

benzaldehyde Essential oil of almond used as a flavoring agent in Medicines.

benzalkonium chloride It is a disinfectant and detergent used as antiseptic solution for external applications. Eye drops contain this as preservative.

benzene It is a colorless volatile liquid hydrocarbon denoted with symbol C_6H_6, obtained from distillation of coal with coal tar It is known to cause bone marrow depression and as carcinogenic.

benzidine It is an arylamine compound formed by the action of acids on hydrazobenzene used in Occult blood testing in the laboratory.

benzocaine Local anesthetic applied topically to the skin and mucous membranes , intubation, dental procedures and in endoscopy.

benzoic acid benzenecarboxylic acid is a fungistatic compound commonly used as a food preservative

benzoin Common topical antiseptic.

benzoxiquine This is a disinfectant.

benzthiazide Diuretic used in hypertension and edema

benzylpenicillin Preparation of Penicillin G

bephenium hydroxynaphthoate An anthelmintic used in the treatment of hookworm infestation.

bereavement In case of death of loved ones person manifests grief and desolation which is a clinical depression.

Berger's disease Diseases of kidney or nephropathy.

beriberi Thiamine deficiency characterized by polyneuritis, heart pathology and oedema and the person is not in a position to do any routine work.

Bernard's duct Other name for pancreatic duct.

Berry's ligament Lateral ligaments of the Thyroid gland.

berylliosis Beryllium fumes cause lung and skin changes which can cause Acute or Chronic Beryllium poisoning manifestations. Beryllium is metal found with coal and is used in the preparation of alloys.

Best Charles Herbert Best Canadian physiologist along with Banting discovered Insulin in 1922. Best also discovered Histaminase.

Best's disease This refers to the clinical condition called Congenital Macular Degeneration.

bestiality Refers to sex with animals called Zoophilia which is a sexual offence.

betacarotene Is a provitamin which is converted into Vitamin A in the body. Named after its colour which is either orange or red. It is present in carrot, sweet potato egg yolk and leafy vegetables.

betahistine hydrochloride A vasodilator used in Vertigo treatment

betaine Present in Sugar beet and other plants and is used in the treatment of Muscular weakness and muscle degeneration.

betel *Pan* or Piper betle leaf used along with areca (betel nut with lime is found to be astringent and stimulant.

Betz's cells These specialized cells are present in the brain in Primary somatomotor area.

Bevan's operation This is the surgical treatment for undescended testicle where the testicle from abdomen is brought down to the scrotum.

Bezold's abscess This is the Sub Periosteal abscess of Temporal Bone.

Bial's test For the detection of pentose in the urine. 5 ml. of Bial's reagent is boiled in a test tube; keeping the test tube away from flame few drops of urine are added. Green colour appearance indicates the presence of pentose.

biallylamicol former name for bialamicol hydrochloride.

biarticular That which is related with 2 joints.

bias This refers to the systemic error in research, survey and clinical trials. There will be gross difference between observed value and estimated value in statistical inferences.

bibliotherapy Treatment of mental illness by reading religious books to the patients.

bicarbonate Salt containing the $\mathbf{HCO_3^-}$ anion.

bicaudal having two tails.

biceps The muscle in the arm which has 2 heads.

biconcave That which has two concave surfaces on it's both side. Refers to lens.

biconvex That which has two convex surfaces on it's both side. Refers to lens.

bicornuate A bicornuate uterus is **a result of a partial fusion of Mullerian ducts resulting in a heart-shaped uterus instead of a pear shape**.

bicuspid It is referable to bicuspid valve of the heart which has two points. Also referable to premolar tooth.

b.i.d. Abbreviation for prescribing drug twice a day.

Bier's amputation By cutting Tibia and Fibula above the stump, osteoplastic amputation of the leg with a bone flap is done.

Bifid That which has or made to two branches.

bifocal Spectacle which has smaller lens for near vision and big lens for distant vision that are called Bifocal Glasses.

bigeminy That which occurs in pairs such as Bigeminal pulse.

bigerminal pertaining to two germs or ova.

bighead Term used for Hydrocephalus and for Osteomalacia changes in skull bone.

bilateral Referrable to both sides of a structure.

bile This is liver secretion passed onto the intestine through bile ducts that contains bile salts and bilirubin. They have alkalizing effect and help in fat digestion.

bile acid They are Steroid carboxylic acid from Cholesterol. Primary Bile Acids are Cholic acid, Deoxycholic acid from liver which go to form bile Salts. Secondary Bile Acids are Deoxycholic acid, Lithocholic acid from Primary bile acids in Intestine.

Bilharzia discovered Schistosoma parasite which cause disease in man.

biliary pertaining to the bile

bilin Yellow pigment produced in bilirubin catabolism of urobilin and stercobilin.

bilirubin This is derived from Red cell haemoglobin and from cytochromes. High level in blood causes jaundice.

bilirubinemia Presence of bilirubin in the blood which beyond the limit value or physiological value..

bilirubinuria Presence of bilirubin in the urine.

biliverdin From the catabolic activity of Haemoglobin this green pigment is produced .

Billroth's diseases Bilroth described these diseases viz., Malignant Lymphoma and Spurious Meningocele.

bimanual Task which is performed by both hands.

bimodal An epidemiological term denoting to have two modes

binary That which is made of two elements or a number system with a base of two.

Binet's test To ascertain mental age, series of standard questions are asked and mental capacity of child or of youth is ascertained. .

Bing's test Test performed to ascertain the lesion of the incus or malleus in case of hard of hearing.

binocular Device which has two eye pieces. Referred to the Microscope.

binomial Mathematical or statistical calculation is done by taking sums of two or differences of two. E.g., Death and Birth, Success and Failure etc.,

binuclear Cell having two nuclei.

bio Denoting relationship with life of living organisms including man.

bioassay Drug vaccine or any medic mentation is examined for its potency as compared with a standard preparation which is called Biological Assy. One of the pharmacological basis for safety, clarity and potency of to be administered medicine.

bioavailability This specify the amount or quantity of drug which is available for action to the target tissue when administered as medicine.

biocatalyst Other name for enzyme.

biochemistry This is the scientific study of chemistry of human body and it's vital processes.

biocompatible That which is adjustable with life and which do not cause any harm on body function.

biodegradation Living organisms make chemicals less dangerous to human surroundings.

biodynamics This is the scientific study of nature of organisms and determinants of deviations in that organism.

bioengineering That deals with Engineering technology that is related with biological system and is called Biomedical Engineering.

bioethics This relates to the moral obligations on Human research or animal research.

biofeedback Information on normal person or of ill person is given that can help that person to act and take a control over the health situation.

biohazard Infectious agents that are present in hospital centre or health care institutions can cause biological hazard to man.

bioinformatics Information on man through computer or data bases .

biologist He is an expert in biology.

biology It is the study of sciences related with man, animal and plant in this universe.

biomarker This refers to Tumour marker where a molecule is used as marker for biological sciences study.

biomass The entire body assembly of man or animal is considered to say as Biomass.

biome In a given geographic region, specified unit is made through biological factors such as vegetation tundra for west grass land etc. Ecological influencing factors around man.

biomechanics In a short form it is called Bionics which implies the Mechanical law application on human beings or living beings. Of late it is name as Kinesiology.

biomedical This is the study of medicine in the background of Zoology, Botany, Biophysics and Biochemistry.. Discipline introduced by Biology and Medicine.

biometry Medical and Biostatistics as applied to Biomedicine in many areas such as Life expectation, life insurance etc.,

biomicroscope Microscope for examining living tissue in the body.

biophysics Modern theories and Modern physical methods are applied to understand Biological situations.

biopsy Surgical removal or excision of tissues from the body for final diagnosis and prompt treatment through Histopathological examination of such removed tissues. If the tissue is removed by aspiration, it is called Aspiration Biopsy.

bioscience Study of Biology through the application of Basic sciences such as Physics Chemistry etc.,

biosis Living transformation or vital events that occur in nature.

biosphere Region of the universe where Biological activity take place which consists of Atmosphere Hydrosphere and Lithosphere.

biostatistics Measurement of biological events through number, facts and figures. Presently it is termed as Biometry.

biotin It is **a water-soluble B vitamin found naturally in some foods and also in supplements**.

biotype Different strains of bacteria which show different identifiable characteristics but belong to same group.

Bird's sign This is the sign seen in Hydatid disease of the lung wherein. In the area of infection Lung sounds are absent and there will be dullness.

Birkett's hernia This refers to Synovial Hernia described by Birkett.

birth Refers to the act of being born in animals and man.

birthmark Nevus or mole present since birth that are identifiable points in identifying the individual, both naturally and legally.

bisexual This refers to Hermaphrodites who exhibit male and female sexual characteristics.

bis in die Prescribing abbreviation meaning twice a day and is written as b.i.d.

bitartrate Salt containing $C_4H_5O_6^-$ which is derived from tartaric acid $C_4H_6O_6$.

Bitot's spots Foamy appearance on conjunctiva in Vitamin deficiency described by Bitot which is early manifestation of vitamin A deficiency.

blackhead This denotes Open Comedo on the skin.

blackout Owing to diminished brain circulation there will be momentary unconsciousness which cause failure of vision.

bland Refers to bland diet which is mild or soothing.

blast Commonly referred to two items No.1 it is an immature cell before definitive characteristics. No.2 it means Air Concussion.

blastocyst In embryological development it is post morula stage which is fluid filled cavity.

blastoma Cancer developed from embryonic cells.

blastomere Zygote which show segmentation called Cleavage Cell.

Blastomycetes They belong to a group of fungus and are called Yeasts.

blastomycosis Fulminating fungal infection caused by Yeast like organisms. Common species which cause Blastomycosis is Blastomyces dermatitidis.

blastula Segmentation differential in a zygote which show blastoderm and blastocoele (layer and fluid)

BLB mask **B**oothby **Lovelace** and **B**ulbulian (inventors) It is Oxygen breathing mask used by Aviators. It contains the following:

- ✓ Inspiratory valve
- ✓ Expiratory valve
- ✓ Rebreathing Bag

bleaching Removing stains or color by chemical means.

bleb (bleb) It is skin eruption called bulla.

bleeding Blood oozing by the cut which is referred to to as haemorrhage.

bleomycin An anticancer drug which is made up of glycopeptide produced by a strain of Streptomyces verticillus.

blepharitis Infection and inflammation of the eyelids.

blepharospasm Spasm of the orbicularis oculi muscle which produce complete closure of the eyelids.

blind One who do not has the sense of sight. In case of blind study it can be single blind, double blind or triple blind studies.

blister This refers to Vesicle.

bloat Distension of abdomen by gas which can be due fermentation and infection.

Bloch Bloch discovered the metabolism of Cholesterol and fatty acids.

block This refers to either an Obstruction or for Regional Anaesthesia.

blockage Refers to the obstruction.

Blom-Singer puncture This refers to Tracheo Esophageal Puncture described by Blom and Singer.

blood Red coloured fluid which circulates through heart, arteries, capillaries and veins that help in the supply of Oxygen to the tissues and organs for vital functions. Blood contains Plasma Red cells and White cells and Platelets.

blood group It is blood typing by antigenic grouping. ABO type of classification describe A group, B group, AB group and O group. Rh blood grouping has major role in blood transfusion.

blotting The act of soaking up with absorbent material.

Blumberg Baruch Samuel. American physician, born 1925; co-winner, with Daniel Carleton Gajdusek, of the Nobel prize for medicine or physiology in 1976 for their discoveries of Hepatitis B virus.

Blumberg's sign In case peritoneal inflammation short acute pain is elicited by pressure over McBurney's point and lifting up suddenly.

blush (blush) Short term acute reddening of face neck due to emotion or heat which is as a consequence of vascular dilatation. **BMA (BMA)** British Medical Association.

BMI Abbreviation for **B**ody **M**ass **I**ndex

BMR Abbreviation for **B**asal **M**etabolic **R**ate.

Bochdalek's duct Thyroglossal Duct described by Bochdalek.

Bock's ganglion Carotid ganglion described by Bock.

Bodansky unit This is Quantitative unit in Biochemistry which measures the quantity of phosphatase required to liberate 1 mg. of phosphorus in the form of ion in one hour of incubation with Sodium Beta glycerophosphate.

Body This is represented with the Trunk of human body which contains many organs. Dead body is called cadaver.

Boeck's disease is a systematised disease of lympho-reticular (reticulo-endothelial) tissue, presenting clinical features of a chronic infectious granuloma..

Bogros' space In this space lower part of External Iliac artery is found and the space is bounded by Peritoneum above and Transversalis fascia below.

boil A type of skin infection which is called Furuncle.

bolus This can be a rounded mass of food. This can be rounded mass of drug ready to swallow.

bomb Radium or radioactive element in a metal shield for Radiation Therapy.

bombard Exposure to Ionising Radiation for therapeutic purpose. It can be Gamma Radiation or Cobalt Therapy.

bonding Make it secured by joining them.

Bondy's mastoidectomy This is radical mastoidectomy.

bone Hard connective tissue containing matrix follagenous fibers and mineral component. Proportion of Calcium Phosphate is 85 % and proportion of Calcium carbonate is 10 %. Because of rigidity it is called osseous tissue.

Bonnet's capsule Posterior two thirds of eye ball is covered by the fibrous sheath which function as synovial capsule for functional purposes.

Bonwill triangle The Triangle of Bonwill is formed by a line drawn from one condyloid process to the other condyloid process; Line from the center of the alveolar ridge of the lower jaw to the condyloid process on left side; line from the center of the alverolar ridge of the lower jaw to the condyloid process of right side.

booster This pertains to the booster dose of vaccine in active immunization.

bootstrap This is a statistical term used for the method of computing distributed values based on random Re-Sampling of observed values.

borborygmus Intestinal Rumbling noise heard with or without auscultation.

borderline A line drawn between two items, between any phenomenon.

Bordet Known personality in the field of Immunology who is also the winner of Noble prize.

Bordet-Gengou agar culture medium This is also called Bordet Gengou Potato Blood Agar medium which has the glycerin potato agar containing blood. The medium is used in the culture of Bordetella pertussis organism.

Bordetella Gram-negative Aerobic minute coccobacilli which are pathogens of the respiratory tract of humans

boric acid This is an acidifying agent has the power of killing germs on the skin mucous membrane and cornea.

boron This is a nonmetallic element which form base for Borax and Boric acid. Boron poisoning is known worldwide.

Borrelia Belongs to Spirochaetaceae that cause Relapsing Fever.

boss Eminence on the surface of a bone

botany The Science that deals with the plant kingdom.

bothrium The sucker in the form of a groove seen on either side of the head of Diphyllobothrium latum parasite.

botulism Human intoxication with Botulinum toxin by Clostridium botulinum bacteria which occurs in Food Poisoning resulting in Neurotoxicity.

bougie Instrument used for dilating urethra or any tubular organ that has flexibility

Bouin's fluid This has the following composition:

- Formaldehyde solution
- Glacial acetic acid
- Saturated solution of Trinitrophenol.

bound Two or more chemicals held in combination. Anything that is confined.

Bourgery's ligament The Oblique Popliteal Ligament described by Bourgery.

Bouveret's syndrome This is Paroxysmal Supra Ventricular Tachycardia described by Bouveret.

bovine Related with ox or cow.

bowel This is referred to the Intestine.

bowleg Knees are abnormally separated and lower legs are bowed inward . Clinically it is called Genu Varum.

Bowman's capsule Globular dilatation which form the beginning of uriniferous tubule within the kidney.

box-note In case of Emphysema, percussion produces a hollow sound heard in the chest

Boyle's law At a given temperature a given mas of gas varies in volume inversely as the pressure.

BP Abbreviation for **B**lood **P**ressure

brace This holds the parts together and in place.

brachial Related with arm.

Bracht's maneuver This is done in case of Breech presentation. At delivery as soon as inferior angle of the scapula appears, the body of the foetus is rotated around the mother's symphysis so that the child's back comes to rest on the mother's abdomen.

brachy It means Short

brachydactyly Abnormal shortness of the fingers and toes.

bracing To hold the parts together and in place.

Bradley's disease Epidemic nausea and vomiting described by Bradley.

bradycardia Slowness of the heartbeat

bradykinin This nonapeptide is produced by activation of the kinin system in human body followed by inflammatory conditions. Bradykinin is a vasodilator, which increase vascular permeability, and stimulates pain receptors.

Bragard's sign Knee is kept in stiff position. Lower leg is flexed at the hip till patient experience pain and at that point the foot is dorsiflexed. If there is increase in pain it is due to nerve involvement. If there is no increase of pain then it indicates muscular involvement.

braille Writing and printing with the help of tangible dots for the use of blind students to develop reading and writing .

brain CNS in the cranium comprising of Forebrain, Midbrain and Mind brain.

brainstem) This consists of Mesencephalon, pns and medulla oblongata which connects the cerebral hemispheres with spinal cord.

brainwashing Against the will of a person installing attitudes and beliefs

bran Soluble and insoluble dietary fiber like oat and wheat respectively .

branch Ramification of vessels, nerves and lymphatics.

brash Refers to heartburn.

Braun's anastomosis To prevent recurrence, in Gastro Enterostomy, anastomosis between afferent and efferent intestinal loops are formed.

Braun's canal Neurenteric canala described by Braun.

Braune's muscle Puborectalis muscle named by Braune.

Braxton Hicks vertion Cervix is dilated to admit only two fingers, combined external and internal manipulation are done to change the position of foetus

braxy This is Malignant Oedema produced by Clostridium septicum infection.

breadth Horizontal measurement from side to side which is called diameter.

break Discontinuity in the structure or some sort of interruption in continuity.

breakdown When biological function stops, When there is sudden collapse of health.

breast Mammary gland in females which are milk producing glands for the newborn.

breast-feeding Feeding breast milk by the nursing mother.

breath This refers to inspiration and expiration which are combined acts of Respiration.

breech This refers to breach presentation in delivery. Breach means buttocks.

bregma The point where Coronal suture and Sagittal sutures meet .

Brennemann's syndrome As a sequel to Throat infection, mesenteric and retroperitoneal lymphadenitis occurs.

Brenner tumor Tumor of the ovary which show epithelial cells and stromal cells.

Brewer's infarcts In case of Pyelonephritis, cut section of kidney show dark red wedge shaped infarcts like area.

Bricanyl tradename for preparations of Terbutaline Sulphate used as Bronchodilator.

bridge Anatomical structure that connects two structures. e.g., Nasal bridge.

Bright's disease Kidney diseases which are manifested by Albuminuria and oedema.

Brill's disease Among people suffered with epidemic typhus, recurrence of mild form of epidemic typhus fever.

Brill-Symmers disease It is Gaint Follicular Lymphadenopathy

brim (brim) The upper edge of a basin such as Pelvic Brim.

Broca's amnesia Pathology of Motor speech area leading to Clinical Amnesia or Forgetfulness.

Brodie's abscess Chronic Synovitis of the knee with pulpy degeneration of affected parts.

Brodie's ligament The Transverse humeral Ligament described by Brodie.

Brodmann's areas The areas described by Brodie in cerebral cortex in specific occipital and preoccipital area that are identified by numbers. Specific functions are found to be seated in these areas.

bromatology Field of Dietetics.

bromatotherapy Field of Diet Therapy.

bromelain Cysteine Endopeptidases enzyme present in fruits like pineapple which has anti-inflammatory property.

bromhexine hydrochloride This is an expectorant and mucolytic agent used in respiratory disorders, Keratoconjunctivitis sicca and in Sjögren's syndrome.

bromoderma Skin eruption due to the use of bromides.

bronchiectasis Destruction and dilatation of bronchiole which may be congenital or acquired.

bronchiolitis Infection and inflammation of the bronchioles in children.

bronchitis Infection and inflammation of a bronchus or bronchi

bronchocele Localized dilatation of a bronchus.

bronchoconstriction Asthma due to bronchial smooth muscle contraction.

bronchodilator Drug that cause expansion of lung passage and avoids bronchoconstriction.

bronchogenic That which originates from Bronchus.

bronchogram The radiogram obtained by bronchography.

bronchopneumonia Infection and inflammation of the lungs that begins in the terminal bronchioles

bronchopulmonary Pertaining to the lungs or air passages viz., Bronchi and Pulmonary

bronchoradiography Radiographic visualization of the bronchial tree.

bronchoscope This is an instrument for inspecting the interior of the tracheobronchial tree and carrying out endobronchial diagnostic and therapeutic maneuvers, such as taking specimens for culture and biopsy and removing foreign bodies etc.,

bronchospasm Spasmodic contraction of the smooth muscle of the bronchi Asthma.

bronchospirometry Doing Lung Function Tests by determining vital capacity, oxygen intake, and carbon dioxide excretion of a single lung, or simultaneous measurements of the function of each lung separately.

bronchostenosis stricture of the caliber of a bronchial tube.

bronchus This is the larger air passage in the respiratory system which show the arranged fibrous coat, hyline cartilage, smooth muscles and inner mucous membrane containing ciliated columnar ciliated epithelial cells to perform specialized function.

Brooke's tumor This is an Epithelioma called Epithelioma Adenoides Cysticum.

broth This is liquid culture medium for the culture of micro organisms.

Broviac catheter It is a Central Venous Catheter which has a small lumen.

brown Reddish yellow color.

brownian movement This refers to the dancing movement or dancing motion of minute particles suspended in a liquid.

Browning's vein The upper portion of the great anastomotic vein which connects the middle cerebral vein with the superior sagittal sinus.

Bruce's tract This is septomarginal tract which is termed as Fasciculus Septomarginalis.

Brucella Pathogenic microorganism causing Brucellosis which is Gram negative Aerobic and Coccobacilli.

brucellosis One of the Zoonotic infection in Man through sheep or goat and is known from time immemorial as Malta fever or Undulant fever.

Brugia Described by *Brug*—a genus of filarial worms of the superfamily Filarioidea, which produce Filaria in man.

bruise This refers to Contusion.

bruit Refers to the sound produced in auscultation at clinical examination.

Brunati's sign In advanced stages of Pneumonia or in Typhoid patient show the opacities in the cornea which is sign of severe complications or it points to impending death.

Brunn's membrane This refers to the epithelium of the olfactory region of the nose.

Brunner's glands Mucous glands in submucous membrane of duodenum which are of the nature of racemose mucous glands.

Brunnstrom method Volatilising 8% formaldehyde to prevent polymerisation.

Brunschwig's operation This is Pancreatoduodenectomy described by Brunschwig.

brushite This refers to colorless type of acid calcium phosphate present in renal calculi and dentum of teeth.

Bruton's agammaglobulinemia This is Sex linked disease called X- linked Agammaglobulinaemia.

brux A type of tics which makes man to grind the teeth rhythmically

bruxism This is involuntary, nonfunctional, rhythmic grinding of teeth related dwith emotion, anger, fear, frustration.

Bryant's line The line refers to the vertical side of Iliofemoral triangle.

bubo Tender enlarged and inflamed lymph node in the axilla or groin following infections. This is specifically termed for Bubo of plague.

bubonic Related to Bubonic plague.

buccal Fleshy portion of the cheek

buccinator The name of a muscle.

Buck's fascia This is the continuation of the dep layer of the superficial perineal fascia.

Buckley's syndrome This is the clinical condition called hyperimmunoglobulinemia.

buckling Crumpled or warped.

buclizine hydrochloride An antihistamine

Buerger's disease This s condition is referred to as Thromboangiitis Obliterans .

buffer Maintaining physiological constancy which can be chemical buffer or physiological buffer.

Buhl's disease Clinical condition associated with Desquamative Pneumonia

bulb Rounded mass

bulbar Related with Bulb like structure or to Medulla Oblongata.

bulla Large elevation on the skin called Vesicle.

Buller's shield A Watch glass fitted over the eye to guard the eye from eye infections.

bumps Clinical conditions of Erythema Nodosum and Primary Coccidioidomycosis.

BUN Abbreviation for **B**lood **U**rea **N**itrogen.

bundle Collection of muscle fibres or nerve fibers

bundle branch pertaining to the Bundle branch of the heart.

Bunge's amputation A periosteal Amputation described by Bunge.

bunion Abnormal prominence of the inner aspect of the first metatarsal head associated with bursa and lateral displacement of great toe.

Bunsen burner A gas burner in which the gas is mixed with air before ignition to give complete oxidation process to occur.

Bunsen Coefficient This is Absorption Coefficient.

buphthalmia Clinical condition called Hydrophthalmos.

buphthalmos Enlargement and distention of the fibrous coats of the eye in cases of congenital Glaucoma.

bur Dental instrument to remove carious material from cavity of decayed tooth.

burette It is a glass tube with graduated column for the use in Volumetric Analysis in chemistry.

Bürger-Grütz syndrome This is Familial hyper-lipoproteinemia described by Burger and Grutz.

Burkitt's lymphoma Large Osteolytic lesion in lower jaw with a mass form which Epstein-Barr virus is isolated and found to be associated with. First identified in Central Africa and later observed in other parts of the world.

burn Fire, steam heat, hot liquid, chemicals, electricity, radiant etc. cause injury to tissues which is called Burn. Partial thickness burn include first and second degree burns and Full thickness burns include third degree burns.

burner Flame issuing stove or furnace.

Burnett's syndrome Milk Alkali Syndrome described by Burnett.

bursa In friction developing areas a sac filled with viscid fluid is present to overcome friction.

bursitis Infection and inflammation of a bursa

Burton's line Gray line at the gingival margin in lead poisoning which is also called as Lead Line.

Buruli ulcer Skin infection by Mycobacterium ulcerans which will be nodular in the beginning and later becomes ulcerated.

busulfan This is cytotoxic and antineoplastic agent used for palliative treatment of advanced cases of leukaemia and polycythemia vera.

butane Aliphatic hydrocarbon with the formula C_4H_{10} from petroleum

Butazolidin Phenyl butazone preparations in the market.

Butcher's saw Amputation saw with a blade which can be set from various angles at surgery.

butoconazole nitrate A topical antifungal for vaginal application in candida infection.

buttocks named for Nates.

butyl The chemical with a hydrocarbon radical C_4H_9

butylene The gaseous hydrocarbon with the formula C_4H_8.

butyric acid Saturated fatty acid present in animal fat or in rancid butter.

bypass This refers to the Shunt which help for an auxiliary flow as in the case of circulatory system or alimentary tract

by-product During the processing of a primary product, we get by products which are called secondary product.

byssinosis Cotton dust inhalation among textile workers produces Pneumoconiosis called Byssinosis which is an occupational hazard .

Bywaters syndrome This is also called Crush syndrome because of development of symptoms following muscle crush that precipitates acute renal failure. The syndrome is manifested with oedema, oliguria and other renal failure manifestations. Pathological features of acute tubular necrosis are observed in the syndrome.

C

cachexia Ill health and malnutrition. Common causes are cancer, heart diseases, fluorosis, pan hypopituitarism, malaria and uraemia.

CAD Abbreviation for Coronary Artery Disease.

cadaver Latin word meaning a dead body; particularly dead body preserved for dissection in anatomy.

cadaverine Produced in decaying protein by bacteria which is Pentamethylene diamine a four smelling chemical.

cadmium Chemical used in photography, lithography that can cause cadmium poisoning if precaution is not taken.

caecum A blind pouch of intestine into which ileum, colon and appendix open.

caffeine Coffee, tea contain methylxanthines which is CNS stimulant.

Caffey's disease Infantile Cortical Hyperostosis described by Caffey.

calamine An astringent and protectant used in the treatment of skin diseases. Main ingredient can be zinc oxide or zinc carbonate

calcaneonavicular That which is related with calcaneus and navicular bone.

calcaneus Irregular quadrangular bone at the back of the tarsus

calciferol It is cholecalciferol containing vitamin D

calcification By the process of calcium salt deposit, tissue becomes hardened.

Calcitonin Used in Paget's disease of bone. An antagonist to parathyroid hormone. It is secreted by parafollicular cells of thyroid gland.

calcium Common and abundant element of human body. With phosphorus it is present in bone and tooth. This also acts as coagulation factor IV in blood physiology.

calculus Abnormal concretion in the body by mineral salts and is called stone. Gall stone, kidney stone, urinary stone etc.,

Caldwell's position A radiological positon where patient puts his forehead and nose against the X-ray plate. It is used in Caldwell's projection.

calibration It is the measurement of the caliber of a tube.

Call-Exner bodies Dark staining of granulose cells in maturing ovarian follicles.

callus Hyperplasia of the horny layer of the epidermis due to pressure or friction.

calor A cardinal signs of inflammation.

calorie It is the heat required to raise the temperature of 1 kilogram of water 1 degree Celsius at a specified temperature.

calorimeter Instrument for measuring the amount of heat produced by an individual.

Calot's triangle It is called cystohepatic triangle and the triangle is formed by cystic artery above, cystic duct below and hepatic duct medially.

calpain It helps in maintaining shape of RBC. They are calcium-activated 7*-+ '1oteinase of eukaryotic cells that itself activates several cellular enzymes.

Calvé-Perthes disease Osteochondrosis of the capitular epiphysis of the femur described by Cavle and Perthes.

calx Hindmost projection of the foot called heel.

calyx Cup shaped cavity such as renal calyx.

Campbell's ligament Suspensory ligament of the axilla described by Campbell.

Camper's fascia It is the superior fascia of the urogenital diaphragm described by Camper.

camphor A ketone obtained from cinnamomum camphora.

Campylobacter Rod shaped gram-negative motile with polar flagella. They cause enteritis.

canal Narrow tubular passage such as adductor canal, anal canal, haversian canal etc.,

Canavan's disease Spongy degeneration of CNS described by Canavan.

cancellous Said of bone tissue which will be spongy and reticular.

cancer Latin word meaning 'Crab' refer to cancerous tissue. Cancer is a disease in which some of the body's cells grow uncontrollably and spread to other parts of the body.

Candida Fungus of cryptococcaceae that cause various infections like vaginitis, meningitis, pulmonary infection

candidiasis infection with a fungus Candida that attack immunocompromised patients causing endocarditis and systemic infections.

cane Wooden stick or metal rod used for support in walking. Common in use are:

- English cane called forearm crutch
- Adjustable cane
- Quadripod cane which is four legged
- Tripod cane with three legs

canker Ulceration of the mouth and lips.

Cannabis Hemp plant from which marijuana the dried leaves and flowers are taken that contains tetra-hydrocannabinol. This produces hallucinations and euphoric effects in the body.

Cannon's ring A narrow of contraction at the mid third of the transverse colon representing the junction of the primitive midgut and hindgut and marking an area of overlap between the superior and inferior nerve plexuses; a finding in the radiograph after a barium meal.

cannula With the help of a trocar, a tube is inserted into a duct, a cavity or a vessel. Common cannula that are used are:

- o Nasal cannula
- o Perfusion cannula
- o Washout cannula

canthoplasty Surgical restoration of a defective canthus by plastic surgery.

canthorrhaphy Suturing of the palpebral fissure at either canthus.

canthus Angle at either end of the fissure between the eyelids.

Cantrell's pentalogy This is associated with

- Midline abdominal defects
- Defective pericardium
- Communication between pericardial and peritoneal cavities
- Cardiac anomalies
- Cleft in inferior part of the sternum.

capacitance This is the property of being able to store an electric charge.

capacitor Device for holding and storing charges of electricity.

CAPD Abbreviation for **C**ontinuous **A**mbulatory **P**eritoneal **D**ialysis.

capillary Hair like minute vessels that connect either arterioles or venules.

capitulum This refers to a small eminence on a bone by which it articulates with another bone.

Caplan's syndrome Pneumoconiosis associated with rheumatoid arthritis called rheumatoid pneumoconiosis.

capping To put a protective or obstructive covering. E.g., pulp capping.

capric acid This is a saturated fatty acid occurring as a minor constituent of numerous fats and oils.

capsid Shell of protein that protects the nucleic acid of a virus

capsule Anatomical structure enclosing an organ or a coating of a drug ready for medicamentation.

caput Refer to cranium and face that contain brain and special sense.

caramel By heating sugar we get concentrated solution which is used as colouring agent.

carbachol Cholinergic agonist used in the treatment of glaucoma and after cataract surgery.

carbamate Ester of carbamic acid which is an insecticide and parasiticide.

carbamazepine Drug used in epilepsy and trigeminal neuralgia as an anticonvulsant and antineuralgic agent.

carbarsone Antiamoebic arsenical compound is a pentavalent organic arsenical , not used nowadays.

carbide Carbon with an element or radical.

carbohydrate They are proximate principles of diet. They are pentahydric and hexahydric alcohols. Hydrogen and oxygen are in the proportion to form water $C_n(H_2O)_n$ as in monosacchaaride, disaccharide, polysaccharide, starches and glycogens.

carbolfuchsin It is a mordant containing carbolic acid and basic fuchsin for routine stains.
carbolic acid Other name for carbolic acid.
carbonic acid Chemically H_2CO_3 that exists in chemical equilibrium with lved carbon dioxide in water
carbonyl Chemical group occurring in aldehydes, ketones, carboxylic acids, and esters.
carboxyhemoglobin Hemoglobin bound to carbon monoxide,
carboxyhemoglobinemia In CO poisoning carboxy-haemoglobin is present in blood.
carboxyl —COOH, present in organic acids and are termed carboxylic acids.
carboxylase This is an enzyme that catalyzes the addition of a molecule of carbon dioxide to another compound to form a carboxyl group. E.g., Amino acid Carboxylase.
carboxylation Chemical process of the addition of a carboxyl group
carboxymyoglobin Carboxymyoglobin is formed from myoglobin on exposure to carbon monoxide,
carbuncle Infection of skin and subcutaneous tissue composed of a cluster of boils
carcass Dead body of animals.
carcinogen Cancer-producing substance such as epigenetic carcinogen that cause alterations to predispose to cancer. This can be genotoxic carcinogen that reacts directly with DNA to predispose to cancer.
carcinogenic That which produce cancer.
carcinoma Malignant new growth made up of epithelial cells tending to infiltrate the surrounding tissues and give rise to metastases. Common types are:

- o Adenocarcinoma
- o Basal cell carcinoma
- o Bronchogenic carcinoma
- o Endometrial carcinoma
- o Hepatocellular carcinoma
- o Papillary carcinoma
- o Squamous carcinoma

Carden's amputation Amputation just above the knee and is transfemoral with a single flap surgery.
cardia Portion of the stomach immediately adjacent to and surrounding the cardiac opening of the esophagus
cardiac That which is related to heart.
cardinal Anything that is of prime importance such cardinal signs
cardiogram Tracing of a cardiac event made by means of the cardiograph which can be apex cardiogram, precordial cardiogram or vector cardiogram.
cardiologist Consultant in Internal medicine or a physician skilled in the prevention, diagnosis, and treatment of heart disease.
cardiology Scientific study of the heart and its functions.
cardiopathy Referable to any disorder or disease of the heart.
cardiopulmonary Related to heart and lungs.
cardiorrhaphy Operation of suturing the heart muscle.
cardiorrhexis Rupture of the heart.
cardiovascular Related to the heart and blood vessels.
carditis Inflammation of the heart. Common types of carditis are:

- Rheumatic carditis
- Streptococcal carditis
- Non bacterial carditis which is called verrucous carditis

care This refers to services rendered by Health professionals including nursing professionals. Common medical situation where care is emphasized are:

- Critical care
- Coronary care
- Intensive care
- Palliative care
- Primary health care
- Comprehensive health care
- Total health care
- Secondary care
- Tertiary care

caries Latin word meaning rottenness normally referred to caries tooth. It also mean the molecular decay or death of a bone According to Block dental caries is classified into 6 categories. They are:

- cavities in pit and fissure = Class I
- cavities in bicuspid and molars=Class II
- cavities in incisors = Class III
- cavities in incisors and cuspids that require removal of incisal angle=Class IV
- cavities in gingival=Class V
- cavities even at the height of contour =Class VI

carminative Medicine that relieves flatulence and assuages pain.
Carnett's sign A test done by palpation while the patient holds the anterior abdominal muscle tense, a test for parietal tenderness. Tenderness present is parietal in location, and not outside the abdominal cavity.
Caroli's disease This refers to congenital dilatation of the intrahepatic bile ducts described by Caroli.
carotene Commonly refers to β carotene present in many dark green, leafy, and yellow vegetables. It is the major precursor (pro-vitamin) of vitamin A in humans
carotid Refers to the principal artery of the neck .
carpal Related to the wrist.
carpometacarpal Related to the carpus and metacarpus.
Carpue operation This refers to Indian rhinoplasty described by Carpue.
Carrel-Dakin fluid This is Diluted Sodium Hypochlorite solution
carrier Person who harbors the specific organisms of a disease without manifest symptoms and is capable of

transmitting the infection. There are variants like chronic carrier, healthy carrier, convalescent carrier described by epidemiologist.

cartilage Fibrous connective tissue which form most of the temporary skeleton of the embryo that providac for bones to develop.

Carus curve Normal axis of pelvic outlet which is also called circle of Carus.

Carvallo's sign Inspiration causes augmentation of the pansystolic murmur and is present in tricuspid regurgitation.

case Used to designate the patient with the disease. Common terms in day-to-day practice are:
- Index case
- Primary case
- Borderline case
- Secondary case.

caseation Latin word meaning cheese. Tissue becomes a soft, dry, crumbly mass resembling cheese as in the case of tuberculosis

case history Data concerning an individual, his family, and environment, including his medical history and any other information that are useful in analyzing and diagnosing his condition or for instructional purposes.

casein This is a phosphoprotein, the principal protein of milk, the basis of curd and of cheese.

Casoni's intradermal test Done for the diagnosis of Hydatid cyst which is a non specific test. Hydatid fluid prepared for skin test is injected to forearm and appearance of wheal and flare denotes positive; that can be immediate or delayed.

Casselberry's position A prone position used after intubation which will allow patient to swallow without danger of fluid entering the tube.

cast Accurate reproduction of an object or part made of plastic that has taken form in an impression or mild. Other terminology used in medical practice are:
- o Bronchial cast
- o Decidual cast
- o Dental cast
- o Epithelial cast
- o Hyaline cast
- o Urinary cast

casting Object formed by the solidification of plastic material

Castle's intrinsic factor Parietal cells of gastric gland secretes a glycoprotein which is necessary for the absorption of vitamin B_{12}

Castleman's disease Abdominal or mediastinal lymphoma without malignant cells

castrate Remove gonads, rendering the individual incapable of reproduction.

castration Removal of the gonads; bilateral orchiectomy or bilateral oophorectomy.

casualty Death or disablement from an accident; also the person so injured or killed.

CAT Abbreviation for **C**omputerised **A**xial **T**omography

catabolic Pertaining to or of the nature of catabolism.

catabolism Destructive metabolic process by which organisms convert substances into excreted compounds.

catalase Haemoprotein enzyme of the oxidoreductase class that catalyses the conversion of hydrogen peroxide to water and oxygen

catalysis Greek word meaning dissolution. Chemical reaction of a process when positive is called positive catalysis. Inhibition of reaction of a process is called negative catalysis. Catalysis by adsorption power of contact surface it is called contact catalysis. When absorbed onto the surface of the catalysis it is called surface catalysis.

catalyst It is referred to a substance that brings about catalysis

cataract Opacity on or in the lens or in the lens capsule of the eye, which impairs vision and cause preventable blindness.

catatonia Motor abnormalities involving extreme under activity or over activity in schizophrenia and catalepsy.

catecholamine Amines having a sympathomimetic action like norepinephrine epinephrine.

catgut Referred to surgical catgut used in surgery. It can be chromic catgut, chromicised catgut.

cathartic Substance which produce emptying of the bowels. They are called purgatives or evacuates.

catheter rubber material which is a tubular and flexible that is inserted into a cavity of the body to withdraw or to introduce fluid.

catheterization Process of insertion of a catheter. Such as cardiac catheterization,

cathode The negative electrode in an electrolytic cell or a storage battery

cauda Tail like appendage in anatomical nomenclature such cauda equine, cauda epididymitis etc.,

caudal Denoting a position more toward the caudal end.

causal Directed against a cause.

causative Responsible as a cause such as causative agent.

caustic Substance which is destructive to living tissues.

cauterization By using electric current, a hot instrument, a caustic substance tissues are destroyed. Accordingly, terms like chemical cautery, electric cautery etc. are used.

cavernous That which contains hollow spaces.

cavity Refers to potential space within the body such as amniotic cavity, body cavity, buccal cavity, abdominal cavity, cranial cavity, dental cavity, epidural cavity etc.,

CCF Abbreviation for **C**ongestive **C**ardiac **F**ailure.

CCU Abbreviation for **C**ritical **C**are **U**nit.

cecum Refers to blind pouch caecum.

cedar Trees of the genus Cedrus from which cedar wood oil is extraxted.

cefixime Cephalosporin a third-generation antibiotic.

cefotaxime A semisynthetic broad-spectrum cephalosporin antibiotic effective against many organisms

cell Cell is a fundamental structural and functional unit of living organism. It is minute protoplasmic masses that make up organized tissue, consisting of a nucleus, which is surrounded by cytoplasm, which contains the various organelles and is enclosed in the cell or plasma membrane.

cellulitis Acute edematous suppurative inflammation of the deep subcutaneous tissues, with or without abscess formation

cellulose Long chain polymer which is polysaccharide in nature, forming the skeleton of most plant structures and of plant cells. Common types are Hydroxyethyl cellulose, oxidized cellulose.

Celsius scale Earlier it was called degree centigrade with 0^0C as freezing point and 100^0 C as boiling point.

Celsus Roman encyclopedist. His famous classical signs of inflammation are heat, pain, redness and swelling, which he described as calor, dolor, rubor and tumor.

cement Filling material, such as zinc phosphate, used in dentistry to assist in retaining gold castings in prepared teeth and to insulate the tooth pulp from metallic and other fillings.

censor Defence mechanism of ego. Mental faculty that guards the border between the unconscious and preconscious

center Middle point of a body.

centesis Tapping, as with an aspirator, trocar, or needle.

centi- Latin word meaning one hundred

centigrade Consisting of 100 gradations.

centimeter It is the unit of length equal to one-hundredth of a meter 10^{-2} m

centrifugal That which moves away from a center

centrifugation Process of separating the lighter portions from heavier portions of a solution, mixture, or suspension

centrifuge It is a machine by which centrifugation is affected.

centriole Centrioles migrate to opposite poles of the cell during cell division and serve to organize the spindles.

centripetal That which moves toward a center

cephalexin An antibiotic cephalosporin C effective against a wide range of gram-negative and gram-positive bacteria

cephalohematoma Subperiosteal hemorrhage limited to the surface of one cranial bone; common in birth trauma.

cephalosporin Antibiotics originally derived from a species of the fungus Emericellopsis minimum

- Cephalosporin C is parent compound of cefazolin sodium, cephalexin, cephaloridine, cephaloglycin, cephapirin, cephradine.
- First generation cephalosporins are cephalothin, cefazolin, cephaloridine, cephapirin, cephadrine, cephalexin, cefadroxil.
- Cephalosporin N is a dicillin
- Cephalosporin P show five component an antibacterial steroid.
- Second generation cephalosporins are cefamandole, cefoxitin, cefaclor, cefuroxime.
- Third generation cephalosporins are cefoperazone, cefotaxime, ceftriaxone, ceftazidime, ceftizoxime, moxalactam.

cephalothoracic That which is related to the head and thorax.

cephalothoracopagus Conjoined twins united at the head, neck, and thorax.

cera Latin word meaning wax such as cera alba and cera flava which are white wax and yellow wax respectively.

ceramic Porcelain, produced by the action of heat on earthy materials, in which silicon and silicates occupy a predominant position.

ceramics Objects made of ceramic material.

ceramidase It is an enzyme of the hydrolase class that catalyses the cleavage of a ceramide to form sphingosine and a fatty acid anion

cercaria Final free-swimming larval stage of a trematode parasite, consisting of a body and tail.

cereal Related to edible grains such as rice, wheat

cerebellospinal nerve fibres that proceeds from cerebellum to the spinal cord.

cerebellum Brain that occupies the posterior cranial fossa behind brain stem. This is mainly responsible for coordination of movements of the body.

cerebrum This is the main portion of the brain occupying the upper part of the cranial cavity

cerumen Ear wax which is wax like secretion found within the external meatus of the ear

cervical That which is related with neck.

cervicitis Inflammation of the cervix uteri

cervix Constricted portion of a body part or organ particularly referable to cervix of the uterus.

cesarean Latin word meaning to cut. This refers to caesarean operation done in C.P.D.L.

Cestoda It is a subclass of Cestoidea comprising the true tapeworms, which have a head or scolex, and segments.

cestode They are tapeworm

cetirizine hydrochloride an H_1-receptor Antihistaminic that is a metabolite of hydroxyzine. It is used in the treatment of allergic rhinitis and chronic idiopathic urticaria and asthma

CFT Abbreviation for **C**omplement **F**ixation **T**est.

CGS Abbreviation for **C**entimeter **G**ram **S**econd System where units that are based on the centimeter as the unit of length, the gram as the unit of mass, and the second as the unit of time.

CH Abbreviation for **C**rown **H**eel length of foetus.

Chadwick's sign It is positive in pregnancy. Congested and purple blue colour of vaginal and cervical mucosa is positive sign.

Chagas' disease It is trepanosomal infection. Disease is tropical in distribution and can be acute, chronic or sub acute in nature; caused by Trypanosoma cruzi and is transmitted by bite of infected reduviid bugs.

chalasia Greek word meaning relaxation. It refers to the relaxation of cardiac sphincter of the esophagus, a cause of vomiting in infants.

chalazion Chronic inflammation of a meibomian gland and shows a granulomatous reaction to liberated fat

chalk Natural calcium carbonate used in dentifrices and as a polishing agent in dentistry. Varieties are Prepared chalk (native variety), Precipitated chalk (Ca. carbonate) and French chalk (talc).

chamber This refers to an enclosed space or antrum. Examples are:

- Anterior chamber of the eye.
- Counting chamber
- Aqueous chamber

Chamberlen forceps An obstetrical forceps invented by Chamberlen.

Chance fracture Because of flexion distraction force horizontal splitting or the neural arch and body of a vertebra occurs.

chancre French word meaning destructive sore. Primary lesion of syphilis, which is painless.

chancroid S.T.D. caused by Haemophilus ducreyi ulcer on genitalia associated with lymphadenitis.

change An alteration such as fatty change, hyaline change, personality change etc.,

channel Refers to a channel through which a given liquid flows such as blood channel, lymph channel etc.,

character This depicts the nature of a person. This also mean an expression of phenotype of genes.

characteristic Typical of an individual .

Charcot's arthropathy Chronic progressive degeneration of joint in tabes dorsalis, syringomyelia or diabetic neuropathy.

Charcot-Leyden crystals They are present in bronchial secretions of asthma. They are present in stools in some cases of intestinal parasitism. Structurally they are elongated birefringent crystals in the form of two hexagonal pyramids joined base to base. Charcot Leyden crystals are derived from lysophospholipase released from the plasma membranes of disintegrating eosionophils.

charge Charge is a fundamental physical characteristic of elementary particles which can be positive or negative

Charles' law This law states "at a constant pressure the volume of a given mass of perfect gas varies directly with the absolute temperature".

chart Simple graphic representation of the fluctuation of some variable such as pulse, temperature, and respiration.

chaude-pisse French word meaning burning sensation experienced during micturition.

CHD Abbreviation for **C**oronary **H**eart **D**isease

cheek Fleshy protuberance of face.

cheilitis Inflammation of lips.

chemical Substance composed of chemicals or that which is related with chemistry.

chemist Person skilled in chemistry.

chemistry Science that deals with elements and atoms and their relations.

chemokine Cytokines that induce chemotaxis in WBC.

chemoprophylaxis Drugs used to prevent the development of disease. Common example is malaria chemoprophylaxis.

chemoreceptor Receptor adapted for excitation by chemical substances such as olfactory and gustatory receptors.

chemosurgery Destruction of tissue by chemical agents;

chemotaxis Chemical concentration gradient which can be positive or negative chemotaxis. They are released in inflammation.

chemotherapy Treatment of disease by chemical agents

chest Other name for Thorax. Clinically common variants are:

- Barrel chest
- Flat chest
- Flail chest
- Pigeon chest

Cheyne-Stokes This is seen in coma due to failure of nervous centres. This is characterised by rhythmic waxing and waning of respiration rate and depth of respiration with recurring apnoea.

CHF Abbreviation for **C**ongestive **C**ardiac **F**ailure.

chiasm Chiasm (anatomy), **an X-shaped structure produced by the crossing over of the fibers**, with the prefix chiasm- means cross examples include: A nerval chiasm, where either two nerves cross in the body midline.

chiasma Anatomical nomenclature for a decussation or X -shaped crossing, such as of nerves.

Chiba needle This flexible steel needle used in transhepatic cholangiography.

chickenpox Contagious infectious disease caused by virus that affect children, spread by respiratory route via droplet nuclei

chigger Larva of a mite of the family Trombiculidae They attach to the skin and produce a wheal, usually with severe itching and dermatitis

chikungunya Infection by alpha virus transmitted by mosquito of aedes. It produces musculoskeletal symptoms and haemorrhagic fever.

Chilblain Localized erythema by exposure to cold associated with dampness, and accompanied by pruritus and a burning sensation, usually involving the hands, feet, ears, and face

child Period of human cycle from infancy to puberty. This is known as childhood.

childbirth This refers to labor, and delivery also called parturition.

chill Shivering or involuntary contractions of the voluntary muscles, accompanied by a sense of cold and pallor of the skin

chip A small broken bone piece,

chisel Wedge like instrument with a cutting edge at the end of the blade.

chi-square It can be a test of significance or can be a distribution.

chitin Exoskeleton of arthropods

chitinous That which is hard usually referable to chitin.

CHL Abbreviation for **C**rown **H**eel **L**ength.

Chlamydia Gram-negative, coccoid organisms that multiply only within a host cell and have a unique growth cycle. Chlamydia trachomatis is common pathogen that cause trachoma.

Chloral Oily liquid, having a pungent, irritating odor; it is used in the manufacture of chloral hydrate and DDT.

chloramine-T Topical antiseptic to irrigate and dress wounds and as a mouthwash and used to sterilize drinking water.

chloramphenicol Antibiotic, originally derived from Streptomyces used against rickettsia and bacteria.

chlordiazepoxide This is a benzodiazepine used as an anxiolytic in the treatment of anxiety disorders, relief of anxiety, relief of alcohol withdrawal symptoms, to control tremor.

chlorhexidine An antibacterial, effective against a wide variety of gram-negative and gram-positive organisms.

chlorinated That which is charged with chlorine.

chlorine A disinfecting agent and a bleaching agent. In the form of bleaching power it is used in water purification

chloroacetaldehyde Metabolite produced by biotransformation of vinyl chloride in the liver.

chloroacetic acid Strong acid which has the formula $CH_2ClCOOH$, used as a laboratory reagent.

chlorobutanol Antimicrobial preservative in various pharmaceutical solutions, especially injectables. It is also used as a local dental analgesic, hypnotic, antipruritic, sedative, somnifacient, and antiseptic.

chlorofluorocarbon Group of hydrocarbons in which hydrogen atoms are replaced by chlorine or fluorine. It was used as aerosols.

chloroform It is trichloromethane with formula $CHCl_3$. It is a colourless, volatile liquid with a strong ethereal odor and a sweetish, burning taste, a common laboratory solvent; it is hepatotoxic and nephrotoxic when ingested. It was used as an inhalation anaesthetic

chloroquine It is a 4-aminoquinoline compound used in the treatment of malaria.

chlorothiazide It is a thiazide diuretic, used for treatment of hypertension and edema

chlorothymol Topical antibacterial and fungicide.

chlorpheniramine It is an antihistaminic derived from Pheniramine. Common preparation is Chlorpheniramine maleate.

chlorpromazine It is a phenothiazine derivative, used as an antiemetic and tranquilizer,

chlorpropamide This is a sulfonylurea used as hypoglycaemic agent in diabetes.

choana Funnel-shaped cavity or infundibulum.

choke Difficult condition resulting from interruption of respiration. It is also called strangulation.

cholangiocarcinoma Adenocarcinoma arising from the epithelium of the intrahepatic bile ducts

cholangitis Inflammation of a bile duct. This can be non suppurative, sclerosing, or pyogenic .

cholebilirubin Pigment occurring in gallbladder bile which gives a direct reaction to the Van Den Bergh Test.

cholecalciferol By irradiation of 17 dehydrocholesterol called vitamin D_3 is produced. This occurs as synthesis on the skin.

cholecystitis Inflammation of the gallbladder which can be:

- Acute
- Chronic
- Emphysematous
- Follicular
- Proliferative
- gaseous

cholelithiasis Formation of gallstones either in gall bladder or in bile duct. (choecystolithiasis or choledocholithiasis respectively)

cholelithotripsy process of crushing of gallstones.

cholera Endemic enteritis in India due to Vibrio cholerae which produce copious secretions to cause acute diarrhoea (rice watery stool) that cause massive fluid loss, saline depletion, acidosis and shock. Summer cholera, Asiatic cholera, dry cholera, are known.

cholesteatoma Benign tumor lined with stratified squamous epithelium with debris and cholesterol in middle ear.

cholesterol Sterol which is the precursor of bile acids and steroid hormones and a key constituent of cell membranes. It is synthesised in liver, transported in plasma in the form of lipoproteins. Cholesterol is responsible for atheroma and gall stone.

choline Water-soluble compound from animal and vegetable tissues. It is considered as vitamin B complex. Acetyl choline form is essential for transmission of nerve impulses.

cholinergic Sympathetic and parasympathetic nerve fibers that liberate acetylcholine at a synapse when a nerve impulse passes.

cholinesterase Enzyme of the hydrolase class that catalyses acetylcholine. It is present in liver, serum and pancreas.

chondral Related with cartilage.

chondritis Inflammation of cartilage.

chondrodystrophy Abnormal development of cartilage.

chondroma Benign tumor mature hyaline cartilage. Within the bone it is called enchondroma and on the surface of the bone it is called juxtacortical chondroma.

chondromatous Related with the nature of cartilage.

chondromyxosarcoma Malignant mesenchymoma containing myxoid and cartilaginous elements.

CHOP Anti cancer drug combination which contain Cyclophosphamide, hydroxydaunomycin, Oncovin and Prednisone.

Chopart's amputation The Chopart amputation is **an amputation at the junction of the midfoot and hindfoot** and is a procedure that preserves full limb length.

chorea (k[schwa]-re?[schwa]a) Rapid, highly complex, jerky, dyskinetic movements that appear to be well coordinated but are performed involuntarily. Types of chorea are:

- Huntington's chorea
- Acute chorea
- Chronic chorea
- Chorea gravidarum
- Hyoscine chorea
- Hysterical chorea
- Sydenham's chorea
- Senile chorea

choriocarcinoma Malignancy of trophoblastic cells, formed by the abnormal proliferation of cuboidal and syncytial cells of the placental epithelium

chorion Outermost extraembryonic membrane composed of trophoblast lined with mesoderm which develops villi about 2 weeks after fertilization. This gives rise to Placenta.

choroid Thin pigmented vascular coat of the eye extending from the ora serrata to the optic nerve. This helps in blood supply to the retina and conducts arteries and nerves to the anterior structures.

choroiditis Infection and inflammation of the posterior portion of the uveal tract.

Christmas disease Name of Englishman who was the first patient with the disease. This is called Haemophilia B and there is deficiency of Factor IX

chromaffin Cells that take up and stain with chromium salts

chromatin Network of nuclear fibrils which stains readily. Chromatic is DNA attached to a protein.

chromatin-negative Cell lacking sex chromatin;

chromatin-positive Cell having sex chromatin called Barr body in the nuclei of somatic cells which is a characteristic of the normal female or of other individuals with two (or more) X chromosomes.

chromatography Techniques used to separate mixtures of substances based on differences in the relative affinities of the substances for two different media. One media is moving fluid and the other is stationary gel.

chromosome Linear thread of DNA in animal cells which transmits genetic information Each organism of a species normally has a characteristic number of chromosomes in its somatic cells. Man has 46 including the two (XX or XY) which determine the sex of the organism.

chronic Which persist for a longer time.

chronicity The one which is being chronic.

Chrysanthemum Pyrethrum extract from flowering herb, which is used as insecticide.

chyle Turbid and milky fluid resembling that produced during digestion.

chylomicron Lipoproteins that transport cholesterol and triglycerides from the small intestine to tissues after meals.

chyluria Presence of chyle in the urine which is due to the obstruction of the retroperitoneal lymphatics in bancroftian filariasis.

chymase Enzyme of the hydrolase class that catalyzes the hydrolysis of peptide bonds

chyme Homogeneous, creamy or gruel-like material produced by gastric digestion of food

chymotrypsin It is secreted by pancreas. This cleaves peptide bonds of tyrosine, tryptophan, phenylalanine and leucine.

cilia They are eyelashes

ciliary That which is related to eyelashes.

cimetidine Used in the treatment of peptic ulcer. It is an antagonist to histamine H_2 receptors, which inhibits gastric acid secretion in response to all stimuli.

Cinchona The bark cinchona named after a countess of Chinchon. Cinchona has medicinal value giving important quinoline alkaloids like quinine, quinidine, cinchonine and cinchonidine used in the treatment of malaria.

ciprofloxacin Antibacterial effective against many gram-positive and gram-negative bacteria, including some strains resistant to penicillins, cephalosporins, and aminoglycosides.

circular Shaped like a circle

circulation Movement through a circuitous course such as blood circulation in the body.

circumcision Surgical removal of all or part of the prepuce, or foreskin.

circumference Outer limit of a rounded body.

cirrhosis Liver tissue show diffuse interlacing bands of fibrous tissue in some of the liver disorders.

cistern An anatomical closed space serving as a reservoir for fluid

citric acid Citric acid is an intermediate in the Tricarboxylic Acid Cycle or Krebs cycle.

citronella This is a source of citronella oil

Citrus Refers to citrus fruits which are rich in vitamin C. Common citrus fruits are Line, Orange, Bergamot.

clamp To effect compression or to grip a tissue

class Categorisation of variables, items, organisms or population. Socio economic classification, neutrophils classification, serologic classification are known categorisations.

Claude American cytologist who won Novel prize for his discoveries of structural and functional organisation of cell.

Claude Bernard French Physiologist who explored the milieu interieur the basic physiological basis of our body. This internal environment (milieu interieur of Claude Bernard) is essential for the normal life process of living organism. Homeostasis of BP and Diabetes are well known. Nervous control constancy is another example of claude Bernard's homeostasis.

claudication Latin word meaning lameness. Pain and tension of weakness in a limb when walking is seen in intermittent cludication.

Claviceps Parasitic fungi of the family Clavicipitaceae that infest the seeds of various plants; several species are sources of Ergotism in man.

clavicle Name of collarbone.

clawhand Flexion and atrophy of the hand and fingers that is seen in leprosy, in syringomyelia. it occurs in lesions of the ulnar nerve, in leprosy, and in syringomyelia. It is also called as Main Ken Griffe.

clearance Removing a substance. Removal of an obstruction.

cleavage This stage is the mitotic segmentation of the zygote

cleft An elongated opening especially one occurring in the embryo.

Clenching Pressing and clamping of the jaws and teeth together. This is associated with nervous tension.

click Brief sharp sound such as mitral click, ejection click, Ortolani's click,

climacteric A critical point in life. Body changes in women at menopause. In man this sort of change is called climacterium.

climax Period of greatest intensity. Crisis of a disease and sexual excitement called orgasm are examples.

clinic Establishment where patients are admitted for special study and treatment by a group of physicians practicing medicine together. Teaching instruction at the bedside.

clinical Actual observation and treatment of patients, as distinguished from theoretical or basic sciences.

clinician An expert clinical physician who is also a teacher.

clinoid That which resembles bed, usually referred to clinoid process.

clip Metallic device to approximate the edges of a wound

clitoris Small erectile body situated at the anterior angle of the rima pudenda in females.

clitoroplasty Plastic surgery of the clitoris.

clitorotomy Surgical incision of the clitoris.

clock Device by which time may be measured.

clofazimine Drug used in leprosy and in tuberculosis.

clone Genetically identical cells, identical animals, identical human beings derived by vegetative reproduction from a single parent.

clonidine hydrochloride Oral hypotensive drug which is an α_2-adrenergic agonist antagonist.

cloning Clone formation, refers to DNA cloning.

clonorchiasis Liver fluke infection by Opisthorchis sinensis which lead to inflammation of the biliary tree, proliferation of the biliary epithelium, progressive portal fibrosis, and sometimes biliary duct carcinoma

clonus Alternate muscular contraction and relaxation in rapid succession.

clorprenaline hydrochloride An adrenergic used as a bronchodilator.

Clostridium Oligate anaerobic bacteria which is gram positive spore forming that produce exotoxins. They are present in soil, water and intestine.

closure This is occlusion or an obstruction such as velopharyngeal closure.

clot Semi solidified mass of blood. Blood clot, laminated clot, post mortem clot etc.,

clotrimazole Broad-spectrum antifungal agent, applied topically to the skin in the treatment of candidiasis and various forms of tinea, and administered intravaginally in the treatment of vulvovaginal candidiasis.

clotting Refers to coagulation.

clouding When there is loss of clarity.

cloxacillin sodium Semisynthetic penicillinase-resistant penicillin, used primarily in the treatment of infections due to penicillinase-producing staphylococci, administered orally.

clubbing Proliferation of the soft tissues about the terminal phalanges of the fingers with no bony changes present in chronic disease of the thoracic organs.

clubfoot Other name for Talipes.

clubhand Twisted and changed position of hand due to congenital absence of the radius or ulna.

clump Aggregation as of bacteria caused by the action of agglutinins

Clutton's joint Joint of congenital syphilis where knee joints are having painless symmetrical hydrarthrosis.

CMI Abbreviation for **C**ell **M**ediated **I**mmunity

C-MOPP Drug regimen for cancer which contains **C**yclophospha**m**ide, **O**ncovin (vincristine), **P**rocarbazine, and **P**rednisone

CMV Abbreviation for **C**yto**M**egalo**V**irus **(CMV)**

CNS Abbreviation for **C**entral **N**ervous **S**ystem.

coagglutination Aggregation of particulate antigens combined with agglutinins of more than one specificity.

coagulant That which make it possible for the coagulation of blood.

coagulase Enzyme that reacts with a cofactor found in blood plasma to catalyze the formation of fibrin from fibrinogen.

coagulation Solidification of a sol into a gelatinous mass called clotting of blood.

coarse That which is not fine.

coat In latin it is called tunica that means the layer of protein that protects.
Common coat in medical vocabulary are:

- Albugineous coat
- Adventitial coat
- Dartos coat
- Graafian follicle coat
- Fibrous coat
- Sclerotic coat
- Seroud coat
- Submucous coat
- Subserous coat
- Uveal coat
- Vascular coat
- Villous coat
- White coat

CoA-transferase Enzymes of the transferase class that catalyze the transfer of coenzyme A from one molecule to another.

Coats' disease This refers to Exudative Retinopathy described by Coats.

cobalamin Term used generically to denote any substituted derivative of this compound, including cyanocobalamin, particularly one with vitamin B_{12} activity.

coca A central nervous stimulant used in South America from leaves of E. coca.

cocaine An alkaloid from coca leaves use of which has been under drug abuse.

Coccidia Parasitic protozoa from Sporozoa which has the life cycle through merogony, gametogony, and sporogony

coccidioidomycosis Fungal disease caused by infection with Coccidioides immitis.

cochlea Spiral shaped anatomical organ in inner ear which is an essential organ of hearing.

cocoa Caffeine and theobromine present in cocoa seeds, which is a flavouring agent in pharmacy.

code In Latin it means something written as a set of rules governing one's conduct.

codeine Narcotic alkaloid obtained from opium used as antitussive and analgesic.

codex Authorized medicinal formulary called *Codex medicamentorum.*

Codman's sign It is a sign of rupture of supraspinatus tendon. During abduction of upper limb, when there is no support deltoid muscle contracts and pain occurs. But when a support is given upper limb can be passively abducted without pain.

codon There are 64 different codons which are seen as a set of three adjacent bases on a single strand of DNA or RNA.

coefficient **A** unit less statistical parameter indicating the amount of change in an outcome under given conditions. Examples are Biological coefficient, correlation coefficient, phenol coefficient, osmotic coefficient, Pearson's correlation coefficient, product moment correlation, Rank correlation, Spearman's rank correlation coefficient, coefficient of variation,

coenzyme A phosphorylated derivative of water soluble vitamin binds with protein molecule to form an active enzyme which is an organic nonprotein molecule Co enzyme A, Co enzyme B are known co enzymes.

cofactor An element with which another must unite to function. Examples are:
Platelet co factor, heparin cofactor etc.,

cognition Latin word meaning to know. All aspects of perceiving, thinking, and remembering.

cognitive Related with cognition.

cohort Term used in epidemiology. Cohort is a group of individuals who share a common characteristic, such as individuals born in one year (a birth cohort) or a group of individuals entered in a clinical trial.

coital That which is related to coitus.

coitus Sexual intercourse between male and female. Coitus interrupts and coitus reservatus are commonly used words, which denote withdrawal before ejaculation, and ejaculation is suppressed respectively.

colchicine Alkaloid obtained from Colchicum used in the treatment of gouty arthritis.

COLD Abbreviation for **C**hronic **O**bstructive **L**ung **D**isease.

cold Catarrhal disorder of the upper respiratory tract which may be viral or allergy in nature. Such viral infection is called common cold.

Cole's sign A sign of duodenal ulcer where in deformity of the duodenal contours in radiograph is seen.

colectomy Surgical excision of a portion of the colon *(partial)* or of the whole colon *(complete)*.

colic Acute abdominal pain characterised by intermittent visceral pain with fluctuations corresponding to smooth muscle peristalsis. Appendicitis, gall stones, Renal colic, intestinal colic, lead colic are known clinical entities.

colicky That which is related to colic.

coliform Enteric fermentative gram-negative rods restricted to the lactose-fermenting gram-negative enteric bacilli such as *Enterobacter Escherichia and Klebsiella*

colistin Polypeptide antibiotic of the Polymyxin group. Against pseudomonas, E.coli and klebsiella.

colitis Infection and inflammation of the colon.

collagen Proteins occurring as a major component of connective tissue, giving it strength and flexibility. On boiling it becomes collagen.

collagenase an enzyme that catalyses the hydrolysis of peptide bonds in triple helical regions of collagen.

colloid Small, insoluble particles called glue which can in dispersed phase or in continuous phase.

coloboma Absence of tissues in ocular tissue due to mall closure of the foetal intraocular fissure. This can be atypical, bridge type, of ciliary body, complete, fundal, of iris, of optic disc.

colon Part of the large intestine which extends from the cecum to the rectum; anatomically ascending, transverse and descending colon are present.

colony Collection of bacteria in a culture derived from the increase of an isolated single organism.

colour This is the property of a surface of a substance resulting from absorption of certain of the incident light rays and reflection of others falling within the range of wavelengths.

colorectal Related to colon and rectum.

colorrhaphy Repair of the colon.

colostomy Creation of an opening between the colon and the surface of the body called stoma.

colostrum This refers to yellow, milky fluid secreted by the mammary gland before or after parturition. It contains Immunoglobulin, less fat.

colpitis Refers to vaginitis.

colpocele Refers to vaginal hernia.

colporrhaphy Suturing of the vagina.

colporrhexis Laceration of the vagina.

colposcope Instrument for examination of the vagina and cervix by means of a magnifying lens.

column Referable to gray column of the spinal cord

comatose That which is related to coma.

comedo Plug of keratin and sebum in hair follicle which is called non-inflammatory lesion of acne. Open and closed comedo are two varieties known

commensal Living on another organism to derive benefit without injuring other individual.

commensalism Phenomenon called symbiosis in which one gains from the association and the other is neither harmed nor benefited.

communicable Capable of being transmitted from one person to another

comparator It is a simple colorimeter consisting of a block of wood with holes in which to place the test tubes to be compared

compartment Small enclosure within a larger space. Examples are vascular compartment, muscular compartment

compatible Capable of harmonious coexistence as in transfusion, histocompatible etc.,

compensation Counterbalancing of any defect of structure or function.

competence Organ function in an adequate way.

complaint This refers to symptoms elicited by the patient.

complement A heat-labile factor in serum that causes immune cytolysis. It is now used to refer to the entire functionally related system comprising at least 20 distinct serum proteins, their cellular receptors, and related regulatory proteins. They are designated C1 through C9.

complementary That which supply the defect to make it complete.

complex Collection of various things or related factors or it can be group of interrelated ideas that have a common emotional tone and strongly influence a person's attitudes and behavior.

complexion Colour and appearance of the skin of the face.

Compliance Quality of yielding to pressure without disruption.

complicated Associated with other injuries, lesions, or diseases.

complication Simultaneous presence of many diseases or many lesions that occur as a sequel of one disease.

component It is one of the constituent of a part.

compound A substance that consists of two or more chemical elements in union.

concave Hollowed inner surface of a segment of a sphere.

concentrate To gather together at one point. It can be the strength of a drug or chemical

concentration This refers to increase the strength of a solution or chemical .

concept This is the image of a thing as held in the mind.

conception This is the onset of pregnancy with pregnancy signs and symptoms.

concha That which resembles a shell or sea shell.

condensation Act of compression, Conversion from the gaseous state to the liquid or solid state.

condenser An apparatus for condensing gases or vapours. Such as Abbe's condenser, mechanical condenser, back action condenser etc.,

condition An item or a structure which is subjected to conditioning.

conditioning Pavlovian conditioning. Learning through stimulus that is repeatedly done on tissue, organ or animals.

condom A cover for the penis, worn during coitus to prevent impregnation

conduction Transfer of sound waves, heat, nervous impulses, or electricity. Air conduction, bone conduction, synaptic conduction, A.V. conduction,

conductivity Capacity of a body to transmit a flow of electricity .

conductor Material that possesses conductivity, Director for surgical use.

conduit a pipe, channel or tube through which liquid, gas or electrical wires can pass.

condylar Pertaining to a condyle.

condyle Rounded projection on a bone

condyloma Central core of connective tissue covered with epithelium . Known ones are C.acuminatum, C.latum,

condylus Rounded projection on a bone, usually for articulation with another.

cone Solid body with a circular base tapering to a point such as acrosomal cone, cerebellar pressure cone, medullary cone, implantation cone, pressure cone, retinal cone, visual cone and Tyndall cone by Tyndall effect.

confabulation Unconscious filling in of gaps in memory with fabricated facts and experiences

confidentiality One of the principle in medical ethics that the information a patient reveals to a health care provider is private and has limits on how and when it can be disclosed to a third party. Permission from patient is required to reveal it.

configuration Arrangement done of parts of a thing to give a shape. It can be arrangement ofa tom in chemistry.

conflict An unconscious psychic struggle due to impulses, drives and demands. Extra psychic, intra psychic and intra personal conflicts are common known conflicts.

confluence This refers to gastrulation in embryology. To run together as stream.

confounder This refers to a third variable that can indirectly distort the statistical relationship between two variables under observation.

confounding This in statistics refers to the interference by a third variable so as to distort the association being studied between two other variables

confrontation Act of face to face interaction about attitude and shortcomings.

confusion Disorientation or the disturbed orientation in regard to time, place, or person, sometimes accompanied by disordered consciousness.

congenic Bred with the intention of maintaining the desired genetic differences by selection of progeny. Related to two inbred strains of animals.

congenital The conditions that are present at birth, regardless of their causation.

congested The state of congestion as seen with blood congestion.

congestion The state of hyperaemia such as:

- Pathological congestion
- Functional congestion
- Active congestion
- Passive congestion
- Pulmonary congestion
- Venous congestion

congestive Pertaining to congestion.

conjugate Latin word meaning yoked together. Referable to chemical coagulation.

conjugation Act of joining together. It can be exchange of material during fusion of two cells.

conjunctiva Delicate membrane that lines the eyelids and sclera called palpebral and bulbar conjunctiva respectively.

conjunctivitis Infection and inflammation of the conjunctiva giving rise to hyperaemia and discharge.

Conn's syndrome This refers to Primary aldosterone's described by Conn.

Connell's suture Continuous U shaped suture used in intestinal anastomosis.

conoid Shaped like a cone.

consanguineous When related by blood.

consanguinity Related by blood.

conscience This is the moral faculty of the mind

conscious State of awareness

consciousness Responsive to the environment with clear sensorium.

consent To grant permission.

conservative That which is designed to preserve health

consistency State of coherence among parts or it can be reliability of results.

consolidation Condition of being solid such as consolidation of lung.

constant That which remain unaltered

constipation Difficult evacuation of the faces.

constitution Make-up of man which is determined by the genetic, biochemical, and physiologic endowment of the individual, and modified in great measure by environmental factors.

constitutional That which is related with constitution.

constriction Refers to a stricture such as pyloric constriction.
consult To get a second opinion about sickness of a patient.
consultant Physician who give advice and counsel a patient and his relative.
consultation Patient is referred to specialist who gives his opinion on diagnosis and treatment.
contact Mutual touch. A person is near to an infectious case.
contagion Communication of disease from one person to another.
contagious Disease which is capable of being transmitted from one person to another
contaminant That causes contamination.
contamination Introduction of organisms into a wound
continence Self-restraint with respect to urination or to sexual indulgence.
contra- Latin word meaning opposed.
contraception Prevention of impregnation.
Contraceptive Agent that diminishes the likelihood of conception. Common types are chemical contraceptive, IUCD, barrier contraceptive and oral contraceptive.
contract Shortening of muscle.
contractile That which has ability to contract in response to a stimulus.
contraction Shortening of muscles by contraction which implies development of tension.
contracture Fibrosis and passive stretch of a muscle.
contraindication Condition of a disease, which renders some particular line of treatment not desirable.
contralateral Situated or affecting the opposite side, as opposed to ipsilateral.
contrast Pattern of an image which differ in different brightness because of optical density.
control Standard against which experimental observations may be evaluated
contuse This refers to bruise.
contusion Injury of a part without a break in the skin and with a subcutaneous hemorrhage. Brain, Myocardium and spinal cord contusion are known contusion.
conus Con shaped organ or part, anatomical description. Medullary conus, Myopic conus are known clinical entities.
convalescence Recovery stage following an attack of disease, an operation, or an injury.
convalescent That which is related with convalescence.
convection Heat transmission in liquids or gases by a circulation carried on by bulk movement of the heated particles to a cooler area.
convergence The coordinated inclination of the two lines of sight toward their common point of fixation
convergent Meeting at a common point.
convex Elevated surface which is a segment of the external surface of a sphere.
Convex concave Convex on one surface and concave on the other.
Convexo convex Convex on each of two opposite surfaces.
convoluted That which is coiled.
convolution Elevation caused by a structure being infolded upon itself such as in Cerebral gyri.
convulsant Agent that causes convulsion.
convulsibility Capability of being convulsed.
convulsion Involuntary and series of contractions of the voluntary muscles. Common entities are Febrile convulsion, puerperal convulsion, convulsion of tetanus, uremic convulsion and tonic epileptic convulsion.
Cooley's anemia This refers to Thalassaemia described by Cooley.
cooling Process of reducing the temperature of body or in experimental animals.
Coombs' test It is an antiglobulin test done in autoimmune and drug induced haemolytic anaemia and haemolytic disease of the new-born.
Cooper's breast Irritable breast described by Cooper is also called neuralgia of the breast.
Coopernail's sign It is positive in Fracture of pelvis where ecchymosis on perineum and scrotum or labia is present.
coordination Harmonious functioning of brain or any other part of the body where there is definite adaptive useful responses.
COP Abbreviation for **C**yclophosphamide, **O**ncovin and **P**rednisone, the combination of drugs used in cancer treatment.
COPD Abbreviation for **C**hronic **O**bstructive **P**ulmonary **D**isease.
Copolymer 1 Polypeptide used in multiple sclerosis. Copolymer 1 contains alanine, lysine, tyrosine and glutamic acid.
COPP Abbreviation for **C**yclophosphamide, **O**ncovin, **P**rocarbazine and **P**rednisone used in cancer treatment.
copula Latin word meaning a connecting part.
copulation Sexual union between male and female animals.
Coracidium Ciliated embryo of tapeworms of the order Pseudophyllidea.
coracoacromial Related with coracoid and acromion processes.
coracoclavicular Related with coracoid process and the clavicle.
coracohumeral Related with coracoid process and the humerus.
coracoid An anatomical structure which looks like a beak.
Coramine This contains Nikethamide.
cord Long, rounded, flexible structure
corditis Infection and inflammation of the spermatic cord.
corneal That which is related with cornea.
cornu Hornlike projection in anatomical nomenclature

corona Anatomical nomenclature to designate a crown like structure.

Coronavirus (Covid) COVID-19 affects different people in different ways. Most infected people will develop mild to moderate illness and recover without hospitalization.

coronal Crown of the head, the crown of a tooth

coronary Structure which is encircling in the manner of a crown such as coronary artery.

corpse Dead body of human body.

corpulency Other name for obesity.

corpus Other name for body of man.

corpuscle Small mass or small body.

corpuscular Pertaining to corpuscles.

correlation Degree to which one phenomenon or random variable is associated with or can be predicted from another. Correlation usually refers to the degree to which a linear predictive relationship exists between random variables, as measured by a correlation coefficient (r).

cortex External layer of a tree, of a fruit. Or of an organ

cortical Related to the nature of a cortex

corticospinal Related to cortex of the brain and the spinal cord.

corticosteroid Steroid of adrenal cortex in response to ACTH. They can be mineralocorticoids or mineralocorticoids. It is anti-inflammatory , antiallergic and suppresses immune response.

corticosterone Similar to cortisol, it is glucocorticoid without anti-inflammatory action.

corticotropin ACTH from animals for diagnostic testing of adrenocortical function, as an antiemetic in cancer treatment.

cortisol Glucocorticoid from zona fasciculate of adrenal cortex has effect on metabolism of glucose, protein, and fats

cortisone It is cortisol from glucocorticoid. Human adrenal cortex secretes only minute amounts

Corynebacterium They are gram-positive, nonsporulating, nonmotile, straight to slightly curved rods. C.diphtheriae is known to cause diphtheria.

coryza The other name is Acute rhinitis.

cosmetic Substance or preparations that are used for beautifying purpose.

costa Latin word meaning Rib. There are 12 pairs of ribs in human beings. They are numbered as Costa I to Costa XII. They're grouped under true and false ribs (connected with sternum and not connected with sternum respectively).

co-trimoxazole This is the combination of a mixture of trimethoprim and sulfamethoxazole.

Cottes operation This is the surgical removal of the presacral nerve devised by Cotter.

Cotting's operation Surgical treatment for Ingrowing toenail. Here ingrowing edge of the nail and side of toe down is excised.

cough Expulsion of air from the lungs to keep the airways of the lungs free of foreign matter or as a result of irritation.

coulomb SI unit of electric charge by a current of one ampere in one second. This is represented as under:
$C = 6.24 ? 10^{18}$ electrons

coumarin Dicumarol the ingredient present in coumarin is used in thrombophlebitis, pulmonary embolism and cardiac embolism. Coumarin is extracted from tonka bean.

count A computation by numbers. Common count of medical importance and Lab.

counter An apparatus for counting values in laboratory procedures. It also can be an apparatus for counting values of ionising radiation.

counterimmunoelectrophoresis Double electro immuno-diffusion in which antibody and antigen are placed in separate wells in an agar plate and driven toward each other by an applied electric field. It works on the ground that the gel is buffered at a pH between the isoelectric points of the antigen and antibody.

countertraction Traction opposed to another traction employed in the reduction of fractures.

couple Forces operating on an object in parallel but opposite directions. This produces a difference in electrical potential.

coupling Joining together of two things. Occurrence on the same chromosome in a double heterozygote of the two mutant alleles of interest. This also means the serial occurrence of a normal heart beat followed closely by a premature beat.

covariance Word used in statistics which means a measure of the tendency of two random variables to vary together. This expresses the expected value of the product of the deviations of corresponding values of the variables from their respective means. Co variance values can be positive, negative or zero.

covariate A variable that is related to a second variable.

coverslip Lab. Glassware called coverglass used in microscopic examinations.

Cowper's gland are **pea sized glands present inferior to the prostate gland in the male reproductive system**. They produce thick clear mucus prior to ejaculation that drains into the spongy urethra.

Cowper's ligament This refers to Pectineal fascia or the public portion of the fascia lata explained by Cowper.

cowpox Eruptive skin disease caused by a pox virus. **Edward Jenner** first demonstrated vaccination **in 1798** when he showed that inoculation with material from cowpox lesions conferred immunity against smallpox.

coxalgia Pain in the hip.

coxsackievirus This was discovered in Coxsackie, New York, and hence the name. Many types are present and described in virology.

CPC Abbreviation for **C**linico **P**athological **C**onference.

CPD Abbreviation for **C**ephalo **P**elvic **D**isproportion.

cps Abbreviation for **c**ycles **p**er **s**econd

cradle For the purpose of protecting the body of a patient from heat, cold or burns, a frame called cradle is placed.

Cramer's splint This is a wire splint which is flexible and has parallel stout wires. Between these parallel stout wires it has smaller wires are stretched.

cramp Tonic spasm of muscle which is a painful spasmodic muscular contraction

Crampton's test This test elucidates physical resistance of a patient. Difference between Pulse and BP in recumbent position and in the standing position are measured & recorded.

cranial Head end of the body. Cephalic or superior is used for cranial end.

craniopagus Conjoined twins united by the heads

craniotabes Reduction in the mineralization of occipital and parietal bones giving rise to abnormal softness of the bone

craniotomy Operation on the cranium

cranium Upper part of the head

crease Linear depression on the palm

creatine Amino acid in muscle which is formed by methylation of guanidinoacetic acid that is energy source for muscle contraction.

creatine kinase This enzyme of the transferase class that catalyzes the phosphorylation of creatine by ATP to form phosphocreatine. Phosphocreatine in muscle and brain tissue help in the muscle concentration of ATP nearly constant during the initiation of exercise.

creatinine It is the final product of decomposition of phosphocreatine. It is excreted in the urine and is an indicator of kidney function.

crèche French word denoting day nursery for infants.

Credé's method Following are the Crede's methods in clinical practice:

1. Placenta expression by forcing the uterus down into the pelvis along with squeezing uterus from all sides.
2. In urinary bladder paralysis, crede's method is followed for expressing urine from urinary bladder.
3. Putting 2% $AgNO_3$ to the new-born to prevent ophthalmia neonatorum.

creep Strain in a tissue as a result of application and maintenance of a stress

cremaster Name of the muscle cremaster.

cremation Burning or incineration of dead bodies.

crematorium This is an establishment for the burning of dead bodies.

crepitation This is an auscultation sound which is like throwing salt into a fire. In case of fracture of bone, fractured ends make sound called crepitation.

crepitus Latin word meaning discharge of flatus from the bowels.

crescent Any organ shaped like a new moon. Examples are Glomerular crescent, malarial crescent, Myopic crescent, and sub lingual crescent.

cresol Coal tar derivative containing not more than 5 per cent phenol

crest Projecting structure such as alveolar crest, anterior crest of fibula, buccinator crest, deltoid crest, femoral crest, gluteal crest, iliac crest, neural crest, occipital crest, orbital crest, pubic crest, sacral crest, tibial crest, ulnar crest, zygomatic crest.

cretin Child which is affected with cretinism.

cretinism Clinical condition of hypothyroidism.

criminology Latin word meaning scientific study of crime and criminals.

crisis Disease condition getting worse by sudden change indicated by raised intensity of symptoms. E.g., Aplastic crisis, addisonian crisis, cardiac crisis, gastric crisis, hepatic crisis, haemolytic crisis, hypertensive crisis, identity crisis etc.,

crista Ridge on a bone or its border. E.g., Ampullary crest, ethmoid crest of maxilla, crista femoris, crista frontalis etc.

criterion For the purpose of judgement, a standard is maintained. E.g., Ranson's criteria for the assessment of severity of acture pancreatitis.

cRNA Abbreviation for complimentary **RNA.**

Crohn's disease is **a type of inflammatory bowel disease (IBD)**. It causes swelling of the tissues (inflammation) in your digestive tract, which can lead to abdominal pain, severe diarrhea, fatigue, weight loss and malnutrition.

crossbreeding Mating of animals or plants of different strains or species called Hybridisation.

crossing over Description of combination of genes during pachytene stage of meiosis cell division. Here exchange of genetic material takes place.

crossmatch Test for compatibility of blood of donor and recipient for blood transfusion. RBC of the donor are placed in serum of the recipient ***(major crossmatch)*** and red cells of the recipient in serum of the donor ***(minor crossmatch)*** and antiglobulin is added to increase reactivity; the presence of agglutination indicates incompatibility. Nowadays **Petra transplant crossmatch** is done for transplantations.

croup Tracheitis in infants that produce cough, hoarseness and stridor, usually caused by parainfluenza virus or Staph aureus bacteria.

Crouzon's disease This refers to Craniofacial Dysostosis described by Crouzon.

crowning Second stage of labor when fetal scalp is visible at the vaginal orifice
CRP Abbreviation for **C** **R**eactive **P**rotein.
crucial Latin word meaning serious, referred to a disease.
cruciate Cross like anatomical structure.
crus Portion from knee to foot.
cry Involuntary and sudden vocal sound. Types of clinical entities are:
- Joint cry
- Epileptic cry
- Arthritic cry
- Cephalic cry

cryosurgery Destruction of tissue by extreme cold, used in intracranial and cutaneous surgery.
cryotherapy Treatment with cold.
crypt Latin word meaning a blind pit or tube on a free surface.
Cryptosporidium Protozoa characterized by the presence of oocysts with four sporozoites present in the intestinal tracts.
crystal Homogeneous angular solid from a chemical compound,
CSF Abbreviation for **C**erebro **S**pinal **F**luid.
CT Abbreviation for **C**omputed **T**omography.
Ctenocephalides Genus of fleas often found parasitic
cubital That which is related to elbow.
cubitus It refers to the joint between the arm and forearm.
cuboid That which resembles a cube.
cuff Band like structure encircling a part made of muscle and tendon fibers.
cul-de-sac Referred to caecum which is a blind pouch
culdoscopy Visual examination of the female pelvic viscera by means of an endoscope introduced into the pelvic cavity through the posterior vaginal fornix.
Culex Culicinae mosquitoes which are differentiated with anopheles mosquitoes. They are vectors in the transmission of diseases.
cult a system of treating disease based on some special and unscientific theory of disease causation.
culture Propagation of microorganisms in microbiology laboratory. Cell culture, blood culture, enrichment culture, primary culture and secondary culture are known.
culture medium Substance used for the cultivation of living cells.
cumulative To increase by successive additions,
cuneiform Wedge shaped bone.
cupula Small inverted dome-shaped cap over some structure.
curare Strychnos plant derivative which is used as arrow poisons in South America. It is used as muscle relaxant in tetanus, and in G.A.
curative To overcome disease and promote recovery.
cure Successful treatment of a disease
curettage Removal of material from the wall of a cavity or other surface
Curie's law This law states "All chemical substances can be rendered radioactive by influence of the emanations of radium. These chemicals hold radioactivity longer"
curie This is a unit of radioactivity which contains the quantity of any radioactive nuclide in which the number of disintegrations per second is 3.700 ? 10^{10}.
curing Process of hardening through the use of dampness, heat, cold, chemical agents, electromagnetic radiation, or other agents.
curriculum An established course of study.
curvature Deviation from a rectilinear direction.
curve Nonangular deviation from a straight course in a line
Cushing's disease Hyper adrenocortical secondary to hyper secretion of corticotrophin from anterior pituitary.
Cushing's suture continuous inverting suture used in G I tract surgery.
cusp Latin word meaning a tapering projection such as cardiac valve.
cut Wound made by a sharp edge.
cutaneous Pertaining to the skin
cutdown Small incised opening over a vein to facilitate phlebotomy.
cuticle Solid layer which covers the free surface of an epithelial cell.
cutis Other name for skin.
C.V. Abbreviation for **C**oefficient of **V**ariation.
CVP Abbreviation for Central Venous Pressure.
Cx Abbreviation for **C**ervix.
cyanmethemoglobin Methemoglobin with the cyanide ion.
cyanosis Bluish discoloration due to excessive concentration of Deoxyhemoglobin in blood.
cyanotic Patient having cyanosis.
cybernetics Science of communication and control processes within systems. Applied to machines and to living organisms
cycle Succession of observable phenomena such as menstrual cycle.
cyclizine This is an antihistaminic antiemetic used in medical treatment.
cyclodialysis Treatment in Glaucoma where a communication between the anterior chamber of the eye and the supra-choroidal space is produced.
cyclodiathermy Glaucoma treatment by the destruction of a portion of the ciliary body by diathermy
cycloplegia Paralysis of the ciliary muscle producing paralysis of accommodation.
Cyclops Crustaceans such as Dracunculus for diphyllobothrium

cycloserine Antibiotic with tuberculostatic activity used against many gram-negative and gram-positive bacteria. It is used in the treatment of tuberculosis and urinary tract infections

cyproheptadine hydrochloride Used for the relief of symptoms of allergy and as an antipruritic for relief of itching associated with various skin disorders.

cyst Pathological closed cavity in the body. This can mean cystic stage of a parasite such as hydatid cyst. Common cysts of medical importance are: Bakers cyst, Dentigerous cyst, Alveolar cyst, Arachnoid cyst, Dermoid cyst, Cervical cyst, Retention cyst, Sebaceous cyst, Urinary cyst, Synovial cyst, Seminal cyst, Umbilical cyst, Pancreatic cyst, Hydatid cyst, Epidermoid cyst, Bronchogenic cyst, Amoebic cyst, Bartholin's cyst, Odontogenic cyst, Sublingual cyst

cystadenoma Adenoma characterized by epithelium-lined cystic masses that contain mucous or serous material. This is common in ovary, salivary glands, pancreas.

cystectomy Excision of a cyst.

cysteic acid This is precursor of taurine which is formed by oxidation of the thiol group of cysteine to a sulfo group .

cysteine Sulfur-containing nonessential amino acid produced by the enzymatic hydrolysis of proteins. Sometimes found in the urine

cysticercoid Larva of tapeworm which resemble cysticercus.

cysticercosis Infection with cysticerci. Man who eats incompletely cooked pork may become infected with larval forms of Taenia solium. Man who eats incompletely cooked beef may become infected with Taenia saginata.

cysticercus Larval of tapeworm with a single scolex enclosed in a bladder-like cyst

cystine Amino acid produced by the digestion or acid hydrolysis of proteins. Found in the urine and in the kidneys in the form of minute hexagonal crystals

cystinuria This is a hereditary condition of persistent excessive urinary excretion of cystine, lysine, Ornithine and arginine. Clinically urinary calculi will be the manifestation.

cystitis Infection and inflammation of the urinary bladder

cystocele Protrusion of the urinary bladder through the vaginal wall

cystolithiasis development of calculi in the urinary bladder.

cystoplasty plastic surgery on the bladder.

Cystoplegia Paralysis of the bladder

cystoscope Endoscope for visual examination of the urinary bladder.

cytidine This is a purine nucleoside which is a component of ribonucleic acid

cytidine deaminase Enzyme that catalyzes the deamination of cytidine to form uridine. This is part of the pyrimidine degradation pathway.

cytochemistry Study of the interactions of cellular constituents by electron microscopy, cell fractionation, and immunochemical techniques.

cytokine This is nonantibody proteins on contact with specific antigen, which act as intercellular mediators, as in the generation of an immune response. Examples are Lymphokines and Monokines.

cytokinesis Cell division changes in cytoplasm.

cytokinin They are phytohormones which induce cell division and its differentiation.

cytologist is a specialist in cytology.

cytology Study of cells, their origin, structure, function, and pathology.

cytopathology Study of cells in disease

cytopenia owered cellular elements of blood.

cytophysiology Physiology of the cell.

cytosine Pyrimidine base found in cells, forms nucleosides cytidine and deoxycytidine when it condenses with ribose and deoxyribose.

cytosine deaminase Enzyme that catalyzes the deamination of cytosine to form uracil which is a step in the degradation of pyrimidine nucleotides.

Cytotoxic Exhibiting cytotoxicity.

cytotoxicity Specific destructive action on cells used particularly in referring to the lysis of cells by immune phenomena

D

dacryocystocele Hernial protrusion of the lacrimal sac; called also.

dactyl Means digital.

Dakin's fluid This is diluted Sodium Hypochlorite Solution.

Dale British physiologist and pharmacologist winner of Nobel Prize for Medicine in 1936 for his work on acetylcholine as an agent in the chemical transmission of nerve impulses.

Dale's reaction Antigen added to a tissue bath in which is immersed the excised uterine horn (smooth muscle) of an anaphylactically sensitized guinea pig causes contraction of the sensitized uterine muscle..

Dalton's law This law states "the pressure exerted by a mixture of nonreacting gases is equal to the sum of the partial pressures of the separate components; it holds true only at very low pressures.

Dam Danish biochemist who won Nobel Prize for medicine in 1943 on his work and discovery of vitamin K.

D and C Dilatation of the cervix and Curettage of the uterus called D & C.

dandruff Scaly and dry material desquamated from the scalp

Dandy's operation Trigeminal rhizotomy using an approach through the posterior cranial fossa.

Dane particle This refers to an intact hepatitis B vision described by Dane.

dapsone a sulfone, belongs to the family of medicines called anti-infectives. Dapsone is **used to treat leprosy (Hansen's disease) and to help control dermatitis herpetiformis, a skin problem**. When it is used to treat leprosy, dapsone may be given with one or more other medicines

Darling's disease This refers to Histoplasmosis described by Darling.

dartos Refers to dartos muscle.

darwinism The theory of evolution by Darwin according to which higher organisms have developed from lower ones through the influence of natural selection.

data Material in the form of facts on which an inference is based.

dATP Abbreviation for **D**eoxy **A**denosine **T**riphosphate.

Datura Plants of the family Solanaceae from which alkaloids like hyoscyamine and scopolamine which are anticholinergic in their pharmacological action.

David's disease This refers to tuberculosis of the spine described by David.

Daviel's operation He is the inventor of extraction of lens for cataract. The said operation refers to the extraction of cataract through a corneal incision without cutting the iris.

Davis graft This refers to a pinch graft which is described by Davis.

dB Abbreviation for Decibel.

DCH Abbreviation for **D**iploma in **C**hild **H**ealth.

DDS Abbreviation for **D**iamino **D**iphenyl **S**ulphone popularly called Dapsone.

DDT Abbreviation for Dichloro **D**iphenyl **T**richloroethane a chlorinated hydrocarbon pesticide used as residual insecticide. Because of ecolobical damage it is not used nowadays.

deaf Lacking the sense of hearing

deaf-mute Person who is unable to hear or speak.

deaf-mutism Absence of sense of hearing and absence of faculty of speech.

deafness Hearing loss called anacusis.

deamination chemical reaction wherein amino group — NH_2, is removed from a compound.

dearticulation Dislocation of a joint.

death Life functioning stops with total cessation of cerebral function, respiratory function and circulatory system. Following terminologies are used in this context:

- Cell death
- Brain death

débride Removal of dead tissues or foreign body by dissection.

débridement Removal of dead tissue by dissection where little surrounding healthy tissue also is removed.

debris French word meaning accumulated necrotic tissue.

decarboxylation Chemical reaction wherein carboxyl group from a molecule is removed.

decay Process of decomposition of dead tissue.

decedent Person who has recently died.

decerebrate Brainstem transected animal whose cerebral function is eliminated for experimental purpose.

decibel One tenth of a bell a unit of intensity of acoustic power.

decidua Endometrium of the pregnant uterus which is shed at parturition.

deciduous used to designate deciduous teeth of man or animals.

decoction Process by which a Medicine or tea prepared by boiling

decompression Surgical treatment of release of pressure in human body compartment such as brain, pleura, abdomen etc., Slow reduction of atmospheric pressure among sea divers.

decongestant Drug which reduces congestion or inflammatory swelling.

decontamination To free people from contaminants such as poisonous gas, radioactive material etc.,

decubitus Lying down position of man.

deep situated far beneath the surface; not superficial.

defecation Evacuation of fecal material from the rectum.

defect Failure or absence.

defense Measures taken for self-protection.

defibrillator Apparatus used to counteract atrial or ventricular fibrillation by brief electric shock to the heart

definition Clear determination of the limits of a given item or the description made in specific sense to detail a material.

defloration Rupture of the hymen in sexual intercourse

deformity Distortion of a part in the body or a malformation.

degeneration Lowered Functional and structural activity of an organ or a tissue.

deglutition The act of swallowing.

Degos' disease This refers to malignant Atrophic Papulosis described by Degos.

degree Unit of a measure, an award to the scholars by college or university.

dehydrase They are dehydrogenases and the dehydratases.

dehydration Condition that results from excessive loss of body water.

7-dehydrocholesterol Pro-vitamin of cholecalciferol that help to have vitamin through skin.

dehydrogenase An enzyme hat catalyzes the transfer of hydrogen in chemical reaction.

Deiters' cells The outer phalangeal cells of the organ of Corti.

Dejean's syndrome This refers to Orbital Floor Syndrome described by Dejean.

DeLee catheter The catheter used to suction of meconium and amniotic debris from nasopharynx and oropharynx of newborn.

DeLeeforceps This is modified Simpson forceps.

DeLee-Hillis stethoscope A stethoscope worn on the head of obstetrician to auscultate foetal heart rate.

deleterious That which is injurious to man and animals.

delinquent Person who neglects the legal obligations. Usually the word is referable to Juvenile delinquent who commits a violation of the law within the jurisdiction of the juvenile court.

delirium Acute disturbance of consciousness accompanied by a change in cognition

deliver The process of child birth.

delivery Process of child birth including expulsion of the placenta.

delousing Destruction of lice from the body.

Deltavirus Hepatitis D virus which required a helper hepatitis B for replication.

deltoid Triangular muscle called deltoid muscle a common site for intra muscular injection to the upper arm.

demarcation Latin word meaning marking the boundaries of an anatomical part.

dementia Loss of cognitive abilities, including impairment of memory.

demethylation Removal of a methyl group CH_3 from a chemical compound.

Democritus Greek philosopher of 370 B.C. who was the first to state that any substance including living one is made up of atoms of different sizes and shapes

demography Study of a population including characteristics such as geographical distribution, physical environment, disease, sex and age composition and birth and death rates.

demonstrator Instructor who teaches individuals in small groups

De Morgan's spots They refer to Cherry Angioma described by De Morgan.

demyelination Removal of the myelin sheath of a nerve

dendrite They are threadlike extensions of the cytoplasm of a Neuron. They are receptive surface of a neuron. .

denervation Removal of the nerves to an organ by nerve section.

dengue Acute viral infection caused by Dengue virus which is self-limiting in nature. It is called Break Bone Fever. Severe type is called Haemorrhagic or bleeding Dengue Fever.

Dennie's sign It is positive in Atopic dermatitis. A secondary crease in the lower eyelids is positive sign.

density This refers to compactness expressed per unit space.

dentifrice A paste, gel, or powder, used with a toothbrush for cleaning the accessible surfaces of the teeth.

dentin Hard portion of the tooth surrounding the pulp which is covered by enamel

dentist Doctor qualified to treat dental problems.

dentistry The specialty which deals with diagnosis and treatment of dental ailments, including surgical intervention.

dentition Teeth in the dental arch as a natural teeth. Nowadays artificial dentition is also accepted.

denture Artificial or prosthetic replacement for missing natural teeth

deodorant Cosmetics used to overcome bad offensive odors.

deoxyguanylate a dissociated form of deoxyguanylic acid.

deoxyribonuclease Nuclease catalyzing the cleavage of phosphate ester linkages in deoxyribonucleic acids

deoxyribonucleic acid Called DNA, Nucleic acid present in cell nucleus with side chain by adenine and guanine cytosine and thymine. This is required in the synthesis of RNA.

dependence This is referable to drug dependence or alcohol dependence.

depigmentation Loss of pigment Melanin called hypopigmentation.

depilate Removal of hair for cosmetic purpose.

depolarization Neutralising the polarity in a cell membrane.

depressant Drug which reduces the functional activity of mental make up.

depression A depressed area on a bone or an organ, Mental state of depression.

Dercum's disease This refers to Adiposis Dolorosa described by Dercum.

dermabrasion Abrasion of skin by mechanical means.

Dermacentor Ticks that transmit diseases such tularemia, spotted fevers. Common species is Dermacentor andersoni.

dermatitis Infection and inflammation of the skin.

dermatologist Consultant who treats skin diseases through special diagnosis and treatment.

dermatology The medical specialty concerned with the diagnosis and treatment of diseases of the skin.

dermatome Instrument for cutting thin skin slices for skin grafts.

dermatomycosis Superficial infection of the skin by fungi.

dermatophyte Fungi parasitic on skin, nails, or hair of humans which will infect patients who are immunocompromised.

dermatotropic Preferentially infecting, the skin

dermoid Resembles to skin the structure of which resembles skin.

desaturation Conversion of a saturated compound to unsaturated compound. This is meant, in chemistry as introduction of a double bond between carbon atoms of a fatty acid.

Descemet's membrane This refers to Posterior Limiting Membrance of the Cornea described by Descemet..

descending That which extends inferiorly.

desensitization By administrating low doses of allergens body hypersensitivity is reduced. It is called immunotherapy.

desiccation The scientific procedure of drying a substance.

desiccator Apparatus used for desiccation.

desmography This is the description of the ligaments.

desmoid A Fibrous Tumour.

desquamation Process of shedding of epithelial tissue.

detergent Chemical, agent or a substance which has the action of purifying or cleansing.

determinant That which determines an event like determinants of distribution of the disease.

detoxification Treatment designed to free an addict from his drug habit.

DEV Abbreviation for **D**uck **E**mbryo **V**accine.

development Biological process of growth and differentiation.

deviant That which varies from normal

deviation This is the difference between a sample value and the mean, An item which deviates from normal standard.

Devic's disease This is referred to Neuromyelitis Optica described by Devic.

device When a thing is contrived for a specific purpose.

devitalization Deprivation of tissues from their normal physiological functions.

Dew's sign In case of Hydatid abscess below right diaphragm, resonance tested moves caudally with the patient on hands and knees.

deworming Giving anthelmintic drugs to kill and remove intestinal worms that cause parasitism.

dexamethasone This is a synthetic glucocorticoid used topically as an anti-inflammatory and administered orally in replacement therapy for adrenal insufficiency chemotherapy, in the diagnosis of Cushing syndrome.

dextran Polymer of D-glucose produced by glycosyltransferases on the cell surface of lactic acid bacteria. It is significantly associated with dental caries and dental plaques. Dextran preparations are used as plasma volume expanders which are produced from Leuconostoc mesenteroides.

dextrin They are polysaccharides from starch. Dextrin is used as tablet binder.

dextrocardia Right sided heart which a congenital anomaly. The condition is called Situs inverses

dextroposition Any anatomical structure or any chemical which is said to be displaced to the right.

dextrorotatory Polarisation of rays of light is turned towards right.

Dextrose Chemically it is D-glucose monohydrate. The Glucose commonly called is obtained by the hydrolysis of starch. A common material used in I V infusion.

DHE Abbreviation for **D**iploma in **H**ealth **E**ducation.

diabetes A metabolic disorder characterized by Polyuria, Polydypsia, called Diabetes mellitus.

diagnosis Ariving at one definite conclusion after clinical examination for the purpose of treatment of illness. In practice, clinical diagnosis, laboratory diagnosis, histopathological diagnosis, biological diagnosis and immunological diagnosis are common.

diagram Representation of data in simplest form which can give overall appreciation of observations made in the study or survey.

dialysis By using a semipermeable membrane which produces difference in rates of diffusion, macromolecules are separated from ions and low molecular weight compounds in a solution. Haemolysis through peritoneum is a type of dialysis. Haemodialysis in renal failure is another example of dialysis.

diameter This refers to the length of a straight line passing through the center of a circle that connects the opposite points on its circumference Cranial and pelvis diameters are frequently measured diameters in clinical practice.

Diamond-Blackfan syndrome This refers to Congenital Hypoplastic anaemia described by Diamond and Blackfan.

diapedesis Transmigration of RBC and WBC through intact vessels.

diaphragm the muscle between your lungs and your stomach that helps you to breathe Separating membrane which separates chest and abdomen

diaphyseal That which is related with shaft of a long bone.

diaphysis Greek word meaning the point of separation between stalk and branch. This denotes the long shaft of a bone.

diarrhea Pathological frequency and liquidity of fecal discharges.

diastase Malt enzyme which converts starch to sugars.

diastasis This word is used in the dislocation of following orthopedic conditions;

- separation of pubic symphysis
- separation of ribs
- separation of radius and ulna

Diastasis also means slow ventricular filling in the cardiac cycle.

diastole This is the period of relaxation of the heart in a cardiac cycle. This coincides with the interval between I and II heart sounds.

diathermy Warming, coagulating or destroying the tissue with the help of heat by high frequency electromagnetic radiation.

diatom They belong to diatomaceous family and are microscopic algae with silica coating.

diazepam Drug used in the treatment of anxiety and is chemically benzodiazepine

Dick test Skin test in Scarlet fever. Intra dermal injection of purified erythrogenic toxin from group A streptococci produces reddening of the skin within 24 to 48 hours. This indicates the susceptibility of a person to scarlet fever.

diclofenac sodium Nonsteroidal anti-inflammatory drug used in the treatment of rheumatoid arthritis, osteoarthritis, ankylosing spondylitis and for a variety of nonrheumatic inflammatory conditions.

dicrotic Representing double notch in heart beat called dichrotism.

dicumarol An anticoagulant which inhibits the liver synthesis of prothrombin and Factors VII, Factor IX, and Factor X.

didactic Theoretical and practical. Conveying the instructions through lecture and not through practical's.

dieldrin Insecticide belonging to chlorinated hydrocarbon used in mosquito control and tick control.

diet Food allowance in a day to have calorie and nutrient to the body for a person. It can be normal diet or therapeutic diet.

dietetic Related with food consumed.

dietetics Science that deals with the regulation of the diet.

diethylstilbestrol Synthetic nonsteroidal Estrogen used for the relief of menopausal symptoms; suppression of lactation; treatment of amenorrhea, dysmenorrhea, senile vaginitis, and pruritus vulvae

dietitian Person trained in the scientific use of diet in health and disease.

diffraction When an obstacle is made, waves will bend and again spreads out but with small wavelength waves.

diffusion Movement of molecules in solution owing to their random thermal motion to reach to an uniform concentration throughout the solvent is called diffusion.

digenetic having two stages of multiplication, one sexual in the mature forms, the other asexual in the larval stages; said of flukes and many other parasites.

DiGeorge's syndrome A congenital disorder in which main defect will be with thymus, parathyroid glands.

digestion Metabolism in which food is converted to absorbable forms to give energy after assimilation.

Digitalis Finger like projections of muscles or any anatomical structures.

digitalis Foxglove used in CCF, supra ventricular tachycardia, cardiogenic shock. This is a major cardiac glycoside in pharmacology.

digoxin Action similar to Digitalis used in cardiac diseases.

dihydrotachysterol produced by the irradiation of ergosterol an analogue of ergocalciferol which has an effect in calcium metabolism.

diiodotyrosine It is a by product of Iodo thyroglobulin an Iodine containing compound.

Dilantin Commercial preparation of Phenytoin an anticonvulscent.

dilatation Stretching or dilating an orifice or a tubular structure. In clinical practice we have anal dilation and cervical dilation for therapeutic purpose. Clinical conditions like cardiac dilation, gastric dilation are often observed.

dilator Instrument used in enlarging an orifice or canal such as –

✓ Hegar dilator (uterine)
✓ Anal dilator
✓ Laryngeal dilator
✓ Pneumatic dilator
✓ Starch dilator for cardioesophageal region

diluent Agent that dilutes an irritant.
dimension Unit of expression for linear measurement of an object, an organ of body part
dimercaprol An antidote for poisoning by arsenic, gold, and mercury, and sometimes other metals
dimorphism Existing in two forms example Fungi that grows as yeast or molds.
dinitrobenzene An asphyxiate chemical found in nature.
dinitrophenol A reagent and an indicator used in chemical analysis.
dinitrotoluene Present in dyes and explosives found to be a carcinogen.
dioxide Binary compound containing two oxide ions such as SiO_2, SO_2. or CO_2
diphenhydramine Drug which has Multi actions like antihistamine anticholinergic, antitussive, antiemetic, and sedative actions.
diphtheria An acute infectious disease caused by toxigenic strains of C. diphtheria bacteria which produce false membrane. Common organs involved are tonsils, uvula, soft palate, pharynx. Cutaneous form is also known.
Diphyllobothrium Tape worm family and common one is D. latum.
diplegia Bilateral paralysis of the body.
diplobacillus Bactria occurring in pairs joined end to end. Gonococci, Neisseria gonorrhoeae, are common pathogen in human beings.
diploid Normal in somatic cells which have two sets of chromosomes.
diplomate A holder of a certificate of National Board of Examinations of India, America or Britain.
diplopia If a person perceives two images of a single object called double vision.
diplotene One of the stages of Meiotic prophase like Pachytene, leptotene, zygotene. In this phase, two chromosomes in each bivalent begin to repel one another and a split occurs between the chromosomes, which are held by chiasmata during crossing over.
dipping Examination of liver by a quick depressing movement of the fingers with the hand flat across the abdomen.
dipstick Strip of cellulose chemically impregnated to render it sensitive to protein, glucose, or other substances in the urine used for routine screening tests.
Diptera Two winged insects like mosquito, flies
director Any person who directs or guides others.
disability Incapacity with respect to physical, mental or physiological functions. For the purpose of Labour organization action it is defined as "inability to engage in any substantial gainful activity by reason of any medically determinable physical or mental impairment which can be expected to last or has lasted for a continuous period of not less than 12 months."
disaccharidase Enzyme that hydrolyzes disaccharides.
disaccharide Sugars composed of two glycosidically linked monosaccharides such as sucrose, lactose, and maltose.
discharge Setting free of a matter or a force or a secretion.
discoid A structure which is disk like in shape such as optic disc, intervertebral disc etc.,
discrete Separate or different parts as in discrete analysis.
discrimination To make a fine distinction.
disease From French word meaning ease from pathos. Deviation from physiological range to produce pathology. This is manifested by symptoms and signs.
disengagement Foetal head which was engaged in pelvic brim is liberated from pelvic brim or vaginal canal.
disinfect To render a material free from pathogen by eliminating microorganisms.
disinfectant Agent which is used for disinfection. The act of disinfecting is called disinfection.
disinfestation Killing wormin which are present on a person, an animal, or clothing
disintegration The process of decomposing.
disjunction This refers to the moving apart of bivalent chromosomes at first anaphase of meiosis or the moving apart of daughter chromosomes at the second anaphase of meiosis or anaphase of mitosis.
dislocation Bony displacement .
dismemberment Refers to amputation of a limb
disorder Morbidity as it is called which is the derangement or abnormality of function
disorganization Too much of a change in anatomical or functional aspect of tissues.
disorientation It is the state of mental confusion as to time, place, or identity.
dispensary Place where treatment for illness given or the place where medical or dental remedy are provided.
dispersion scattering of elements or substances. This can be colloid dispersion for unstable colloid system, temporal dispersion for desynchronisation of components in an action potential.
displacement This can be replacement of an atom in a chemical reaction, This can mean the malposition of a crown in dentistry, This can also mean a defence mechanism in case of emotions. In orthopaedics it can mean abnormal position of a bone or articular surfaces.
disposition Physical or mental ill-being.
disproportion There is no proper relationship between two elements or factors.
dissect Cadaver dissection for the anatomical study. To cut and separate tissues or a part in surgical treatment.
dissection The act of dissecting.
dissolution One substance is dissolved in another.
distal Anatomical depiction to show a structure is in distant position.

distillation Chemical means of separating volatile substance from another less volatile substance.

distortion Disguising unconscious ideas . Deviation of an image in radio imaging, That which is twisted and not normal in position.

distraction Attention is diverted from main point. Joint surfaces are separated with ligaments intact. Surgical separation of two bones in surgery.

distribution Arrangement of continuing or successive events in space or time.

disulfiram Drug used in chronic alcoholism. Disulfiram is an antioxidant that inhibits the oxidation of the acetaldehyde metabolized from alcohol, resulting in high concentrations of acetaldehyde in the body that gives rise to uncomfortable symptoms

diurnal That which occurs during the day.

DM abbreviation for **D**iabetes **M**ellites.

DMRD Abbreviation for **D**iploma in **M**edical **R**adio-**D**iagnosis

DMRT Abbreviation for **D**iploma in **M**edical **R**adio-**T**herapy

recombinant DNA, DNA molecule composed of linked sequences

DNB Abbreviation for **D**iplomat of the **N**ational **B**oard

doctor Person who receives highest degree PhD from University. Person qualified in Medicine and who treats illness.

domiciliary Related to house such as domiciliary treatment.

dominant Capable of expression when carried by only one of a pair of homologous chromosomes.

donor Person who gives blood to others, a person who gives tissues to other. Person who donates organs to others.

Donovan bodies *Calymmatobacterium granulomatis.*

Donovania granulomatis This refers to *Calymmatobacterium granulomatis.*

Dopamine It is a neurotransmitter in CNS. Chemically it is 3,4-dihydroxyphenylethylamine that occurs by decarboxylation of DOPA. Dopamine is an intermediate product in the synthesis of norepinephrine.

Doppler Refers to Doppler USG.

dormant That which is not dominant and is inactive in nature.

dorsal Latin word meaning back. This denotes the position in anatomical sense.

dorsolumbar That which is related to back and the loin.

dosage To regulate the size, frequency, and number of doses for a medicamentation.

dose Drug to be administered as a single dose.

Dossier Cumulative records of a patient's case history.

double blind Clinical trial in which neither the subject nor the person administering treatment knows which treatment the subject is receiving.

douche Water wash of a cavity.

Douglas bag A bag like receptacle worn over the mouth to collect exhaled air.

Down syndrome This is clinical manifestation associated with chromosomal aberration which Trisomy is trisomy 21. . This is associated with late marriage and late child birth.

doxycycline Methacycline derivative a broad-spectrum antibacterial of the tetracycline group

DPH Abbreviation for **D**iploma in **P**ublic **H**ealth.

DPM Abbreviation for **D**iploma in **P**sychological **M**edicine

DPT Abbreviation for Triple antigen used in Immunisation. **D**iphtheria-**P**ertussis-**T**etanus

Dracunculus Nematode parasites of the family Dracunculidae.

dragée A medicated confection.

dream During sleep images, emotions, and thoughts are experienced

dressing Material used which is sterilized for protecting a wound. Also called bandage.

drift Relatively minor changes in antigenic structure of a virus called antigenic drift.

drip Drop by drop infusion of a liquid.

droplet Moisture expelled from the mouth in coughing, sneezing, or speaking, which y carry infection to others through the air.

drowning Suffocation and death resulting from filling of the lungs with water

DrPH Abbreviation for **D**octor of **P**ublic **H**ealth.

drug Medicaments given in the treatment of illness. Drug administration can be oral or aboral.

DT Abbreviation for double antigen. **D**iphtheria and **T**etanus

Dubin-Johnson syndrome A familial chronic form of Non haemolytic jaundice due to defect in the secretion of conjugated bilirubin.

Duchenne's disease This refers to Pseudo muscular Dystrophy described by Duchenne.

duct Duct is a passage with well-defined walls

dull On percussion the note is not resonant

dullness Diminished resonance on percussion

Dumdum fever Visceral leishmaniasis first seen in Dum Dum in Kolkata in India hence the name.

duodenum Pylorus to jejunum proximal portion of small intestine.

dupp Syllable that represent the second sound of the heart in auscultation

Dupuytren's contracture refers to contracture of Palmar Aponeurosis. Described by Dupuytren.

dura mater Outermost, tough and most fibrous of the three membranes covering the brain and spinal cord

Durham rule A definition of criminal responsibility which says "an accused is not criminally responsible if his unlawful act was the product of mental disease or mental defect". This 1954 Rule was reversed in 1972.

Durham's tube Small inverted test tube used in determining bacterial gas production.
dwarf Short person which will be invariably by dysfunction of endocrine glands such as pituitary gland or thyroid gland.
azo dye are organic compounds bearing the functional group RHN=NHR2, in which R and R2 are usually aryl.
vital dye Dye that penetrates living cells and colors its structures without injury to the cells.
dynamic Related to manifesting force.
dynamics Mechanics which deals with the motions of material bodies
dyne Unit of force which when acting continuously upon a mass of 1 gm. will impart to it an acceleration of 1 $cm \cdot s^{-2}$.
dysarthria No good articulation due to loss of muscular control which is neurological in origin.
dysbasia Difficulty in walking caused by nerve lesion.
blood dyscrasia Disease and disorder s of the cellular elements of the blood.
dysdiadochokinesia Impaired ability to perform the rapid alternating movements of diadochokinesia.
dysentery Frequent stools containing blood and mucus caused by bacteria and protozoa. They are referred to as Bacillary dysentery and Amoebic dysentery.
dysgerminoma Most common malignant ovarian germ cell tumor
dysgnathia Abnormality of the oral cavity and teeth that also involves the jaws.
dyslipidosis Disturbance of fat metabolism
dysmenorrhea Painful *menstruation.*
dyspareunia Painful coitus.
dyspepsia Impairment of the power or function of digestion
dysphagia Difficulty in swallowing
dysplasia Abnormality of development
dyssebacia Greasy scaling lesions involving the alae nasi, malar areas, canthi of the eyes, and earlobes and sometimes the scrotum or vulva.

E

e This is the symbol for electron
EAHF This a clinical complex described which contains **E**czema, **A**sthma and **H**ay **F**ever
Eales' disease Recurrent bleeding tendency in retina and vitreous which is predominant among males and common age group being 30 to 40 years of life.
ear Sensory organ of hearing and also the organ of equilibrium which consists of the external ear, the middle ear, and the internal ear
eardrum Part of hearing organ called Tympanic membrane through which sound magnifies and enters.
earwax Waxy secretion called cerumen is normal process of secretion for protection. Otherwise, it can be a source for hard of hearing and infection if not properly attended.
eating Act of ingestion.
Ebner's gland They are gustatory glands situated in the posterior part of the tongue.
Ebola virus This is the causative agent under Filovirus with four sub types.
ebonation When bone fragments are removed from wound.
ébranlement Surgical removal of a polyp by twisting the pedicle
Ebstein's angle Cardiohepatic angle described by Ebstein.
ebullition When any liquid reaches the boiling point we notice vibratory movement of liquid which is called ebullition.
eccentric Meaning away from the centre of a circle.
ecchymosis Bleeding spots on the skin which or round, purplish and not elevated.
ECG Abbreviation for **E**lectro **C**ardio **G**ram, an investigation for noting the function of heart.
echinococcosis Refers to Hydatid disease.
Echinococcus They are small tapeworms under Taeniidae family studied in Helminthology.
echo A Returned sound, Reflection of ultrasonic waves, Radio waves and radar waves.
echocardiography By directing the ultrasonic waves through chest wall we get the graphical representation of position and movement of heart
echogenic That which produces reflections referred in ultrasonography
echopraxia Clinical manifestation of Schizophrenia wherein stereotyped imitation of the movements of another person is seen.
echovirus Viruses that produce Fever, Rashes and Aseptic meningitis in man. They are about 29 serotypes
Eck's fistula This is created while treating oesophageal varices by an artificial communication between portal vein and inferior vena cava.
Ecker's fissure Transverse fissure of the occipitalis.
eclampsia Fits during pregnancy due to toxaemia of pregnancy along with other signs of pre eclampsia. (Fits, High blood pressure, Protein in urine and pedal oedema).
ecologist An expert in ecology.
ecology The scientific study of the surroundings of an organism as affected by environment.
econazole nitrate A broad-spectrum antifungal agent against skin candida infection and tinea infections.
écorché Inner parts particularly muscles of the body are exposed for it's understanding or for the study.
ecosystem This is the major system in the universe where interaction between living and non living is occurring.

écouvillon French word which denotes a swab for swabbing wounds or lesions.

écouvillonage French nomenclature which means scrubbing a cavity or a lesion.

ECT Abbreviation for **E**lectro **C**onvulsive **T**herapy

ectasia Refers to distension such as arterial ectasia, papillary ectasia or corneal ectasia.

ecthyma Bacterial infection on shin or dorsal feet which go to form an ulcer. Common causative organism of this type of pyoderma is Streptococci.

ecto A prefix meaning situated on the outside.

ectoderm This is the outermost layer of cells of the three primary germ layers of the embryo which is the germinal area for the development of nail, hair, teeth, skin, nervous system ear, eye, mucous membrane of mouth and mucous membrane of anus.

ectodermal That which is related to ectoderm.

ectomy This meaning the surgical excision

ectopagus Birth defect where conjoined twins are connected along the side of the body

ectoparasite Parasite that lives on the outside of the body of the host.

ectopia Congenital malformation or malposition.

ectopic That which is located away from is normal position such as ectopic pregnancy.

ectostosis This is bony ossification below the perichondrium of a cartilage or the periosteum of a bone.

ectrodactyly Birth defect with absence of fingers or toes which is normally seen in a syndrome

ectropion Eversion of the eyelid

ectrosis Medical management to halt a disease process in man.

eczema Caused by endogenous or exogenous agent, eczema is a type of dermatitis where papule or vesicle are manifested with itching sensation. On examination usually we observe erythema, oedema serous exudates crusting or scaling.

eczematous Affected with eczema.

ED Abbreviation for **E**ffective **D**ose

ED_{50} This denotes the median value for the effectiveness of a testing substance. It is also called Medial Effective Dose, which produces the desired effect in 50 % population.

Eddowes' syndrome This refers to Osteogenesis Imperfecta Type I described by Eddowes.

Edebohls' position This is also called Simon's position. It is the dorsal position with knees and thighs drawn up, lower limbs flexed on thighs, thighs flexed on to abdomen, hips are raised and thighs abducted.

Edelman American biochemist winner of the Nobel prize for medicine 1972 for his work on antibody molecule.

edema Fluid in intercellular space and subcutaneous tissues. Types are local and generalized oedema.

edematous Related to oedema

edentulism Person not having teeth may be complete or partial.

edge This refers to border such as cutting edge or denture edge.

Edinger's nuclei The Accessory Nuclei of Oculomotor nerve described by Edinger. It is also known as Edinger-Westphal Nuclei.

Edsall's disease This refers to Heat Cramps described by Edsall.

EDTA Abbreviation for **E**thylene **D**iamine **T**etra **A**cetic **A**cid a chelating agent.

Edwards' syndrome This refers to Trisomy 18 Syndrome described by Edwards.

EEE Abbreviation for **E**astern **E**quine **E**ncephalomyelitis.

EEG Abbreviation for **E**lectro **E**ncephalo **G**ram

EFA Abbreviation for **E**ssential **F**atty **A**cids.

effacement At labour thinning of external os and obliteration of cervix take place for an effective labour which is a natural phenomenon.

efferent Referable to efferent nerve fibers which convey nerve conduction away from its root.

effervescent That which give rise to gas bubbles.

efficacy It denotes to the ability of a drug to produce the desired effect in man.

effuse That which spreads out

effusion Fluid escaping from tissue which can be an exudation or a transudation such as Pleural effusion or pericardial effusion.

egestion Undigested material is thrown out the casting out of material which is indigestible.

egg Egg before fertilization is called ovum and after fertilization is called Zygote. Always-referable to female reproductive cell.

ego A dominated personality. In Latin term it mean 'I' that is 'self' in first person.

egocentric One who looks after one's own interest or a person who is self-centered

Ehlers-Danlos syndrome This is one of the inherited disorders of connective tissue with major clinical manifestations of Hyperextensible skin Hyperextensible joints .

Ehrenritter's ganglion Ganglion of superior Glossopharyngeal nerve described by Ehrenritter.

Ehrlich's reaction This reaction is a diagnostic reaction in liver disease which is called Diazo reaction.

EIA Abbreviation for **E**nzyme **I**mmuno **A**ssay

Eicken's method In clinical examination, Cricoid cartilage is drawn forward and Hypopharynx is examined.

Eijkman He discovered Thiamine for which he was awarded the Noble Prize in the year 1929.

Einhorn string test 1953 Test devised to find out the site of bleeding in upper Gastro Intestinal Tract particularly in oesophagus, stomach and duodenum.

Einthoven Physiologist who discovered Galvanometer which produce E.C.G. He received Nobel Prize in 1924.

Eisenmenger's complex Interventricular septal defect producing following complex:
- Pulmonary Hypertension
- Hypertrophy of Right Ventricle
- Cyanosis

ejaculate To eject Semen in a single shot at the climax of intercourse. Common types in clinical practice are a) Premature ejaculation b) Defective ejaculation

ejaculation Sudden act of expulsion of semen.

ejecta Refers to stool.

ejection Discharge of blood, Discharge of body secretion, Discharge of body secretion.

EKG Abbreviation for **E**lecltro **K**ardio **G**ram

Ekman's syndrome Type I Osteogenenis Imperfecta described by Ekman. This is also referred to as Ekman Lobstein Syndrome.

elaboration Detail establishment, Expansion of dreams.

Elant's triangle Base is Sacral Promontory, One side is by Left Common Iliac Artery and the other side is by Right Common Iliac Artery.

elastic Force applied for compression and stretching such as elastic tissue.

elasticity Quality of being elastic.

elastosis Changes that have occurred in skin tissue.

elation Tendency to be optimistic and with extreme joy.

elbow This anatomical area is called Cubitus which is the joint formed by the distal end of arm bone and proximal ends of forearm bones.

elective Choice taken to undertake surgery at appropriate time with all arrangement as opposed to emergency surgery.

electrocardiogram Graphical representation of deflections of heart contraction and relaxation, a common laboratory investigation called E.C.G. A diagnostic test for the diagnosis of heart diseases.

electrocautery Heated metal wire is used to produce coagulation of tissue which is called cauterization of tissues.

electroconvulsive Electric shock is given to produce induce convulsion as a part of psychological treatment.

electrocution Electric shock and burns that produce death of a person.

electrode It is the medium of electrical conduction where a needle or a metal plate is used. They are called Lead in E.C.G.

electroejaculation Electrical probe is used to induce ejaculation by inserting probe into rectum to collect semen from patients of spinal cord injury.

electroencephalogram (EEG) This is the graphical representation of brain waves for diagnostic purposes of neurological conditions.

electrolysis In a solution chemical disintegration is done. In beautification hair is removed from unwanted place

electrolyte This referred to an Ionic solute that is a substance that dissociates into ions when fused and produce electricity

electromyography (EMG) By using electrodes, skeletal muscles' action potential and evoked potential are found out as a diagnostic test. This test is done as a comparison during rest period, during contraction period and during electrical stimulation.

electron They are negatively charged elementary particle of atom which can be in its free state or in combined state. Combined state are; a) Radioactive substance b) Beta rays c) in a conductor as electrical current

electronic Related to electron.

electronics Scientific study of electric conduction in media like liquid, gas, solid or vacuum.

electron-microscopic organism or material which are made visible under the electron microscope.

electrophoresis By creating an electric field ionic solutes are separated which is based on their rate of migration.

electrophotometer Instrument used for the determination of calorie wherein the measurement is made possible through the equipped photoelectric sensor

electroplating By using electroplated die in a process coating of an object is done. .

electroshock E C T through which shock produced by application of electric current to the brain for therapy.

electrovalence This suggests the transfer of electrons to make an ionic bonding in case of chemicals. This also indicate the number of charges an atom acquires (either loss of electrons or gain of electrons)

element Generally it is primary constituent of a substance or material. Specifically it is a foremost unit which cannot be further broken by any means. In chemical notation each element has symbol and its own atomic weight.

elephantiasis Filarial infection caused by Wuchereria bancrofti and Brugia malayi that cause obstruction of lymphatics and hypertrophy of skin and sub cutaneous tissue giving rise to big elephant leg.

elimination This refers to the physiological processes like defecation and urination

ELISA **E**nzyme **L**inked **I**mmuno **S**orbent **A**ssay; This is a laboratory technique in which a material to be tested binds with immunosorbent and labeled antibody that can measure the material tested concentration is determined. Presently ELISA is the common screening test for HIV/AIDS.

elixir Clear sweet Hydroalcoholic liquid with a flavouring agent used for the prescription of drugs or medicaments.

Elliot's operation Surgical relief for Glaucoma by sclerocorneal trephining.

Elliot's position This position is allows the surgical operative procedures for gall bladder surgery. Here ldower chest is elevated with a support under lower costal margin.

Elliot's sign Edge of the Syphilitic skin lesion has an indurated edge. Another Elliot's sign is that scotoma extending from blind spot has many spots at observation.

Ellis-van Creveld syndrome This is Chondro Ectodermal Dysplasia described by Ellis and Van Creveldee

Eloesser flap For open drainage of chronic empyema, a flap is created over the ribs as described by Eloesser .

Elsberg's test In case of tumous of brain, intra cerebral or extra cerebral is assessed by the rate of fatigue and variations in function.

Elschnig's bodies Proliferation of epithelial cells seen in cataractous lens after its removal that are found to be gralpelike clusters or pearls.

El Tor vibrio This is a biotype of Vibrio cholerae that was identified in *El Tor*, in Egypt in the year 1960

Ely's test This test is positive in contracture of the lateral fascia of the thigh. In prone position, flexion of leg on thigh causes buttocks to arch away.

emaciation Body wasting or leanness due to malnutrition.

embalming Embalming is done to dead body with antiseptics and preservatives which helps to prevent putrefaction.

embedding Tissue fixation in a firm medium in histology or histopathology section.

Embelia Fruit of a plant which has anthelminthic property.

embolism Blood clot or air block of an artery which produce sudden blocking of an artery .

embolus Blood clot, air, a mass or any other material runs in blood stream can get lodged and produce obstruction. Such a material goes to form an embolus. The process of formation of embolus and subsequent changes is called embolism.

embrocation Liquid medicine for external application.

embryo This refers to a foetus which is aged 4 days to 64 days . The terminology is also used among animals and plants in different version.

embryoblast In human embryology this refers to Inner Cell Mass.

embryogenesis Development of an embryo through the stages of early development.

embryology Scientific study of human development from early stage to subsequent stages of development.

embryoma Cancerous growth from embryonic tissue such as teratoma, dermoid cyst, nephroblastoma.

emergence Coming back to earlier status for example patient coming back to normal after general anaesthesia.

emergency This means Medical emergency and cases are attended in Emergency Medicine in Casualty. National level alert for outbreak of acute communicable and infectious diseases

Emery-Dreifuss muscular dystrophy It is Scapulo Peroneal muscular dystrophy described by Emery and Dreifuss which is X linked disorder of Muscular dystrophy involving weakness of upper arm and pelvic girdle muscles.

emesis Process of vomiting.

emetic Substance which cause the process of vomiting.

emetine This is an alkaloid obtained from ipecac

EMF Abbreviation for **E**lectro **M**otive **F**orce

EMG Abbreviation for **E**lectro **M**yo **G**ram.

eminence It is the bone surface prominence. E.g., Thenar eminence, Collateral eminence of lateral ventricle, Frontal eminence, Occipital eminence, Thyroid eminence, Ulnar eminence etc.,

emission Semen discharge which can be involuntary or voluntary in nature.

emmenia This means Menstruation.

Emmet's operation This surgery is lacerated perineal repair devised by Emmet.

emmetrope Normal vision or no refractory error.

emollient External application which softens the skin

emotion An instinct drive that leads to a state of tense that are seen in situations as excitement, sadness, hate, fear etc.,

empathy Understanding other's feelings as opposed to sympathy which suggest sharing of other's feeling.

Empedocles According to this Greek Philosopher the disease is due to imbalance of four roots Earth, Air, Fire and Water.

emphysema Large quantity of air collected in lungs or any organs. Common ones are pulmonary emphysema and cutaneous emphysema.

emphysematous of the nature of or affected with emphysema.

empirical Treatment based on experience and not by training.

emporiatrics The Branch of Medicine which deals with Health problems of Travelers.

empyema Presence of pus which can be an abscess, a pleural effusion or prothorax.

EMS Abbreviation for **E**mergency **M**edical **S**ervice.

emulsion This is the chemical phenomenon of one liquid distributed in another liquid. Two main known emulsion are: a) Water in Oil emulsion b) Oil in Water emulsion.

enamel Smooth glossy coated enamel, The Baked porcelain.

enantiomerism When chemicals which have molecules that are mirror images of each other , they are called stereoisomers. When they show identical chemical and physical properties they are called Enantiomers. The chemical process is called enantiomerism.

en bloc Any structure as a whole when described.
encapsulated That which is enclosed within a capsule.
encephalitis Infection and inflammation of the brain.
encephalo That which is related to the brain.
encephalocele Hernia of brain tissue through skull defect.
encephalography Radiological diagnosis of CSF running spaces for lesion, space occupying lesions or leakage after trauma.
encephalomeningitis Infection and inflammation of brain and brain coverings.
encephalomyelitis Infection and inflammation involving brain and the spinal cord.
encephalomyelopathy Diseases of brain and spinal cord.
encephalomyopathy Diseases involving brain and muscles.
encephalon The Forebrain, Mid brain and Hind brain which are called Prosencephalon, Mesencephalon and Rhombencephalon.
encephalopathy Degenerative diseases of brain.
enchondroma Benign tumous of cartilage tissue.
endemic Disease is always present in a population residing in a geographical area.
Enders John Franklin Enders an American microbiologist who discovered Polio virus culture and showed the world the possibility of polio vaccine.
endoarteritis Meaning Endarteritis.
endocarditis Infection and inflammation of endocardium involving valves.
endocardium Innermost lining of the heart which are made of collagen fibers and elastic fibers.
endocrine Glands which produce and release the hormones into blood stream.
endocrinologist An endocrinology specialist or consultant.
endocrinology Scientific study of hormones, the endocrine system, their physiological functions that help in diagnosis and treatment of endocrine dysfunctions.
endoderm In embryo the innermost primary germ layer from which following structure develop a) Pharyngeal epithelia, Respiratory tract except nose, G I tract, Urinary bladder and uretha.
endodontics The branch of Dentistry which deals with the diagnosis and treatment of Dental pulp, Root of tooth and Periapical tissue.
endogamy consanguineous marriage leading to inbreeding.
endogenous Cause of illness found within the organisms.
endolymph This is the fluid in Membranous labyrinth of the ear.
endometriosis Presence of Endometrial tissues in other places of the body. This is an aberration that produce clinical conditions.
endometritis Infection and inflammation of the endometrium.
Endomycetales They are Saccharomycetaceae of the order of yeasts.
endomyocarditis Infection and inflammation of the endocardium and myocardium.
endophlebitis Infect ion and inflammation of the intima of a vein
endophthalmitis Infection and inflammation of ocular cavities and their adjacent structures
endoplasm Main or central portion of the cytoplasm of a cell.
end-organ Terminal nerve endings which are endings of sensory nerves.
endorphin It is a neuropeptide which combines with opioid receptors in brain to produce total pain relief. It is responsible for potent analgesic activity.
endoscope To examine hollow viscus endoscope is used. Usually it is flexible type used in endoscopic examination or in endoscopic surgery.
endoscopy Visual inspection of a cavity by an endoscope.
endosome Intra nuclear organelle of a cell that persists during mitosis.
endosperm Food reserve in embryo sac of plants.
endospore Protective thick wall in certain bacteria to withstand adverse environmental conditions.
endosteum It is the tissue lining of medullary cavity of a bone.
endothelioma They are hemangioendothelioma, a benign tumour of blood vessels.
endothelium This is from mesoderm in its development and is present in heart, blood vessels , and serous cavities.
endotoxin They are bacterial toxin from Brucellae, Enterobacteria, Neisseriae and Vibrio Cholerae. Endotoxin is released when the organism is disrupted. Endotoxin is of complex lipopolysaccharide.
endotracheal Refers to endotracheal tube which is passed through the lumen of trachea.
endovascular This refers to Intra Vascular.
end plate This means a flat termination such as Motor End Plate.
end-pleasure The Climax in Sexual intercourse.
end point In Qualitative Analysis by titration, the highest dilution of a substance that produces a reaction with a given volume of another substance is called end point.
end product Fully completed sequence of metabolic reaction which gives rise to a chemical compound.
endrin An insecticide which belong to chlorinated hydrocarbon group.
enema Liquid preparation pushed into the rectum to treat constipation, to prepare for surgery of rectum.
energy Work, movement, motion and resistance require energy which is called capacity

enervation Nerve is cut due to natural means, surgical means and by trauma and is called Neurectomy.

engagement When foetal head particularly biparietal head is below the plane of the pelvic inlet and constitute a presenting part in delivery.

Engel-Recklinghausen disease Recklinghausen disease of the bone called Osteitis Fibrosa Cystica described by Engel and Recklinghausen

Engelmann's disease Diaphyseal Dysplasia described by Engelmann.

engorged Organ distended with fluids.

engorgement Because of more blood supply and local congestion an organ in question is distended by fluid accumulation

enlargement This refers to hypertrophy or hyperplasia of tissue or an organ. E.g., cardiac enlargement, Cervical enlargement, Atrial enlargement etc.,

enophthalmos Backward displacement of the eyeball

enrichment This may mean Food enrichment or culture media enrichment as the case may be, in Nutritional science and in Microbiology.

Enroth's sign Changes due to Grave's disease with the manifestation of abnormal fullness of eyelids.

ENT Abbreviation for **E**ars, **N**ose and **T**hroat The discipline is also called Otorhinolaryngology.

Entamoeba A protozoal parasite which causes Intestinal amoebiasis and amoebic hepatitis in man which comes under order amoebida.

enterectomy Surgical excision of a part of the intestine

enteric That which is related to small intestine.

enteric-coated Special coating to tablets and capsules which can allow it's dissolution in intestine and not in stomach.

enteritis Infection and inflammation of the intestine

Enterobacter They produce Nosocomial infections and belong to Enterobacteriaceae which are Gram negative and motile organisms.

enterobiasis Thread worm infection by nematode which belong to Enterobius genus.

Enterococcus They are common intestinal flora in humans.

enterocolitis Infection and inflammation involving both the small intestine and the colon

enterocolostomy Anastomosis done between the small intestine and the colon

enterogastrone Hormone that inhibits gastric secretion and gastric motility.

enteroglucagon Gllicentin and Oxyntomodulin are called enteroglucagon which are Gut glucagons

enterology Scientific study of diseases of intestine.

enterorrhaphy Repair of the intestine.

enterostomy Surgical opening is provided to intestine on the abdominal wall for therapy.

enterotoxin Intestinal pathogenic bacteria like clostridium, Escherichia, vibrio produce toxin which affect the cells of intestinal mucosa manifesting in G.I. symptoms like vomiting and diarrhea.

Enterovirus They are human enteroviruses that are numbered with numbers or figures such as human entero virus 68. Polio virus, Coxsackievirus and echovirus are common enteroviruses. Big family under this genus is Picornavirus group.

entoderm Inner layer of embryonic tissues which are called primitive entoderm or Primordial entoderm.

entomologist An expert or a larned man in Medical entomology which deals with the vectors of disease transmission in man.

entomology Scientific study of insect population which deals with the morphology, life cycle, diseases transmitted and their prevention. It denotes Medical Entamology.

entoplasm This is other name for Endoplasm.

entrainment This is the technique for the control of cardiac arrhythmia with the help of an external stimulus.

entropion Eyelid margin is turned inwards.

enucleate In case of tumour of the eye, surgical removal of total eye and cleaning it.

enucleation Surgical procedure for the tumour of the eye. Eye muscles and optic nerve are cut; whole eye is removed like a nut from its shell and cleaned.

enuresis Commonly called Bed Wetting or Urinary Incontinence.

environment It is the sum of our surroundings may be physical, chemical, biological, social, economical, spiritual which influence the health of an individual in the society.

enzootic Diseases of animals found always present in their groups.

enzymatic That which is related to enzyme.

enzyme Enzymes are protein molecules, they catalyze chemical reactions of other substances but they do not get altered in that reaction.

Enzyme Commission (EC) It was established in 1956 to standardize enzyme classification and nomenclature.

eosin Bromine derivatives of Fluorescin which is used to stain plasma along with haematoxylin and methylene blue. Chemically it is the salt of tetrabromofluorescein $C_{20}H_6Br_4Na_2O_5$.

eosinophil They are granular leukocytes containing coarse round granules in the cells.

EP Abbreviation for **E**voked **P**otential.

ephedrine It is an adrenergic obtained drug which has multiple pharmacological use in clinical practice.

epicanthus This is vertical fold of skin on either side of the nose that is characteristic to given race in mankind.

epicondyle Bony prominence above the condyle.

epidemic Occurrence of a disease which occur more than our expectations. In other words it an outbreak of disease.

epidemiologist An Epidemiology Specialist.

epidemiology The study of determinants and distribution of disease process or of health related events in a community or in a society (defined population)

epidermis Outer layer of the skin which is not vascularised and usually measures to 0.1 mm. In case of palm and sole it will be about 1.4 mm.

epidermoid The structure that looks like epidermis.

Epidermophyton Moniliaceae family fungi which infect skin and nails

epididymal That which related to epididymis.

epididymis Elongated cordlike structure with duct which provides the storage, transit spermatozoa.

epididymitis Infection and inflammation of the epididymis.

epididymo-orchitis Infection and inflammation of the epididymis and testis.

epidural That which is situated outside the dura mater.

epigastrium Upper middle region of the abdomen

epiglottis Lid made up of cartilage that help to close the entrance of larynx during swallowing.

epiglottitis Infection and inflammation of the epiglottis which is often life threatening in children.

epignathus Hard palate tumour in foetus in Rathke's pouch (Hypophyseal pouch) and produce mouthful protrusion. Organised epignathus is called a parasitic foetus.

epilation Removal of hair called depilation.

epilepsy Group of syndromes with paroxysmal transient disturbances of brain function where there is loss of consciousness. It may be major or minor in nature. One episode is seizure.

epileptic Person afflicted with epilepsy

epimastigote Crithidial stage of trypanosome protozoa.

epimenorrhagia Menses which is frequent and excessive.

epimenorrhea Frequently occurring menses which is abnormal.

epimorphosis Cut end of an organism gets regenerated as in the case of tail of lizard.

epinephrine Hormone of adrenal medulla which stimulates the adrenergic receptors of sympathetic nervous system. It is a cardiac stimulant.

epiphora Overflow of tears due to block of lacrimal apparatus.

epiphysis End of long bone which is articular that develops from secondary ossification center.

epiploon It is the Omentum.

episclera The connective tissue of external surface of sclera.

episio Related with vulva.

episiotomy Incision into the perineum and vagina to prevent traumatic tearing during delivery.

episode Refers to episode of illness which denote that it is occurring as a continuous events.

epispadias Urethral opening will be situated on the dorsum of penis in the form of a groove without a covering.

epistasis Control of bleeding in case of nasal bleeding or in case of menses

epistaxis This refers to nasal bleeding.

episternal That which is situated over the sternum.

epithelioma This can be adenoma, papilloma or carcinoma.

epithelium Covering of external surface of the body as well as of internal surface of the body.

epitrochlear Above the trochlea of the hummers.

epizootic Outbreak of diseases of animals among animals which is more than expectations

eponychium the thickened layer of epidermal tissue over the developing fetal fingernail or toenail that disappears before birth except over the base of the nail.

epoöphoron An ovarian vestigial structure corresponding to mesonephric duct.

epoxide Reactive group of an organic compound which is produced by the combination of an atom of oxygen and two atom of carbon.

epsilon A Greek alphabet.

EPSP Abbreviation for **E**xcitatory **P**ost **S**ynaptic **P**otential.

Epstein's disease It is pseudodiphtheria which looks like pearl described by Epstein.

Epstein's nephrosis Nephrotic syndrome described by Epstein.

Epstein-Barr virus It is called Human Simplex virus which causes Infectious mononucleosis and is often found associated with Burkitt's tumour and nasopharyngeal carcinoma..

epulis It is tumour like mass in the gum.

equation This is a chemical expression that make two chemicals connected with the sign of equality. Common usage is Chemical equation

equatorial That which occurs at the same distance from each end of an axis.

equilateral Sides that are equal and identical.

equilibration It is the balance between opposing elements or opposing forces.

equilibrium Producing or creating a situation where opposing forces counteract each other. This also denotes body balance or acid base equilibrium.

equine Anything obtained from a horse such as horse serum.

equivalence In chemical reaction that which has equal Valence. In immunology antigen and antibody are found equal strength

equivalent That which show or has same value as other such as equivalent weight.

Erasistratus Greek physician who described human body function as a mechanical and is by external force. His writings are seen in differentiating cerebrum and cerebellum, sensory nerve and motor nerve. According to him the illness was by indigested food, Hyperaemia and Plethora. His writings suggest diet, exercise steam bath and no violent remedies.

Erb-Goldflam disease This refers to Myasthenia Gravis described by Erb and Goldflam.

Erben's reflex When head or trunk is bent forwards with force, pulse slows down. This is positive in vagal excitability

ERBF Abbreviation for **E**ffective **R**enal **B**lood **F**low

erectile That which is capable of erection usually refers to male sex organ

erection Becoming rigid and elevated as in the case of erectile tissue when filled with blood. Usually refers to erection of penis.

ERG Abbreviation for **E**lectro **R**etino **G**ram.

ergasia This term is given by Adolf Meyer for the total activity of a person that include both behavior and mental activity.

ergocalciferol The sterol present in fish oils and synthesized by irradiation of ergosterol It has the therapeutic use in Rickets, Hypoparathyroidism, Hypocalcaemia.

ergonomics Science that fits man to work and fits work to man in occupational health. In industrial health it suggests maximum use of human energy for maximum production.

ergosterol This is a sterol which forms to vitamin D_2 upon irradiation by ultraviolet light

ergot Is a Rye plant Claviceps purpurea an alkaloid that yield ergotamine. This is the combination of lysergic acid, ammonia, praline, phenylalanine and pyruvic acid. Ergotamine is used in the treatment of Migrane.

ergotism This refers to Ergot poisoning by the consumption of ergot from ergotised grain. Ergotism is characterized by spasms, cramps and dry gangrene.

ergotoxine It has oxytocic and adrenergic blocking effect which contain a mixture of three toxic ergot alkaloids, **ergocornine, ergocristine, and ergocryptine .** Now it is not used in medical practice because of too much of vartiation in actions.

Erichsen's sign It is positive in Sacroiliac disease and negative in Hip disease. When iliac bones are pressed toward each other pain is felt in case of positive sign of Erichsen.

erode Means wearing away.

erosion Tissue destruction. Skin erosion

erosive That which produces erosion.

erotic That which produce sexual feelings or sexual desire.

erotism Sex instinct in man or woman

erotomania Sex delusion and hypersexuality in man.

erotophobia Fear of sexual activity.

ERPF Abbreviation for **E**ffective **R**enal **P**lasma **F**low

erratic Deviating from an accepted conduct and thought.

errhine Drug which promote nasal secretion.

error This suggest a defect or a deviation in case of a structure, a function or in statistics.

erucic acid It is present in Mustard oil and Rapeseed oil. It is known to cause damage to heart muscles.

eructation Casting of gas of stomach through mouth called belching.

eruption It refers to skin eruption or tooth eruption.

ERV Abbreviation for **E**xpiratory **R**eserve **V**olume

erysipelas It is a form of Cellulitis by Group A streptococci. Colloquially it is called St. Anthony's Fire.

erythema Due to congestion of capillaries skin show the manifestation of redness or flush.

erythematous Clinically characterized by an erythema.

erythroblastic That which is related with erythroblasts.

erythroblastoma Tumor like mass produced by Erythroblasts.

erythroblastosis More nucleated red cells present in the blood. Common clinical entity is Erythroblastosis Foetalis.

erythroclast Ghost cells are called erythroclast.

erythrocyanosis Cold exposure produces swelling and pink colour of legs and thigh among women and girls.

erythrocyte It is the blood element. It is called R B C which is non nucleated, biconcave in shape. The haemoglobin content help in the transport of oxygen supply to vital organs and parts of body.

erythrocythemia This is the other name for Polycythemia.

erythrokinetics Kinetics of erythrocytes by describing the measurements of total red cell volume, rate of red cell production, and red cell life-span

erythroleukemia Blood cancer showing proliferation of erythroblastic and myeloblastic elements of blood. Severe anaemia, liver and spleen enlargement and haemorrhagic tendence are common.

erythrolysis Haemolysis is called erythrolysis.

erythromycin A Macrolide derivative antibiotic effective against Gram positive and Gram negative organisms. Useful in Penicillin resistant cases and in patient who show allergy to penicillin

erythropenia Deficiency in the number of erythrocytes causing Anaemia in patients.

erythrophyll Red coloring matter found in plant kingdom.

erythropoiesis RBC production in spleen and bone marrow in young ones and in bone marrow in adults.

erythropoietin This is responsible for RBC production. It is a glycoprotein hormone secreted chiefly by the kidney in the adult and by the liver in the fetus that acts on the bone marrow cells to stimulate Erythropoiesis.

eschar Slough produced from Burns and Corrosive.

Escherich's bacillus E.coli discovered by Escherich. They are Gram negative, facultative anaerobic and rod shaped. E.coli are indicator of water pollution.

ESIS Abbreviation for Employees State Insurance Scheme for the welfare of industrial workers, comes under occupational health.

Esmarch's tourniquet A rubber bandage used to make a limb avascular during surgery.

Esophageal speech In case of cancer of larynx, removal of larynx produces speech less owing to loss of vocal cord, in such situations person learns to talk with the help of stomach and oesophagus which is in the place of wind-pipe.

Esophagus Anatomical structure stretching from pharynx up to stomach, it is a musculo mem-branous canal which measures about 9 inches.

ESR Abbreviation for Erythrocyte Sedimentation Rate.

Essence Refers to volatile oil in alcohol used for fragrance, also refers to an item which is an indispensable part.

Essential newborn care Under RCH this component is intended to reduce perinatal and neonatal mortality in the community, this includes:
- Resuscitation of newborn with birth asphyxia.
- Prevention of hypothermia.
- Prevention of infection.
- Exclusive breastfeeding.
- Referral of sick newborn.
- Care of low birth weight babies.

Essential obstetric care This refers to basic maternity service to all pregnant women in the country to ensure:
- Registration of pregnancy at 16 week.
- 3 antenatal check ups by ANM (MPW).
- Safe delivery either at home or at health centre.
- 3 postnatal check ups.

Essential Very much required or indispensable, like
- Essential amino acid.
- Essential fatty acid.
- Essential nutrients.
- Essential oils.
- Essential obstetrics.
- Essential paediatrics.
- Essential tool.

Ester Ester is the outcome by the elimination of water when acid and alcohol reacts.

Esterase It is an enzyme which is used in hydrolysis of esters, helpful in breaking ester into acid and alcohol.

EST Abbreviation for Electro Shock Therapy.

Estimates They are observed values of a sample or of a popu-lation, types are:
- Point estimates.
- Range estimates.

Estrogen They are female hormones responsible for female sexual characteristics.

Ethanol Other name for alcohol.

Ether An anaesthetic agent which is highly inflammable, a liquid anaesthetic which evaporates readily and is inhaled during anaesthesia.

Ethical issue Components of medical professional ethics which is in vogue e.g., ethical issues in genetic engineering include the following:
- Patenting of the biological system by big industries.
- Use of Human Genome Project for genetic discrimination.
- Genome based information used for LIC.
- Misuse of technology in general.

Ethics It is the regulation for moral obligation in nursing profession, this code of ethics controls the nurse's behaviour with patients and in management procedure, specific area of ethics for nurses is called *nursing ethics*.

Ethmoid It is a bone of the base of the skull which contains ethmoid sinuses, ethmoid sinus is situated between the eyes.

Ethnic This is a group with a social structure and functions forming a cultural group, a social group with common characteristics.

Ethnology Study of human race, human evolution and human relationships including his origin

Ethos Particular social and cultural characteristics and norms of a group.

Ethyl chloride It is a liquid anaesthetics, this evaporates rapidly, it produces cooling effect, used as local anaes-thetic.

Ethyloestrenol It is an anabolic steroid used in the treatment of weight loss, debility, osteoporosis

Etiology Deals with the causation of illness and it's perpetuating factors, pathogenesis of a disease is studied.

Etiquette professional Rules of behaviour laid down in nursing profession,code of manners in nursing profession,ceremonial observed in profe-ssional duties of a nurse.

Eucalyptus oil Oil from eucalyptus tree which is antiseptic and a mild stimulant used in nasal catarrh.

Eugenics In the prevention of genetic disorders, measures taken to improve physical and mental environment, helpful to get good future generation.

Eunuch Male whose testes are removed, castrated.

Euphoria A good perceivable feeling of well being, usually by a drug.

Eustachian tube Partially collapsible canal which admits air from the throat into the middle ear, this helps to equalise the pressures on the eardrum.

Euthanasia Euthanasia is the Act of deliberately ending the life of a patient which can be active or passive, " it is unethical procedure of taking life of a patient, with or without consent of the patient in irreversible/terminal illness"

Euthyroid Thyroid which is normally functioning, normal thyroid gland.

Evacuation Making discharge from natural orifices, bowel movement, removal of any material from the body organ.

Evaluation Critical appraisal of a clinical condition, assessment of a clinical condition, in nursing practice evaluation of patient is the later procedure.

Evidence based medicine Decision on diagnosis and treatmentor management is done based on descriptive study and appraisal of research findings upto date, it is also called McMaster university approach since it was developed there, McMaster criteria for evidence based medicine are:

- available evidence of patient and population is taken
- patient's problem is taken than patient's protocol
- epidemiology, statistics, pathophysiology and clini cal experience is best taken
- patients outcome is regarded as prime factor.

Evisceration It means removal of entire internal organ from its place, commonly used in case of evisceration of the eye.

Evolution Changes in the characteristics of an organism over a few generation is called evolution, this can refer to physical, mental and cultural aspect of the given organism.

Ewing's tumour It is sarcoma of the long bone.

Exacerbation This refers to the increased severity of clinical signs and symptoms in a patient who is suffering from an illness, acuteness of a clinical condition.

Examination of lower eyelid it is done to find out redness, congestion, watering, foreign body or any ulcer.

Exanthem Skin rashes occurring in case of infectious diseases.

Exanthematous Related to the disease with skin rashes

Excavation Surgical scooping of material from a cavity, refers to dental excavation before dental filling of caries cavity.

Exception If there is a variation in clinical case, unusual than usual in case of illness, sometimes refers to rare entity.

Excision Surgical cutting and removal of part of tissue or part of organ tumour excision.

Excitation Stimulated, overwhel-med, it is an act of stimulating.

Excitement It is a response to a stimulus which is emotional and physiological in nature.

Exclusion Taken out or rejected, surgical separation of an organ from the main organ in human body.

Exclusive breastfeeding Only breastfeeding till 4 months and no other feed at that time constitute *Exclusive Breastfeeding.*

Excrement Metabolic secretions of the body like faeces, urine and sweat.

Excreta Discharge of excretory system like stool, urine and sweat.

Excretion Waste material which is thrown out of the body or expelled from the body.

Exdwelling catheter Other name for male urinary collection catheter, condom catheter, Texas catheter; it is used for clients with renal urinary disorders by applying an external urinary device (with a leg drainage system).

Exercise For correcting deformity or for maintaining health physical exercise or physical exertion is done, types of exercises are:

- Active exercise.
- Passive exercise.
- Isometric exercise.

Exflagellation This is seen in the life cycle of malaria parasite in the body of mosquito where microga-metes are transformed into microgamestocytes.

Exfoliation Thin flaky layer coming out of surface of the tissue, this is referable to dead tissue peeling off

Exhalation The act of expiration or giving out of breath, giving off of a vapour.

Exhibitionism To show off, one who is showing off for attention, under unacceptable circumstances a person exposes genitals in the public.

Exocrine Glands that have ducts to secrete their secretion like salivary gland.

Exogenous The origin is from outside, opposite of endogenous.

Exomphalos It is referred to congenital umbilical hernia, herniation of abdominal viscera into the umbilical cord.

Exophthalmometer Ophthalmic instrument which can measure the protrusion of eyeball.

Exophthalmos Abnormal protrusion of the eyeball seen in cases of thyrotoxicosis and injury.

Exostosis Bony growth from the surface of the bone.

Exotic That which is not native, that which is foreign.

Exotoxin Bacterial poison which is released to tissues around it.

Exotropia Outward turned eyes of a person, strabismus which is divergent.

Expanded role This word is used in nursing profession when the nurse takes the role play in her duties outside the duties and responsibilities of her working institution.

Expected outcome In nursing practice planning is done to have an expected result in case of case management.

Expectorant Drug which produce expulsion of phlegm or sputum in a patient who is having lung inflammation due to infection.

Expectoration Phlegm or sputum coughed out of lung passages.

Experimental design It is part of nursing research, used to fulfil the requirement of procedure and good design in research or experiment.

Characteristics of experimental design are:

- Random allocation of patients.
- No arbitrary correction.
- No bias in result noting down.
- Use of control with similar characteristics.

Common experimental designs are:

- One way approach.
- Two way approach.
- Latin square approach.
- Factorials design.
- Split plot design.
- Use of analysis of co-variance.

Experimentalism It is a philosophy of Nursing Education, it teaches that every thing is changing continually including man, mortality, democracy and education, according to this philosophy the experience is the only reality.

Experiment To demonstrate truth or fact, a procedure is followed in science.

Expiration Moving the inspired air out of the lung by the way of breathing.

Exploration Surgical opening of any tissue, part, organ for coming to final diagnosis, opening of abdomen to find out cause of acute abdomen.

Expression Facial expression during emotion in man, breast milk removal by manual pressure, prominent character seen in future generation in case genetic characters.

Extension traction It is indicated for patients who require presurgical immobilisation of a fractured hip or for patients with fractured femur, pelvic injury sciatica, muscle spasms degenerative arthritis of knee or knee injury which require immobility; extension traction is also known as buck's boot with the help of adhesive straps or a sponge rubber boot.

Extension Name given to the movement which cause straightening, like:

- Extension of the arm.
- Extension of the leg.
- Extension of the back.

Extensor It refers to a muscle which helps in the straightening of limb, muscle which extends the limb.

External respiration Regular breathing of man, this is visible form of expiration and inspiration.

External skeleton Bony framework which is carried by the organism on outside of its body, crayfish has an external skeleton.

External urinary device When prolonged use of indwelling catheter is needed external urinary collection device is used, male urinary collection system also called Texas catheter or condom catheter.

Extracapsular this refers to a type of cataract operation, it also refers to fracture of long bone which is outside the capsule.

Extracellular It refers to extra-cellular fluid, which means outside the cell.

Extramedullary situated outside medulla oblongata.

Extrasensory Thoughts coming out about future happening without any available means of communi-cation, occurring beyond usual ordinary senses, extrasensory perception called ESP.

Extrasystole Contraction not occurring in cardiac cycle but occurring before regular contraction, premature contraction of the atrium or of the ventricle

Extrasystole or premature VPB Ventricular premature beat

Extrauterine Refers to events occurring outside the uterus such as ectopic pregnancy.

Extra It is a prefix meaning additional such as extramural, extracellular, extracalorie, etc.

Extract Any substance when steeped in water or alcohol and then evoporation of fluid is done; it gives a concentrate which is called extract, e.g., belladonna extract, opium extract, etc.

Extraction When a concentrate is taken out from plant by extract, when breech is pulled out in breech extraction, when a thing is removed by applying vacuum called vacuum extraction.

Extrapyramidal When a thing is outside the pyramidal tract, nerves outside the pyramidal tract is called extrapyramidal system.

Extravasations Escape of fluid to its abnormal position, blood leak as in case of bruise or contusion.

Extremity Distal part of feet or the hand.

Extrinsic The origin is from outside, common usages are extrinsic muscle, extrinsic factors in disease causation.

Extroversion When an organ is turned inside out, extroversion of uterus.

Extrovert Is a type of personality where person mixes well in society, socialable and outgoing, opposite of introvert.

Extubation Tube is removed which is inserted for intubation.

Exudate Substance which is thrown out, substance which is deposited.

Exudation Discharge of serous fluid around tissue, discharge around RBC, WBC or any cell, discharge due to cell wall permeability.

Eye bandage It is used to retain a dressing on the eye.

Eye bank Since 1944 we have eye banks which help in availability of qualified hospitals and surgeons a sup-ply of fresh or preserved cornea for the corneal graft operation, they are for sight restoration.

Eye It is the organ of sight, special sense organ of human body or any living organism.

Eyedrops Medicamentation to the eye in case of infection or inflammation put through dropper.

Eyelid lids which cover eye is made up of connective tissue and muscle, lower and upper eyelid which protects the eye, the special sense organ.

Eye tooth This is the name given to upper canine tooth.

F

F° Symbol for degree Fahrenheit.

fabella Sesamoid bone found in Gastrocnemius muscle and is detectable in X-ray as a bony shadow behind knee joint.

Faber's syndrome Hypochromic anemia described by Faber.

Fabricius Italian anatomist and surgeon who lived during the period 1537–1619 was the first person to demonstrate the valves of the veins in human body.

Fabry's disease Lysosomal storage disease in man, which is X linked disease. Ceramide trihexoside accumulates in heart and kidney causing various clinical manifestations like telangiectases, burning in sole and palm, oedema of legs, retarded growth.

FACD Abbreviation for **F**ellow of the **A**merican **C**ollege of **D**entists.

face Anatomical area from forehead to the chin that include eyes, nose, mouth, cheeks, and chin.

face-bow Instrument used in dental cast development in dentistry.

facet Plane surface on a bone such as articular facets.

facial Any structure that is directed toward the face.

facilitation Hastening of natural process such as proprioceptve neuromuscular facilitation,

FACOG Abbreviation for **F**ellow of the **A**merican **C**ollege of **O**bstetricians and **G**ynecologists.

FACP Abbreviation for **F**ellow of the **A**merican **C**ollege of **P**hysicians.

factitious Not natural.

factor This refers to either a substance or an activity in science. Hereditary factor refers to gene, Chemical factor where mechanism of action is not known such as coagulation factor, Hormonal factor in endocrinal functions in the body, Co efficient factor and conversion factor are known in scientific field.

facultative This refers to bacterial growth in the presence of air or in the absence of air that signify that they can adapt to any odd situations.

faculty This pertains to teaching faculty like professors and Instructors in an Institution. This also denotes to mental faculty which works normal or abnormally.

Fahrenheit This is a temperature scale to measure heat in a substance. 0 degree centigrade (Celsius) is equal to 32 degree Fahrenheit. 100 degree centigrade (Celsius) is equal to 212 degree Fahrenheit.

failure Not able to perform a desired function. E.g., Heart failure, Kidney failure, Respiratory failure

faint Fainting is called Syncope in medical terms.

falciform Any structure which looks like a sickle such as Falciform malaria parasite.

Fallopian Fallopio described many Anatomical structures among which the main ones are Fallopian or Uterine tube, Inguinal ligament, Uterine artery .

Fallot's logies Fallot's tetralogy: Combination of four defects which are 1) pulmonary stenosis 2) interventricular septal defect 3) dextroposition of the aorta and 4) right ventricular hypertrophy. Fallot's triology: - Combination of three defects which are 1) Pulmonary stenosis 2) atrial septal defect and 3) right ventribular hypertrophy. Fallot's pentology; - Combination of five defects which are 1) Pulmonary stenosis 2) interventricular septal defect 3) dextroposition of the aorta 4) right ventricular hypertrophy and 5) Patent foramen ovale

false-negative When a screening test is done, the test show negative but presence of disease exists denoting false negativeness. Test result that wrongly excludes an individual from a diagnostic category

false-positive When a screening test is done, the test show positive but the disease do not exist denoting false positiveness. Test result that wrongly includes an individual from a diagnostic category.

familial An illness or a disease that affects more members in a family than what is expected.

family It is a group of individuals who are biologically related and live together, and eat from a common kitchen. House and social environment are shared by them and hence a family is called a "Social Unit" When the members are not biologically related the social unit becomes a "Household"

Fanconi syndrome A rare recessive disorder with the manifestations of a) Pancytopaenia b) Bone marrow hypoplasia, c) Melanin pigment deposits on skin producing patchy brown skin discolouration d) congenital anomalies of musculoskeletal system e) congenital anomalies of genitourinary system

fantasy Day dream imaginations by a person which is described as a defense mechanism to overcome repressed emotions or conflicts.

FAPHA Abbreviation for **F**ellow of the **A**merican **P**ublic **H**ealth **A**ssociation.

Farabeuf's amputation Lower limb amputation with a large external flap

Farabeuf's triangle This is an anatomical triangle in the superior aspect of the neck. The base of the triangle is formed by Hypoglossal nerve. One side is formed by internal jugular vein and the other side is formed by facial vein.

Farber's disease Lipogranulomatosis described by Farber.

Farr's law When the incidence of new cases are drawn in a line diagram, It ascends rapidly, levels off to a maximum, and descends rapidly to resemble a bell shaped curve. This Farr's law states "All zymotic diseases have the property of subsidence."

Farre's tubercles This refers to hard mass beneath the capsule of the liver. This can be palpated in Ca. Liver

Farre's white line White line represents the boundary of the insertion of the mesovarium at the hilus of the ovary.

farsightedness Hypermetropia or Distant vision.

fascia Band of fibrous tissue that lie deep to the skin such as abdominal fascia, Anoscrotal fascia, Bulbar fascia, Cervical fascia etc.,

fasciculation Small visible local muscular contraction that can be due to spontaneous nerve impulse.

fasciculus It can refer to f a bundle, a tract of nerve fibers such as Fibrous fasciculus of Biceps, Fronto occipital fasciculus.

fasciectomy Surgical excision of fascia.

Fasciola It is a genus of flukes of the family Fasciolidae.

fasciola This denotes to a small band

fascioliasis Getting infected with Fasciola hepatica fluke.

Fasciolopsis Trematodes of the family Fasciolidae Fasciolopsis buski is common in Asia.

fast Fasting or Abstention from food.

fat Soft pads by fat in the body, Chemistry of fat tells this as an ester of glycerol with fatty acids.

fatal That which causes death, that which is lethal.

fate Ultimate outcome, Outcome can be of life, death, of a drug etc.,

fatigability Person gets fatigue easily.

fatigue Prolonged exertion leads to lowered efficiency , power of a muscle seems lowered.

fatty That which is related with fat .

fatty acid They are straight chain monocarboxylic acids, that can be saturated or unsaturated in nature. Fatty acids leads to hypercholesterolemia and is found related to heart disease. Common fatty acids are:

- Palmitic acid
- Stearic acid
- Oleic acid
- Linoleic acid
- Linolenic acid
- Butyric acid

Fauchard's disease Marginal periodontitis described by Fauchard.

faucitis In common terminology it is the sore throat or inflammation of the fauces.

fauna Group of animals or the animal life present in a geographical region. Big and small animal kingdom are called Macrofauna and Microfauna respectively.

Favredisease Lymphogranuloma Venereum described by Favre and his associates.

favus This is colloquially called white head or honeycomb ringworm in man caused by Trichophyton. Hair loss and skin atrophy are common.

Fay method American physical therapist of 20th century who deviced physiotherapy exercises. Re educating the nervous system by starting simpler exercises followed by progressive movements and then advanced pattern s of coordination. .

Fazio-Londe atrophy Progressive bulbar palsy of children described by Fazio and Londe.

Fe Symbol for Iron element.

fear Response to external danger which is not a pleasant emotional state of the person. Fear is a psycho-physiological response.

febrile That which is related to fever . It is also calle Pyrexial.

fecal pertaining to the nature of human excreta.

fecalith Human excreta in lower intestine in the form of hard matter.

feces Excreta of man which consists of food residue, exfoliated cells and discharges of small intestine.

fecundate To fertilize, process of fertilization is called fecundation.

fecundity The ability of a person to produce offspring

Federici's sign It is positive in intestinal perforation. Gas in the peritoneal cavity makes heart sounds heard on auscultation of the abdomen.

feeblemindedness Other name is Mental Retardation which is clinically can be idiots, imbeciles and morons.

feedback After an action or event, output result is obtained that can be useful in improving a given system. Common types of feedback are Bio Feedback, Positive feedback, Negative feedback, Feedback from consumers, Feedback from health service utilisers.

feeding To consume Food, To give eatables.

fee-splitting When a patient is referred to a specialist, the doctor who refers gets some percentage of money by the specialist at the cost of treatment of case. Fee splitting is unethical practice.

FEF Abbreviation for Forced Expiratory Flow; a measure of lung volume for Forced expiration.

Fehling's solution A reagent used in qualitative analysis of urine for sugar detection. The solution is an alkaline cupric sulphate solution similar to Benedict's solution.

Felderstruktur The name is given to the pattern of cardiac myofilaments, which are continuous field with in between mitochondria.

feline That which is connected with cat.

Felix-Weil reaction Laboratory diagnosis for Typhus fever. It is tested for OXK, OX19 and OX2 strains of Proteus.

felon This is closed space infection of terminal phalanx called Whitlow.

Felton's phenomenon By giving larger dose of antigen in mice, immunological tolerance is produced.

female Latin word meaning a young women who bears the offspring.

feminine That which is related with female sex who has female characteristics.

feminization This can be either normal secondary sex character development in woman or man showing the development of female secondary sex charters.

femoral That which is related with thigh or the femur.

femur The largest bone in the body which articulates with hip bone above and with leg bones below. .

fenestra This refers to a round window such as fenestra cochleae.

Fergusson's operation Surgical removal of maxilla through Fergusson's incision which runs along the junction of the nose with the cheek bisecting the upper lip.

ferment Decomposition of carbohydrates called fermentation which is the anaerobic enzymatic conversion of rganic compounds.

ferritin Iron storage form in liver, bone marrow and R E cells.

ferrokinetics This refers to the process of movement of iron from plasma to RBC. Ferrokinetics helps to know the Erythrocyte Iron Turnover.

ferrous Iron in it's Oxidation state which is denoted as Fe^{2+}

ferroxidase This enzyme catalyses the oxidation of ferrous to ferric ions for the transportation of iron in the body.

fertile Person having the capacity to reproduce. Fertility indicate the capacity to conceive by a person.

fertilization When spermatozoon combines with oocyte, oocyte matures to release polar body. Later stages are zygote formation and the development of cleavage. Other equivalents are Impregnation and Fecundation. Types of fertilisation are:

- Internal fertilization
- External fertilization
- In vitro fertilization
- Cross fertilisation

festination This refers to a type of gait in person who takes short accelerating steps in walking without his knowledge.

fetal That which is related to foetus or growing embryo in the uterus.

feticide Killing the growing foetus through modes of abortion such as female infanticide which is condemnable act.

fetid Sweet disagreeable smell such as seen in hepatic coma.

fetish 1. a material object, such as an idol, charm, or talisman, believed to have supernatural powers. 2. an inanimate object used to obtain sexual gratification.

fetoscope Tubular device for listening to foetal heartbeat.

fetus Growing foetus in uterus or womb. This is the period in human life cycle from 9th month to birth.

FEV Abbreviation for Forced Expiratory Volume.

fever Raised body temperature called Pyrexia. Common causes are infection. Physiological reasons are vigorous exercise, Hyperthyroidism, Ovulation etc.,

FIA Abbreviation for Fluorescent Immunoassay.

fiber Any structure which is thread like such as diet fiber, nerve fiber1.

fiberoptics Optics that deals with mode transmission of light, also called Optic fibers.

fibra Anatomical structure which looks like a thread.

fibril A fiber component such as collagen fibrils, nerve fibrils etc.

fibrillation Involuntary contraction of muscle fibre which gets activated by spontaneous stimuli. Atrial and Ventricular fibrillation are commonly known pathology.

Fibrillin structure Opposite of folder structure where separate myofibrils are present in skeletal muscles.

fibrin Main constituent of blood clot which is formed from fibrinogen by a proteolytic action.

fibrinogen It is a Coagulation Factor from which fibrin is formed.

fibroadenoma An adenoma containing fibrous tissue such as Fibroadenoma of breast.

fibroangioma An angioma containing fibrous tissue such as Nasopharyngeal fibroangioma.

fibroblast This is a connective tissue cell from which chondroblasts, osteoblasts are formed for binding connective tissue.

fibrocartilage Cartilage made up of chondrocytes

fibroid Fibrous structure containing organ such uterine fibroid.

fibrolipoma This refers to a lipoma containing an excess of fibrous tissue.

fibromatosis Condition of formation of multiple fibromas seen in colon or gingiva.

fibroplasia Fibrous tissue formation which can be normal or abnormal.

fibrosarcoma Cancer containing fibroblasts which are aggressive and metastasizing forms.

fibrosis This denote to the formation of fibrous tissue which is seen in healing process.

fibrositis Inflammation of the muscle sheaths and fascial layers of the locomotor system

fibrothorax As a consequence of pleural effusion adhesion of the two layers of pleura occurs which is nothing but a non expansible fibrous tissue.

fibula One of the smaller and outer bone of

FICS Abbreviation for **F**ellow of the **I**nternational **C**ollege of **S**urgeons.

field This can be an operational field, a visual field, an area of specialization by a person.

figure It can be a number , a sketch of a person

filament a delicate fiber such as glial filament, actin filament, muscle filament etc.,

Filaria One of the nematode worm which causes elephantiasis in man.

filariasis Infestation by filarial worm.

Filatov's disease This refers to Infectious Mononucleosis described by Filatov.

Fildes enrichment agar This is used in the culture of Haemophilus influenza wherein sheep blood is used.

file This is dental instrument used for smoothing rough teeth surface; Common files used in dentistry are endodontic file and root canal file.

filling In dental restoration process of cavity, cement, gold , resin, amalgam are used to fill dental cavities. The types of dental filling are;-

- o Direct filling
- o Permanent filling
- o Root canal filling
- o Temporary filling

film This is a thin layer of coating. Such as blood film X-ray film etc.

film badge This is called Dosimeter used by Radiologist and Radiology technicians to check the radiation absorption in the body.

Filoviridae This is RNA virus called Marburg virus and Ebola virus:

filter A device with porous item to separate particulate matter from a liquid. E.g., Collodion filter, Rapid sand filter, Slow sand filter, Trickling filter, etc.,

filtrate This refers to a liquid that has passed through a filter. The process of filtering a liquid, a gas or photons of longer wavelengths.

fimbria The edge of an organ or the border of an organ.

finding A scientific observation or a discovery in science.

finger Any digit of the hand like index finger, middle finger, ring finger, little finger or thumb. Common pathological variants are:

- Clubbed finger
- Hammer finger
- Webbed finger
- Gangrened finger

fingerprint Skin ridges impression from palmar surface of distal portion of a finger for the purpose of identification in Forensic Medicine.

Finkelstein's feeding It is a therapeutic infant liquid feeding or semisolid feeding wherein milk sugar or lactose is avoided.

Finsen Danish physician who won Noble Prize for the discovery of U V rays use in Lupus Vulgaris in the year 1903.

first aid Aid given to a patient before the start of actual medical or surgical treatment. Trauma, Injury, Acute medical emergencies, Acute surgical emergencies are attended to by first aid.

Fischer American biochemist who won Nobel Prize for the discovery of Protein Kinases in Cell Metabolism in the year 1992.

fission Splitting process in cell division which is asexual type of reproduction which can be binary fission or multiple fission.

fissura A cleft or an organ or a groove of an organ such as anal fissure, Cerebral fissure, Pterygomaxillary fissure etc., The other name is fissure.

fistula An abnormal communication created between two organ or two structure such as:

- Vesicovaginal fistula
- Rectovaginal fistula
- Abdominal fistula
- Bronchial fistula
- Oroarterial fistula
- Urethrovaginal fistula
- Perineal fistula
- Pilonidal fistula
- Anal fistula
- Genitourinary fistula
- Oroantral fistula
- Tracheoesophageal fistula

fistulectomy Surgical treatment of fistula.

fitness Refers to physical fitness, genetic fitness and mental fitness in day to day medical examinations.

fixation Latin word meaning to hold in a fixed position. It can be chemical removal in film processing, It can be Eye fixation, It can be Histological specimen fixation in pathology, It can be Mother or father fixation in psycho analysis. It can be complement fixation in immunology.

fixative Common chemicals used as fixatives are Osmium tetroxide, glutaraldehyde, acetic acid, alcohols, picric acid. In histology or Histopathology these fixatives are used.

flaccid Latin word meaning absence of tone such as flaccid paralysis condition.

Flack's node This refers to Sinoatrial Node described by Flack.

flagellum Whip like projection of a cell meant for locomotion.

Flagyl Preparation of Metronidazole which is the chemotherapeutic agent in amoebiasis.

flail When there is an abnormal mobility of an organ in the body such as flail joint, flail chest, or flail valve.

Flajani's disease Grave's disease described by Flajani.

flame Fire produced by the combustion of chemicals like spirit that is commonly used to sterilise an object.

flank This refers to the portion of the body on the sides from ribs to ilium.

flap This is skin tissue for grafting which gets it's blood supply from it's original place even at transfer. It is a technique in plastic surgery for repair of a defect. Common types of flaps are:

- Full thickness flap
- Local flap or sliding flap
- Pedicle flap
- Delayed transfer flap
- Direct transfer flap
- Flap for closing open drainage of chronic empyema called Eloesser flap
- Flap for repair of upper lip called Estlander flap
- Tube flap
- Rotation flap
- TRAM (Transverse Rectus Abdominal Muscle) Flap for Breast reconstruction.
- Z flap

flare In case of Urticaria (triple response) the outermost red zone .

flasking This is a type of molding of denture.

flat When even surface is there for an organ the word flat is used.

flatfoot When the arch of the foot is flat and lowered which is also called as Pes planus.

flatulence When stomach or intestine is filled with excess quantity of air that leads to distension of stomach or intestine.

flatus Fermented gas is expelled from anus.

Flavivirus They are group B viruses that cause clinical conditions like Dengue fever, Yellow fever, J.E., K F D

flea Common disease producing is Rat flea, Other known fleas are dog flea, cat flea, human flea

Flechsig's tract This refers to Posterior Spino Cerebellar Tract described by Flechsig.

fleck This refers to a spot in medical description.

Flegel's disease Hyperkeratosis due to lenticular cause described by Flegel.

Fleischner's disease Osteochondritis of middle phalanges of hand described by Fleishchner.

Fleming Alexander Fleming a Scottish bacteriologist who won Noble Prize for the discovery of Penicillin in the year 1945.

flesh Colloquial term denoting muscle and skin.

flexion This is an act of bending such as flexion of knee, flexion of elbow.

Flexner's bacillus This is the name given to Shigella group of pathogens that cause dysentery described by Flexner.

Flint's murmur This is popularly called as Austin Flint Murmur which is heard in case of aortic regurgitation.

floaters Vitreous protein in the form of deposits produce spots before the eyes.

flocculation In case of coagulation where visible particles are separated from invisible particles. Small mass formation in chemical coagulation is called flocculus.

floor Inferiors aspect of a cavity such as floor of oral cavity, floor of fourth ventricle.

flora In Latin Flora means the name of Goddess of Flowers. This is plant life in earth, which can be macroflora or microflora for a given geographical area.

florid Full blown and having bright red colour.

flow This refers to the movement of liquid such as blood flow, air flow etc.,

Flowers index It is craniometric index obtained by the following formula:

$$\text{Dental Index} = \frac{(\text{Dental length}) \times (100)}{\text{Basinasal length}}$$

flowmeter This is an apparatus for measuring the rate of flow of liquids or gases. Common flow meters used in medical practice are:

- Doppler flowmeter
- Blood flowmeter
- Ultra sound flowmeter

floxacillin This is a semi synthetic preparation of Penicillin used against resistant strains of staphylococci

floxuridine This is a metabolite of 5-fluorouracil used in the treatment of cancer of stomach, cancer of intestine and secondary's of liver cancer.

fl oz Abbreviation for Fluid Ounce.

flu Influenza viral infection in man.

fluctuant Wavelike motion of a liquid, It can denote variations in occurrence.

fluid Fluid is a substance which is composed of elements which change their positions and do not allow separation of elements or particles. Common fluids in medical practice are:

- Tissue fluid
- Seminal fluid
- Pericardial fluid
- Synovial fluid
- Bleaching fluid
- Cerebro spinal fluid
- Intra cellular fluid
- Extra cellular fluid
- Amniotic fluid
- Allantoic fluid
- Zenker fluid
- Ventricular fluid
- Ascitic fluid
- Follicular fluid
- Candy's fluid
- Labyrinthine fluid
- Interstitial fluid
- Serous fluid

Fluid extract This is prepared by the process of percolation from vegetables for therapeutic purposes such as senna fluid extract (laxative) and Cascara fluid extract (cathartic)

fluke They are Trematodes under Helminths causing intestinal infestations. Blood fluke, Intestinal fluke, Liver fluke, Lung fluke are common flukes of public health importance.

fluorescein Fluorine dyes such as FITC (Fluorescein Isothiacyanate) or Fluorescein sodium that are used in the assessment of corneal injury and for subsequent contact lenses fixation.

fluorescence It was first observed in fluorspar and hence the name fluorescence. This is the property of emitting light when exposed to light.

fluorine Bone and teeth contain fluorine. Fluorine is a halogen compound which is gaseous in nature and not a metal. F_{18} (Fluorine 18) is a radioactive isotope used in tomography.

fluoroscope X-ray device used for examining deep structures

fluorosis Clinical conditions like Dental fluorosis and Skeletal fluorosis caused by consumption of excess quantity of fluorine that can be a public health problem.

flush Redness occurring due to heat, emotion, physical exertion and drugs. Histamine flush, atropine flush, carcinoid flush and breast flush are well known in medical practice.

flutter Appreciable vibration in a tissue which can be pathological or physiological. Mediastinal flutter, Atrial flutter, Diaphragmatic flutter and Ventricular flutter are common flutters in clinical practice.

fly They are two winged insects of public health importance . Musca domestica or house fly is common vector in the transmission of diseases by mechanical means. Other types are Sand fly, Black fly and Tsetse flies in Medical entomology.

Flynn-Aird syndrome This is a rare autosomal dominant syndrome characterised by the following manifestations:

1. Retinitis pigmentosa
2. Cataract
3. Skin atrophy
4. Dental caries
5. Myopia
6. Ulcerations
7. Peripheral neuropathy
8. Ataxia
9. Deafness

foam Frothy character of a substance. Chemically it is the dispersion of gas in liquid giving rise to foam.

focus Point of light convergence. This can also mean main area of pathology.

fog Mass of water droplet spread in the air

Fogarty catheter Catheter with balloon tip that is used to remove blood clot in a vessel.

fogging In eye examination for refractive error, patient is made myopic before using cylinders. In mosquito control Malathion fogging is done to control mosquitoes.

foil This refers to thin pliable sheet such as Gold foil, Platinum foil, tin foil etc.,

Foix syndrome This refers to Cavernous Sinus Syndrome described by Foix.

folate Anionic form of Folic Acid.

Foley catheter It is an indwelling bladder catheter. This has a balloon filled with air to fit in to bladder.

folic acid This is a water soluble vitamin B complex that is used in Folic acid deficiency and in megaloblastic anaemia.

Folin's method Done for the detection of acetone, amino acids, creatinine and for urea in a given biological substance.

follicle A pouch like depression in an organ or a structure. Graafian follicle, Dental follicle, Lymph follicle, Hair follicle, Ovarian follicle, Primordial follicle, Thyroid follicle are known follicles.

Foltz's valve Fold made of mucous membrane that help reflux of contents at lacrimal canaliculus.

fomentation A poultice treatment through warm and moist applications

fomite Any object like table, chair, cot, clothing etc., which can serve as an agent in disease transmission which when gets contaminated.

Fontan procedure Functional correction by surgery for Tricuspid valve atresia with a nonvalue prosthesis.

fontanelle Soft spot on vertex of infant which is due to incomplete ossified skull portion. This is popularly known as Anterior fontanelle or bregma

food Naturally available food consumed as such or by cooking which can provide nutrient and calorie.

foot Distal portion of leg to stand and to walk in man and in animals. Common terminology in usage are:

- Burning feet
- Athlete's foot
- Club foot
- Charcot foot
- Immersion foot
- Madura foot
- Trench foot

foot-candle A unit of illumination (1 lumen per square foot)

footdrop Lesion of tibial nerve and or peroneal nerve gives rise to paralysis of anterior muscles of leg producing footdrop.

foramen A passage or opening in a bone such as auditory foramen, carotid foramen, Styloid foramen, cribroethmoid foramen etc.

Forbes' disease This refers to Glycogen Storage Disease Type III described by Forbes.

force Force is an action that can change the rate of motion or direction of motion or both of an object. This is commonly known as gravitational force.

forceps Instrument used to grasp and handle tissues in surgical operation.

forearm Upper limb part from wrist to elbow which is called antebrachium.

forensic That which is applied in legal proceedings. This refers to Medical Jurisprudence or Forensic Medicine in medical practice.

foreplay This denotes to pleasurable activity before actual intercourse in man.

fore-pleasure Sexual pleasure before orgasm.

foreskin This is the name for prepuce of glans penis

Form Externally how a structure looks like in terms of size and shape.

formaldehyde It is in gas form and made available in solution form. This is a disinfectant, a preservative and fixative. Other name is methanal. Formalin is solution form of formaldehyde.

formation When a structure, an organ gets a shape in its development it is called formation.

Formica Ant like creatures that are domestic pests of man.

formic acid An irritating pungent and caustic chemical with the formula "HCO_2H" Sodium salt of formic acid is used as food preservative.

formication Hallucination of ants crawling on the body in a person who has cocaine intoxication. Magnan has described this and hence it is called Magnan's name.

formula With the help of symbol and number a statement can be made or structure of a chemical can be written. When medication is done to a patient with specific dose and duration it can be called formula. Formula gives one single concept. Common terminologies are;

- Chemical formula
- Dental formula
- Molecular formula
- Structural formula

formulation Dose and duration of drug prescription to patient.

fornix This refers to a structure which is an arch like or a vault like in shape.

Forssell's sinus On radiological examination stomach wall show a smooth space which is surrounded by folds of mucosa.

Forssman's antigen This antigen produces antisheep haemolysis that can be established in RBCs and in organs

Forssmann German surgeon who won Noble Prize for the invention of cardiac catheterisation in the year 1956.

Foshay's test It is a skin test done for Tularaemia infection. Suspension of Pasteurella tularensis is injected into the skin, a positive reaction similar to tuberculin test is seen.

fossa This refers to a hollow place such as Cubital fossa, Acetabular fossa, Cerebellar fossa, Condylar fossa, Cranial fossa, Glenoid fossa, Hyaloid foss, Ilieocolic fossa, Intercostal fossa, Lacrimal fossa, Navicular fossa, Olecranon fossa etc.,

Fothergill operation Surgical procedure adopted lby Fothergill for Prolapse of the uterus. The procedure include:

- D and C
- Anterior repair
- Vaginal portion of cervix is amputated
- Cardinal ligaments are shortened
- Posterior colpoperineorrhaphy

Fouchet's test Qualitative test for bilirubin in urine. With Fouchet's reagent urine give green colour is positive.

fourchette French word meaning a fork-shaped object such as pudendal lavial frenulum.

fovea Refers to small pit in an organ or in a structure. Fovea of head of femur and fovea of fourth ventricle are examples.

Foville's syndrome Crossed paralysis where same side limb paralysis and opposite side face paralysis occurs, paralysis of outward movement of the eye is present. Paralysis of conjugate movement is also present.

Fowler's position This refers to patient's position wherein his head is raised by 50 cms. And knees are elevated

Fowler's solution Potassium Arsenite Solution described by Fowler.

foxglove Colloquial word used to denote digitalis.

Fracastorius Fracastoro an Italian physician also a poet wrote a medical poem in which 'syphilis' was first mentioned

fraction A small portion of a unit such as plasma protein fraction. This also denotes to a dose.

fracture This is a break in a bone which can be due to fall, truma or accident.

Common clinical types of fractures are:

- Simple
- Complicated
- Complete
- Incomplete
- Epiephyseal
- Extra capsular
- Spiral
- Hair line
- Potts
- Colles
- Axial Neck
- Blow out

- Closed
- Open
- Compression
- Avulsion
- Linear
- Secondary
- Greenstick
- Multiple'
- Pathological
- Impacted
- Depressed
- Le Fort I, II and III
- Complicated
- Butter fly

fracture-dislocation This is the bone fracture occurring near a joint which involves dislocation.

fragility Continuity is lost due to the susceptibility. Capillary fragility and erythrocyte fragility are known property.

fragment A small piece of a fractured bone.

fragmentation Division to small pieces.

framework This gives the basic totality of a unit or of a system.

Franceschetti syndrome Mandibulofacial Dysostosis which is complete in occurrence.

Francis' disease This refers to Tularaemia described by Francis.

Franco's operation This refers to Suprapubic Cystotomy described by Franco.

François' syndrome Oculomandibulofacial Syndrome described by Francois.

Frank's operation A type of gastrostomy where a cone of stomach is pulled through an incision in the left rectus muscle and suturing it to the skin.

Frankel Classification This is classification of spinal cord injury considering motor and sensory loss. Frankel grouped into A to E five types.

Fränkel's sign It is positive in Tabes dorsalis where muscular tone is decreased. The positive sign is excessive range of passive movement of the hip joint in Tabes dorsalis.

Fränkel's test Nasal cavity is examined by bending head down between knees and rotated so that side to be examined is turned upward. If pus is present in middle meatus, suppuration in sinuses is indicated and expressed as positive sign.

Frankenhäuser's ganglion This refers to cervical ganglion of the uterus.

Fraser syndrome This is an autosomal recessive disorder (known as Cryptophthalmos syndrome) characterised by the following manifestations:

- Disorganised ocular globe
- Laryngeal stenosis
- Cleft palate
- Malformation of ears
- Imperforate anus
- Syndactyly
- Cardiac defects
- Maldeveloped kidneys

***F*-ratio** This is the ratio between Group Variation and Within Group Variation. This approximates to one if two measures of variance yield similar results. F ratio is used in F test as a statistical test comparing the means of more than two groups simultaneously by comparing two different measures of variance of the observations. F distribution describes the simultaneously distribution of two independent estimates of a population variance. It is expressed as ratio.

$$F \text{ ratio} = \frac{\text{Greater Variance}}{\text{Lesser Variance}} = \frac{S_1^2}{S_2^2}$$

FRCP Abbreviation for **F**ellow of the **R**oyal **C**ollege of **P**hysicians.

FRCS Abbreviation for **F**ellow of the **R**oyal **C**ollege of **S**urgeons.

Freckle Small macule which gets darker to sunlight exposure.

freeze-drying This is called Lyophilisation wherein the tissue is frozen and later dehydrated at low temperature in a high vacuum.

Frei's disease This refers to Lymphogranuloma Venereum described by Frei.

fremitus On palpation the vibration due to pathology is felt. Bronchial and Pericardial fremitus are known entities.

frenulum This is a small fold of mucous membrane such as Lingual frenulum, Clitoris frenulum, Frenulum of superior lip etc., This is synonym with frenum.

frequency This can be number of occurrence of an event, can be number of vibrations per second.

Fresnel lens Lens which is thin but has the property of thick lens by giving optical property by stepped setbacks concentrically arranged.

fressreflex Striking lips and cheeks produce sucking chewing and swallowing movements.

Freud Sigmund Freud is a German psychiatrist. He is the founder of Psychoanalysis. Many of his inventions are applied to human behaviour. The major ones are:

- Ego
- Super ego
- Repression
- Infantile sexuality
- Unconsciousness
- Sublimation

friable That which can be easily pulverised or powdered.

friction Act of rubbing on the skin

Friedländer's bacillus The bacteria belonging to Klebsiella that cause pneumonia described by Friedlander.

Friedmann's vasomotor syndrome This refers to Post Concusional Syndrome described by Friedmann.

Friedreich's ataxia This is the pathology of sclerosis of the dorsal and lateral columns of spinal cord It is attended by ataxia and other clinical manifestations described by Friedmann.

frigidity Female sexual arousal disorder also called coldness in females.

Fröhlich's syndrome This refers to Adiposogenital Dystrophy described by Frohlick.

frolement In pericardial disease rustling sound heard in auscultation

frontal That which is related with forehead.

frostbite Tissue damage by very low temperature. This can be superficial or deep frostbite.

fructosazone When Fructose reacts with phenyl hydrazine it produces the osazone

fructose This is present in honey, sweet fruits and is chemically '$C_6H_{12}O_6$'

FSH Abbreviation for Follicle Stimulating Hormone.

fuchsin They are tri amino Tri Phenyl Methane Dyes that are red to purple in colour used in staining. Acid fuchsin, Basic fuchsin and New fuchsin are known fuchsin in laboratory procedures.

Fugl-Meyer assessment An assessment which is standardised by Fugi Meyer for the assessment of motor function of a part following neurological damage.

Fuller's operation see under This is the surgical drain of seminal vesicle abscess. The route of drain is through perineal incision.

fulminate Occurring suddenly with great intensity.

fumaric acid This is an intermediate product of Tri Carboxylic Acid Cycle.

fumigant A substance used in fumigation process.

fumigation Disinfectant fumes are allowed in a given area

function The Physiological action of an organ or of a system in the body. This refers to the process of an action. In chemistry it refers to behaviour of a chemical. In mathematics it can be assigned rule to a set or a value.

fundamental Related with the foundation.

fundus Base of uterus or of any hollow organ.

Funduscope Other name for an ophthalmoscope.

Fungi They are Mushrooms, Yeasts and Molds that are heterotrophic in nature that live as saprobes or parasites.

funiculitis Infection and inflammation of spermatic cord

funiculoepididymitis inflammation of the Spermatic cord and Epididymis.

furazolidone Anti bacterial and antiprotozoal nitrofuran compound used against gram negative organisms.

furuncle Staphylococcal infection of sub cutaneous tissue which is painful and irritable.

fusion Joined adjacent parts, Separate images coordination for vision. Operative procedure of arthritic bones.

G

g Used as a symbol for Gram

γ Gamma letter of the Greek alphabet is used as a symbol for the heavy chain of IgG , Referring to third carbon atom of a chemical structure as in **γ** amino butyric acid, as **γ** band in gamma globulin, in a series of chemical or entity as in **γ** Rays or **γ** Carotene.

GAD Abbreviation for **G**eneralised **A**nxiety **D**isorder

Gaffky scale This provide a table for the correlation of number of tuberculosis bacteria in a field of sputum AFB examination. This is used as a scale in the prognosis of Tuberculosis.

gag This refers to Mouth Gag used to hold the mouth open.

Gaisböck's disease This refers to the Stress Polycythemia described by Gaisbock.

gait (g[amacr]t) Style of walking which is used in clinical diagnosis. Common clinical entities are:

- Charcot gait
- Tabetic gait
- stuttering gait
- Trendelenburg gait
- spastic gait
- scissors gait
- Waddling gait
- Cerebellar gait
- Propulsive gait
- Ataxic gait
- Hysteric gait
- Hemiplegic gait
- Drop foot gait
- Steppage gait
- Swing to gait

Gajdusek American pediatrician who discovered the mode of spread of major infectious diseases and he was awarded Nobel prize in Medicine in the year 1976 for his work in this public health field.

galactagogue Substance that promote the milk flow in a lactating mother.

galacto That which is related with milk.

galactocele Enlargement of mammary gland in the form of a cyst that contains milk.

galactometer Lactometer which measures the Sp.Gr of milk.

galactosazone When phenyl Hydrazine reacts with galactose, osazone is formed which is characteristic and diagnostic to galactose.

galactose Galactose is a component of various glycolipids and glycoproteins . Chemically it is an epimeric with glucose at the 4 carbon atom.

galactosemia It is a genetic disorder showing defective galactose metabolism. Three types of galactosemia are a) Classic galactosemia b) Galactokinase deficiency and c) Galactose epimerase deficiency

galactosuria Presence of galactose in the urine.

galea Anatomical structure is given the name when it is looking like a helmet. E.g., Galea aponeurotica (Aponeurosis of pericranium of scalp)

Galeati's glands Duodenal glands described by Geleati.

galeatus born with a caul.

Galeazzi's fracture [Riccardo *Galeazzi,* Italian orthopedic surgeon, 1866–1952] It is Dupuytren's fracture wherein radium has the fracture above the wrist along with dislocation of the distal end of the ulna.

Galen Galen is known in the history of medicine as Greco Roman anatomist, physiologist and physician. He wrote many epics of which only 83 are available for documentation. His major depictions are importance of pulse in diagnosis, Brain as seat of man's intelligence, Artery carry pure blood. His successors are many among whom Anatomist Vesalius and Physiologist Harvey.

Galen's nerve Communicating branch of superior and inferior laryngeal nerves.

galenic Well known teachings of Galen in the history of medicine way back c. 129 to c. 200

gall It refers to gall bladder and also to a localized swelling on skin by friction.

gallbladder Called biliary vesicle which store bile .

Gallie transplant While doing hernia repair, strips of fascia lata is used as sutures.

gallon This is a measure of volume equivalent to five litres or equivalent to four quarts

gallop Cardiac arrhythmia or disordered rhythm of the heart such as a) Diastolic gallop b) Pre systolic gallop c) Atrial gallop d) Summation gallop e) S_4 gallop f) S_3 gal lop g) Ventricular gallop

gallstone Concretion in gallbladder by cholesterol or Calcium

Galton's law of regression This is the law of acquiring parental peculiarities. Very tall parents will have average or short children, Very short parents will have average or tall children whereas average parents will have average children.

galvanic Refers to unidirectional battery current described by Galvani and hence Galvanic.

galvanization Galvanic current treatment

galvanometer Refers to Einthoven's Galvanometer a fore runner of ECG. Galvanometer measures current, which is produced by Electro Magnetic Action.

Gambusia Mosquito larvae eating fishes called larvivorous fishes used in mosquito control programmes. Common ones are Gambusia affinis.

gamete Refers to either oocyte or spermatozoon. In case of malaria life cycle it refers to Macrogamete or Microgamete

gametocyte This either oocyte or spermatocyte which is capable of dividing to form gamete.

gametogony Reproduction occurring by means of gametes as in case of malaria parasite Plasmodia. Here Merozoites develop to male gametes or to female gamete.

Gamgee tissue Surgical dressing devised by Gamgee which consists of thick layer of absorbent cotton kept in between two layers of absorbent gauze. .

gamic Egg developing only after fertilization or only after sexual process.

gamma Denoted by sumbol γ the third letter of the Greek alphabet.

gamma benzene hexachloride An insecticide made available as Indene.

gamma globulin One of the globulin present in serum

Gamna's disease A type of spleen enlargement due to thickening of splenic capsule.

Gamstorp's disease Familial periodic paralysis II described by Gamstorp.

ganglioblast This refers to an embryonic cell of the cerebrospinal ganglia.

ganglioglioma Benign tumour called ganglioneuroma in the central nervous system

ganglion Greek word meaning any mass which looks like a knot. Known ganglia are Basal ganglia, Acoustico-fascial ganglia, Auditory ganglia, Carotid ganglia, Coeliac ganglia, Cervical ganglia, Thoracid ganglia, Mesenteric ganglia, Nerve ganglia, Paravertebral ganglia, Sino aortic ganglia, Spinal ganglia, Synovial ganglia, Troisier's Ganglia, Wrist ganglia.

ganglioside They are present in nervous tissue which is the nature of glycosphingolipids with glucose residue.

gangrene Tissue undergoing effect of avascularity and bacterial invasion. Finally it goes to the stage of putrefaction which is called necrobiosis or necrosis. Common types are:

- Diabetic gangrene
- Atherosclerotic gangrene
- Epidemic gangrene due to ergotism
- Gas gangrene
- Pressure gangrene
- Senile gangrene
- Raynaud's gangrene
- Trophic gangrene

gangrenous Related with gangrene or tissue necrosis

Ganser's commissure Supra Optic Commissure described by Ganser.

gap (gap) a calculated time interval, a calculated space interval or unoccupied interval in a given time.

Garcin's syndrome Tumour at the base of the skull cussing unilateral paralysis of all cranial nerves.

Gardner's syndrome Familial Polyposis described by Gardner.

Gardner-Diamond syndrome Painful Bruising Syndrome described by Gardner and Diamond.

gargle Rinsing the mouth for medication purpose which will also clean the throat. Common advice for sore throat is mouth gargling.

gargoylism Mucopolysaccharidoses with hypertelorism, depressed nasal bridge, large tongue, dwarfism, short neck, gibbus, liver enlargement and spleen enlargement. Heart failure and severe respiratory infection are usual complications.

Garland's triangle Resonant area in the lower back on the side where Pleurisy with effusion is present

garlic A derivative from the stem base of a flowering plant which has multiple uses in medicine. The main ingredient is Sulphur ester derivative allicin which is used against cough, sepsis, toothache, earache and for some of the nervous conditions.

garnet Silicate of magnesium used on dental disks.

Garré's osteomyelitis Sclerosing non suppurative osteomyelitis described by Garre.

Gärtner's bacillus Salmonella enteritidis discovered by Gartner.

Gartner's cyst Vaginal tumour which is benign and cystic. This is derived from Gartner's duct.

Gärtner's phenomenon This demonstrates the pressure in the right atrium. When the arm is raised above the level of the heart and point at which it collapse is the degree of pressure. The phenomenon depicts the fullness of the veins of upper limb which in turn indicate the degree of pressure in the right atrium.

gas any elastic aeriform fluid in which the molecules are separated from one another and so have free paths. Physiological expression is there for flatus and belching. Common gases of health importance are:

- Mustard gas
- Tear gas
- Inert gas
- Alveolar gas
- blood gas
- Laughing gas
- warfare gas or war gas

Gasser's ganglion Trigeminal ganglion described by Gasser.

Gasser's syndrome Haemolytic uraemic Syndrome described by Gasser.

gaster G.I. part between oesophagus and duodenum which produce Juice containing HCl pepsin that make food digestible in intestine.

gastrectomy Surgical resection of stomach for surgical treatment.

gastric That which is related to stomach

gastrin Polypeptide hormones released from G cells of Pyloric glands of gastric antrum. Gastrin stimulates secretion of gastric acid .

gastrinoma Islet cell tumour in antrum of stomach giving rise to Zollinger Ellison Syndrome.

gastritis Inflammation of the stomach.

gastrocnemius Name of leg muscle.

gastroduodenitis Inflammation of the stomach and duodenum.

gastroduodenostomy Anastomosis between the stomach and the duodenum.

gastroenteritis Acute inflammation of the lining of the stomach and intestines, characterized by anorexia, nausea, diarrhea, abdominal pain, and weakness. Food poisoning by E.coli, Staph aureus and Salmonella pathogens.

gastroenterologist Medical Doctor who specializes in diseases of the digestive tract.

gastroenterology Scientific study of diseases of stomach and intestine.

gastroenterostomy Anastomosis between stomach and jejunum which is done for surgical treatment.

gastrointestinal Related with stomach and intestine.

gastrojejunostomy Surgical operation for anastomosis between stomach and jejunum for chronic peptic ulcer patients.

gastromegaly Big stomach or enlargement of the stomach.

gastrone It is present in gastric mucosa which is responsible for inhibiting gastric acid secretion in the stomach.

gastrophrenic Related with stomach and diaphragm.

gastroscope Instrument called endoscope for inspecting the interior of the stomach also called Fiber optic gastroscope.

gastrostomy Creating an opening in stomach through surgical operation. Common surgical techniques are;

- Glassman's permanent opening from anterior abdominal wall.
- Stamm's method of inserting a tube in to stomach through a stab incision
- Wetzel's creating serosal tunnel of stomach

gastrotomy Incision into the stomach by using gastronome instrument in surgery.

gastrula Succeeding stage of Blastocyst in embryonic development.

Gaucher's disease It is Glucosyl Ceramide Lipidosis due to deficient glucocerebrosidase. There are three clinical entities. They are a) Type I Adult type b) Type II infantile type and c) Type III Juvenile

gauge This is used to measure dimension, pressure or caliber of an item.

Gauss' sign This sign is positive in early pregnancy where mobility of uterus is seen increased. .

gauss This is represented as 'G' which is the cgs unit of magnetic flux density (10^{-4} tesla)

gaussian curve This refers to Normal curve described by Gauss which is bell shaped and symmetrical around the mean of the distribution. This is a frequency curve in normal distribution.

gauze Muslin cloth used in bandages, dressings, and surgical sponges. It is sterilized with antiseptics before use in surgery. The common ones are a) Absorbable gauze b) Sterile absorbent gauze (c) Petroleum gauze and d) Zinc gelatin impregnated gauze.

gavage Eating more than the requirement by a person's overeating, super alimentation. This refers to forced feeding.

Gavard's muscle Oblique muscle of stomach wall.

Gay-Lussac's law The law states at constant temperature and pressure, the ratio of the volumes of two gases that react with each other is always a small whole number.

gaze Study look at one direction.

gear Equipment such as Head gear or cervical gear.

Gee's disease Infantile form of celiac disease described by Gee.

Geiger-Müller counter It detects the presence of ionising particles that can be made use of in diagnosis of diseases of certain organs.

gel A semi solid material which can be called a colloid.

gelatin Hydrolysed product of skin collagen and animal bones.

Gélineau's syndrome Narcolepsy described by Gelineau.

Gell and Coombs classification Immune mechanism after injury under allergic reactions are classified under 4 types, which are as under:

- Type I Immediate hypersensitivity reactions
- Type II antibody mediated hypersensitivity reactions
- Type III immune complex mediated hypersensitivity reactions
- Type IV cell mediated hypersensitivity reactions

geminus It means Twin.

gender This refers to sex male or female .

gene DNA molecule containing the information's required for synthesis of polypeptide chain or RNA molecule. Gene is the biologic unit of heredity with locus on the chromosome map.

generation This is the process of generation or reproduction in animals and man.

generic Name given to a genus and non proprietary such as chemical name of a drug and the trade name of the drug.

genesic Pertaining to generation

genesiology The study of reproduction.

genesis Related with the origin process.

genetics The Scientific study of genes and their heredity. Common areas of interest are:

- Clinical genetics
- Population genetics
- Molecular genetics
- Cytogenetics

Geneva Convention The convention declares that signatory nations pledge to treat the wounded without discrimination. It stipulates that Doctors and nurses are neutral army in the battlefield. This agreement was stipulated in the year 1864

Gengou phenomenon Complement Fixation described by Gengou.

geniculate Any structure which is bent and looks like a bent knee.

geniohyoid Relates to chin and hyoid bone.

genital Genitalia related or reproduction related.

genitalia Organs of genitalia in male and female referable to both external and internal genitalia.

genitourinary Related with genital organs and urinary organs also called urogenital.

genius Special nature such as very high ability and high aptitude of a person. His or her I Q will be above 140

Gennari's line This is prominent band in the region of calcarine sulcus in the brain called striate cortex.

genome Gene set in man which is the haploid set of 3,000,000,000 base pairs of DNA.

genotype This refers to type species of Homo sapiens or man which is nothing but total genetic constitution of man.

gentamicin Antibiotic belonging to aminoglycoside complex derived from Micromonospora purpurea with the mixture of C_1, C_{1A}, C_2 fractions . It is effective against a wide range of aerobic gram-negative bacilli like Pseudomonas and Enterobacteriaceae.

genu Joint which connects threw thigh and leg in the body. Referable to Knee. Genu valgum is deformity of knees abnormally close together called knock knee. Genu varum is deformity of knees abnormally separated together and is called bowleg.

genus Categorization kunder Taxonomy either in Botany or in Zoology.

geomedicine This is Geographical pathology which deals the influence of geographic factors like climate and environment on health and disease.

geotropism Any thing that is growing or moving against gravitational force such as plant root downward and stem of plant upwards growing.

Gerbich blood group Erythrocytic antigen based classification as Ge1, Ge2 and Ge3 that are present in Papua New Guinea area. This is discovered by Gerbich.

GERD Abbreviation for **G**astro **E**sophageal **R**eflux **D**isease.

Gerhardt's disease Erythromelalgia described by Gerhardt.

Gerhardt's test Test for Acetoacetic acid in urine. Also the test done for bile pigments in the urine.

Gerhardt-Semon law In partial paralysis of recurrent laryngeal nerve vocal cord assume a position between abduction and adduction .

geriatric Related to aging or senescence

geriatrician A Consultant in Geriatrics.

geriatrics Branch of medicine that deals with problems of old age called senility problems.

germ Pathogen or microorganism which cause disease in man.

germicidal Drug, chemical or medicaments that kill pathogens or germs.

gerodontology Scientific study of the dentition and dental problems in the aged

gerontology Study of old age people from different aspect such as clinical sociological biological and historical .

Gerota's fascia Renal fascia described by Gerota.

Gesell developmental schedule Infant development assessment called Gesell developmental schedule that include the following:

- Assessment of Motor Development
- Assessment of Adaptive Behaviour
- Assessment of Language Development
- Assessment of Personal Social Behaviour

gestation Pregnancy period which is from the time of fertilization till birth of child.

GFR Abbreviation for **G**lomerular **F**iltration **R**ate

GH Abbreviation for **G**rowth **H**ormone

Ghon's complex This is popularly called Gohn's Primary complex which include the following:

- Parenchymal lung lesion called Ghon Focus
- Lymph node focus called Gohn Tubercle cellular necrosis and calcification at a later stage. Gohn's complex is primary tuberculosis in children.

Ghon-Sachs bacillus Clostridium septicum bacilli described by Ghon

ghost Faint shadow figure in a cell called Ghost cell.

GI Abbreviation for **G**astro **I**ntestinal

Giacomini's band Gray band over the inferior surface of uncus at hippocampus area

Gianelli's sign During extreme lateral fixation, unilateral dilatation of pupil of abducting eye is positive.

giant Man with very great height usually pathological with hormonal overactivity.

giantism Gigantic personality due to over activity of pituitary gland.

Giardia Nonpathogenic, flagellate intestinal protozoa in man.

giardiasis Intestinal infection with parasite Giardia lamblia transmitted through contaminated food or water.

gibbous Hump back of a person. Also called gibbus.

Gibson's murmur It is called machinery murmur present in Patent Ductus Arteriosus. It is described as long rumbling sound in systole and diastole maximum heart in second left inter costal space.

Giemsa stain Stain used to stain protozoan parasites particularly Plasmodium malaria parasite. Pink to purple blue stain is characteristic of the stain. The ingredients are a) Azure II eosin, b) Azure II, c) Glycerin, d) Methanol

GIFT Abbreviation for **G**amete **I**ntra **F**allopian **T**ransfer

giga Unit of measurement which is big such as gigabyte which is one billion time more and is indicated by the notion 10^9

gigantism Excessive growth due to many reasons such as Cerebral gigantism, Acromegalic gigantism, Foetal gigantism

Gigli's operation is a flexible wire saw used by surgeons for bone cutting. A Gigli saw is used mainly for amputation, where the bones have to be smoothly cut at the level of amputation.

Gilbert's sign Manifestation of cirrhosis by opsiuria.

Gilles de la Tourette's syndrome Childhood syndrome with multiple motor tics including vocal tics associated with obsession, compulsion.

Gilliam's operation Gynecological operation for retroversion of uterus.

Gillies' flap Tube flap used in plastic surgery.

Gilman American pharmacologist winner Nobel prize for medicine in 1994 for his research on cell response on G protein to environmental signals.

Gilmer's splint Steel wire fastening in mandibular fracture.

Gimbernat's ligament Inguinal ligament described by Gimbernat.

gingiva Gum which is the part of the oral mucosa overlying the crowns of unerupted teeth

gingival Related to gingivae.

gingivitis Infection and inflammation of the gingivae. Common clinical entities are:

- Senile gingivitis
- Dilantin (anti epileptic drug) gingivitis
- Marginal gingivitis
- Vincent's acute necrotizing gingivitis
- Tubercular gingivitis
- Herpetic gingivitis
- Hormonal gingivitis
- Ulcerative gingivitis
- Eruptive gingivitis
- Haemorrhagic gingivitis

Giraldés' organ Paradidymis described by Giraldés.

girdle Anatomical structure which has encircling zone such as Pelvic girdle and pectoral girdle

glabella Smooth area on the frontal bone between the superciliary arches.

glacial That which is like an ice or white in resemblance or in pure form such as glacial acetic acid

glandular That which is related with gland

glandule It means a small gland.

glans A small round mass such as glans penis, glans clitoris

glare Due to bright light a condition of dimness of vision . This is due to depressed central vision by bright light.

Glasgow Coma Scale

Eyes open	Spontaneously	4
	To speech	3
	To pain	2
	never	1
Best verbal response	Oriented	5
	Confused	4
	In appropriate word	3
	In comprehensible sound	2
	none	1
Best motor response	Obeys commands	5
	Localises pain	4
	Flexion to pain	3
	Extension to pain	2
	none	1
	Total	3 to 14
	Unarousable coma	Score 10
	To be done repeatedly to assess improvement or deterioration.	

Glasgow's sign In case of asymptomatic aneurysm of the aorta, systolic sound in brachial artery is heard.

glass The transparent brittle and hard material which is manufactured by silica, calcium and fused amorphous silicates. Common utility of glass are a) optical glass b) Cover glass.

glasses spectacles used in the correction of refractive errors. Bifocal glasses and contact glasses are common in use.

Glauber's salt This is Sodium Sulfate discovered by Glauber.

glaucoma Eye diseases characterized by an increase in intraocular pressure that produce pathological changes in the optic disk and defects in the field of vision.

gleet Purulent discharge from urethra which is normally by gonococcal infection.

glenoid Socket like such as glenoid cavity.

Gley's glands Accessory Thyroid Gland described by Gley.

glioma Tumour of the brain and spinal cord which include astrocytoma and medulloblastoma.

globin This is the protein of haemoglobin.

globule This can be a small drop or a small mass.

globulin They are serum globulin which belong to plasma protein.

glomerulonephritis Infection and inflammation of the capillary loops in the glomeruli of the kidney.

glomerulus It is renal glomerulus which is composed of blood vessels and nerves.

glossa Name for the tongue

Glossina Glossina palpalis which is called tsetse flies which transmit Trypanosoma infections.

glossitis Infection and inflammation of the tongue.

glossopharyngeal That which is related with tongue and pharynx.

glottis Vocal cord and vocal opening are called the vocal apparatus

glucagon The hormone secreted by alpha cells of islets of Langerhans. It stimulates the relese of insulin. It stimulates gluconeogenesis.

glucan It can be any one of the polysaccharide like glycogen, starch or cellulose which is the polymer of glucose.

glucan transferase This is an enzyme which is responsible for the transfer of chain shifting in glucans from one site to another usually 1-4 glucan transferase.

glucocerebroside They are present in other than nervous tissue. If the glucose is present in nervous tissue it is pathological. Common example is Gaucher's disease.

glucocorticoid They are steroids produced by adrenal cortex which is responsible for the metabolism of protein fat and carbohydrate. They also inhibit adrenocorticotropic hormone. Glucocorticoid are responsible for blood pressure, muscle tone gastric secretion inhibit immune system.

glucogenesis Formation of glucose from products of glycolysis.

glucogenic Producing glucose.

glucokinase Present in microorganisms and is responsible for phosphorylation of D glucose at 6 carbon atom.

glucokinin They are present in yeast and vegetables which act similar to insulin in animals.

gluconeogenesis Glucose production from amino acids also called gluconeogenesis.

glucosamine Generally present in blood group substances and are polysaccharides that is found acetylated.

glucosazone Yellow crystalline substance produced by the reaction of glucose with phenyl hydrazine which identifies glucose.

glucose It is the constituent of fruits, plants, blood usually in the form of D glucose It is an aldohexose monosaccharide that is the chief source of energy in the body. Excess glucose is converted into glycogen and is stored in liver and muscle in the body.

glucose-6-phosphatase It is present in liver kidney intestinal that control blood glucose level. This enzyme catalysed the dephosphorylation of glucose 6 phosphate. Deficiency of this enzyme results in Glycogen Storage Disease.

glucose-6-phosphate dehydrogenase This help in oxidation of Glucose 6 Phosphate to lactone which is the first step in glucose metabolism.

glucoside Any sugar (mon di or poly) that contain glucose is called glucoside which is also called Glycoside.

glucosidolytic causing the splitting up of glucosides.

glue Adhesive preparation of impure gelatin from boiling certain animal substances

glutamic acid his is a nonessential amino acid in the form of α-amino glutaric acid present in in proteins. They function as neurotransmitters of CNS system.

glutaraldehyde Chemically it is $C_5H_8O_2$ and is a disinfectant used to sterilize thermometer, endoscope plastic and rubber catheter and gloves. It is used in the treatment of warts by dermatologists.

glutathione It is a tripeptide present in animal and plant tissue that maintains disulfide bonds in proteins in tern help in transport of amino acids across cell membrane.

gluteal That which is related with buttock.

glycemia Presence of glucose in the blood

glyceraldehyde Oxidation of glycerol produces glyceraldehyde is an aldehyde from triose .

glyceric acid This is a hydroxyl acid derivative that is an intermediate product of glucose metabolism.

glycerin By product of soap with the formula $C_3H_8O_3$ that is commonly used as solvent and vehicle in pharmaceutical preparations. It is used as cathartic (rectal), as diuretic (oral) in Glaucoma

glycerol Intermediate product in carbohydrate metabolism and in fat metabolism. It is trihydroxy sugar alcohol. Glycerin is the commercial preparation available.

glycine This is chemically aminoacetic acid which is a nonessential amino acid present in proteins. It inhibits neurotransmission of CNS system

glycogen Polysaccharide present in plants and animals particularly in liver and muscle. It is used whenever it is required for the body.

glycogenesis This denote the production of glucose.

glycogenolysis By digestion and phosphorylation glycogen is broke down into glucose by the process of hydrolysis.

glycol A solvent and a plasticizer which belong to aliphatic dihydric alcohol.

glycolysis Conversation of glucose to simpler compounds that enabling the body to store energy in the form of ATP.

glycoprotein They include mucoproteins and proteoglycans which are conjugated proteins.

glycoside Any chemical compound that contain sugar molecule. Common glycoside are cardiac glycosides.

glycosuria Presence of glucose in urine is demonstrated by chemical tests.

gm Abbreviation for **gram**.

gnathion Lowest point on the midline of mandible.

Goa powder Goa is the name of a state in South India on the west coast from which Goa power has come. This is brown powder collected in the interspace of large tree trunk which is bitter and used in the preparation of local native medicines.

goiter Swelling in front of neck by thyroid gland .

goitrogen Any substance that can produce goiter

gold An element with the symbol Au . Gold has medicinal value in some of the diseases including arthritis.

Goldberg's syndrome Galactosialidosis described by Goldberg.

Goldenhar's syndrome Oculoauriculovertebral dysplasia described by Goldenhar.

Goldflam's disease Myasthenia Gravis described by Goldflam.

Goldstein American physician won the Nobel prize for medicine in 1985 for the discovery on the cholesterol metabolism and treatment of cholesterolemia.

Golgi Italian neurologist who won the Nobel prize for medicine in 1906 for work on the structure of the nervous system.

Gombault's degeneration Progressive Hypertrophic Neuropathy described by Gombault.

gonad This refers to ovary or testis which produce gamete.

gonadotropic Anterior Pituitary hormone which stimulate the gonads.

gonadotropin Gonads stimulating hormones like F.S.H, L.H, and chorionic gonadotropin.

Gonin's operation Thermocautery treatment for retinal detachment.

goniometer Used to measure the angles of joint motion.

gonion A landmark located on the external angle of the mandible

goniopuncture Filtering operation for glaucoma .

gonioscope Ophthalmic instrument to examining the angle of anterior chamber.

goniotomy Surgical treatment for glaucoma.

gonococcus Neisseria gonorrhoea which cause gonorrhoea.

gonorrhea One of S.T.D which is known to cause Ophthalmia neonatorum, urethritis, salpingitis, oophoritis, arthritis and meningitis

Good's syndrome Immunodeficiency with thymoma described by Good.

Goodell's sign It is a sign of pregnancy which is softening of the cervix of uterus.

Goodman's syndrome Acro Cephalo Syndactyly type IV described by Goodman.

Goodsall's rule A rule for grouping or classifying anal fistulae. Opening in the posterior half of perianal area means fistulae open in posterior half of anus. Opening in anterior half of perianal area means fistulae open in anterior half of anus.

Gopalan's syndrome *Gopalan, an* Indian biochemist who was Director of National Institute of Nutrition Hyderabad India described the syndrome and hence the name. Burning feet syndrome which consists of burning sensation in legs, feeling of pins and needles in distal parts and hyperhidrosis in riboflavin deficiency in malnutrition.

Gordon Scottish obstetrician who first demonstrated Puerperal fever epidemic in Aberdeen in the year 1795 which is the historic even in Public health early to Ignaz Philipp Semmelweis.

Gordon's reflex, sign This sign is positive in case of pyramidal tract disease. Dorsiflexion of all toes occurs when calf muscle is pressed upon.

Gordon's syndrome Increased absorption of chloride by renal tubules produce pseudoaldosteronism with hypertension, hyperkalemia.

Gorham's disease Disappearing Bone Disease associated with multiple haemangioma and trauma described by Gorham.

Gorlin formula Estimating the area of the opening of a cardiac valve by calculating flow through the opening and pressure gradient across the concerned valve.

Goslee tooth Artificial tooth with metal base which can be interchanged.

Gossypium Latin word meaning Cotton.

gossypol From cotton seed which has male antifertility action by affecting the function of seminiferous tubules.

Gougerot-Blum syndrome Pigmented lichenoid and purpuric skin changes described by Gougerot and Blum.

goundou Yaws manifestation producing distortion of face feature due to periostitis of nasal and maxillary bones. It is also called as endemic syphilis.

gout Defects in Purine metabolism producing Hyper uricemia, arthritis crystal deposits around joints and urolithiasis.

Gowers' tract Spino Cerebellar Tract described by Gowers.

GP Abbreviation for **G**eneral **P**ractitioner

G6PD Glucose **6 P**hosphate **D**ehydrogenase

GPI Abbreviation for **G**eneral **P**aralysis of the **I**nsane.

GPT Abbreviation for **G**lutamic **P**yruvic **T**ransaminase

gr Abbreviation for **grain**

graafian follicle Follicle of the ovary described by Graaf

gracile Delicate with reference to a structure.

grade Refers to score obtained such as Nutritional grades, Gleason's cancer grades etc.,

gradient Variation in different variables or different chambers such as mitral gradient, density gradient Electro chemical gradient etc.,

graduate Procurement of a degree from a university by a person. Markings on a measuring cylinder.

Graefe's knife The slender knife used in lens extraction during cataract operation.

graft Usually refers to skin graft which are done in implantation or transplantation procedure. Common grafts in use are:

- Full thickness graft
- Epidermal graft
- Split thickness skin graft
- Cartilage graft
- Nerve graft
- Patch graft
- Bone graft
- Autogenous graft
- Tube graft
- Mucosal graft
- Arteriovenous graft
- Pedicle graft
- Cable graft
- Hyperplastic graft

grafting Process of putting flaps or transplantation of skin graft.

Graham's law The law enunciated by Graham states 'The rate of diffusion of a gas through porous membranes is in inverse ratio to the square root of their density'.

Graham's test This is Radiological test to demonstrate pathology of gall bladder by I V administration (or oral) administration of iodophthalein sodium.

Graham Steell murmur This is heard in Pulmonary Hypertension and is high pitched diastolic murmur. It is best heard in left near space between second and third cartilage.

grain Latin word meaning 1/20th of one scruple i.e., 0.065 gram by weight. This also can mean a crystalline material made of a metal. Common notion is plant seed is called grain.

Gram's stain Is a method staining pathogens for identification and grouping, devised by Gram, as Gram positive and Gram negative organisms. Procedures involve:

- Thin film of suspension is prepared, dried and fixed in usual manner
  Stained with Gentian violet for 3 minutes
- Washed with gentle stream of water, slide is drained, Gram's Iodine is put and allowed to act for one minute.
- Washed and dried.
- Slide is flood with alcohol with gentle rocking. Excess of dye will diffuse into the alcohol. This is repeated till it is no longer colored by the dye. Alcohol is allowed only for two minutes, later washed with water.
- Counter stained with dilute carbol fuchsin for one minute
- washed, blotted and allowed to dry
- Examined under microscope and inferred as Gram positive if stain violet and Gram negative if stain red.

gram Greek word Gramma meaning it is a small weight. This is the basic unit of mass which is equal to 1/1000th of Kg and equal to 1 ml of water at 4°C.

grand mal French word meaning Major epilepsy.

Granger line In skull X-ray it shows the position of optic groove.

Granger sign This sign is positive in cases of extensive destruction of the mastoid among children below 2 years of age

Granit Noble Prize Winner of 1967 who discovered the chemical and physiological visual processes of the eye.

Granit's loop This is gamma loop devised by Granite.

granula This refers to small grain also called as granule.

granule Any small particle, any grain , any small piece of tissue or even a small pill for medicamentation. Common granules of medical importance are:

- Red granules
- Nissl's granules
- Elementary granules
- Zymogen granules
- Sulphur granules
- Cytoplasmic granules
- Schûffner's granules
- Acidophil granules
- Chromatic granules
- Protein granules
- Basophilic granules
- Neutrophil granules
- Paschen's granules
- Metachromatic granules
- Dense granules
- Seminal granules

granulocyte This refers to granular leukocytes.

granulocytopenia Granular leukocytes are less in number in blood count which is pathological

granulocytosis Granular leukocytes are more in number in blood count which is also pathological.

granuloma Collection of macrophages, collection of mononuclear inflammatory cells, This refers to granulomatosis which means there is chronic inflammatory process in the tissue.

granulosa The oophorus cell

graph The diagrammatic representation of data on graph sheet.

-graph Suffix to denote the instrument which writes or records a given thing.

Grasset's phenomenon see under This is positive in incomplete hemiplegia where patient cannot raise both limbs simultaneously.

Grasset phenomenon It is a sign of incomplete hemiplegia where patient is unable to raise both lower limbs at the same time.

Grasset-Gaussel-Hoover sign In case hemiparesis of lower limb there is greater downward pressure on to the examiner's hand with the sound limb.

grating Grill like structure

Gratiolet's radiating fibers Optical radiation fibers described by Gratiolet.

grave Serious in nature such as grievous injury.

Graves' disease An autoimmune disease of Thyroid hyperplasia common in women. Goitre and Orbitopathy are common manifestations.

gravid One who is pregnant

gravida In reference to pregnant women for her pregnancy count such as Primigravida, Gravida II Gravida III etc.,

gravitation Natural Phenomenon of attraction between mass according to law of gravitation force.

gravity Gravitational attraction at the surface of the earth. Common Physical terminology with reference to gravity are; a) Standard gravity and b) Specific gravity.

gray Colour between white and black. It also states the unit of absorbed radiation dose equal to 100 rads.

Greenfield's disease Infantile form of Leukodystrophy described by Greenfield.

Greig's syndrome Ocular hypertelorism described by Greig.

grief Human mourning particularly for the loss of life which is self limited in a reasonable time.

Griesinger's sign Seen in thrombosis of transverse sinus which produce oedematous swelling behind the mastoid process.

Griffith's sign Sign of Grave's disease where lower lid lag on upward gaze.

Griscelli syndrome This is called hypopigmentation immunodeficiency disease which is an autosomal recessive disorder. This has the clinical manifestations of a) hypomelanosis, pyogenic infection, liver enlargement, spleen enlargement, thrombopenia.

Grisel's syndrome Among children subluxation of Atlanto Axial joint occurs after U R I or after adenoidectomy

griseofulvin An antifungal antibiotic used in the treatment of skin and nail fungal infections. It is produced from Penicillium griseofulvum fungus

Gritti's amputation Disarticulation of knee where patella is fused to distal end of femur bone.

Grocco's triangle In case of pleural effusion, dullness on the back which is on a triangular area can be elicited on the side opposite to that of a pleural effusion.

Groenouw's type I and type II corneal dystrophy Granular corneal dystrophy and Macular corneal dystrophy described by Groenouw as type I and type II corneal dystrophy.

groove This refers to a shallow linear depression on any anatomical structure. Common grooves are medical importance are:

- Labial groove
- Infra orbital groove
- Costal groove
- Bicipital groove
- Pharyngeal groove
- Optic groove
- Aortic groove
- Genital groove
- Dental groove
- Inter tubercular groove
- Ulnar groove
- Olfactory groove
- Nail groove
- Vertebral groove
- Carotid groove
- Buccal groove

gross That which is visible to the naked eye or visible one.

ground-glass Hazy radiological appearance

grouping Classification of entities with the criteria of their characteristics. Blood grouping and Haptenic grouping are common clinical grouping.

growth Growth is increase in physical growth and increase in size.

Gruber's reaction Widal reaction described by Gruber , a test used in the diagnosis of enteric fevers. (Typhoid and Para Typhoid)

Grynfeltt's hernia Lumbar hernia described by Grynfeltt.

GTH Abbreviation for **G**onado **T**ropic **H**ormone.

GTT Abbreviation for Glucose Tolerance Test.

guanidine Product of metabolism present in urine. It is used in Laboratory research.

guanine This is purine base which go to form nucleoside by combining with ribose which is the component of nucleic acids.

guard Any protective device such as mouth guard, dental guard etc.,

gubernaculum Any anatomical structure that guides such as Gubernaculum testis,

Gubler's tumor A wrist tumour which is associated with lead poisoning and has paralysi of extensors of hand.

Gudden's commissure Supra Optic Commissures described by Gudden. .

Guérin's fold Valvula fossa navicularis described by Guerin.

guide Passing the sound through bougie, passing a guide in stricture of the urethra.

guillotine French word denoting an instrument which is used in tonsillectomy or uvulectomy.

Guidi's canal Pterygoid canal described by Guidi.

Guillain-Barré syndrome Acute Idiopathic Polyneuritis described by Guillain and Barre.

guinea pig Common laboratory animal used in experiments

Gull's disease Myxoedema from atrophy of Thyroid described by Gull.

gullet Colloquially called for the anatomical part Oesophagus.

Gullstrand Swedish ophthalmologist who won Noble Prize for his discovery on Optical image formation in the eye.

gum Gingival tissue in mouth. Plant secretion used as gum material.

Gumboro disease Infectious Bursal disease first described in Gumboro place and hence the name.

gumma Tertiary syphilis which is the third stage of syphilis disease caused by Treponema pallidum. Any organ may be involved. Usually liver, bone, testes, brain are commonly attacked.

Günther disease Congenital Erythropoietic Porphyria described by Gunther.

Günz's ligament The end portion of Obturator membrane described by Gunz.

gurney Hospital cot which will have wheels

gustation This refers to the taste.

gut Colloquial word for the intestine.

Guthrie's muscle Urethral Sphincter Muscle described by Guthrie.

gutta This refers to a drop in measure of pharmacy preparations.

gymnastics This is an athletic word denoting a systematic muscular exercise.

gynatresia Atresia referable to vaginal atresia.

gynecium As opposed to Androecium, gynoecium is female part of a flower.

gynecoid When a person looks like a woman called feminine.

gynecologic Any thing affecting the female reproductive tract.

gynecological That which is related with gynecology.

gynecologist A person specialized and is consultant in Gynecology.

gynecology Branch of medicine that treats the diseases of the genital tract in women.

gynecomastia Breast development in males because of hormonal imbalance.

gypsum This is calcium sulphate which can get converted to plaster of Paris when calcined.

gyrate That which looks like a spiral ring.

gyrus They are brain convolutions that are seen on the surface of the brain.

H

H Symbol for Hydrogen.

H_0 Symbol for Null Hypothesis.

Habermann's disease This refers to Acute Lichenoid Pityriasis described by Habermann.

habit An established habit of an individual such as food habit, sleeping habit, bowel habit or reading habit.

habitat Natural abode of an animal or plant

Haemagogus It is the name of genus of mosquitoes present in South America which transmits Jungle Yellow Fever.

Haemaphysalis Genus of Hard tick which are responsible in spreading Rickettsial infection, K.F.D. H.spinegera is common in South East Asia.

Haemophilus Gram negative aerobic bacteria common causative organism for U R I.

Hagedorn's needles They are surgical needles flat from side to side. Have straight cutting edge near the point and have a large eye.

Hagner's disease This refers to Hypertrophic Pulmonary Osteoarthropathy which was first studied in a family of Hagner and hence the name.

Hahnemannian pertaining to Christian Friedrich Samuel *Hahnemann*, German physician, 1755–1843, founder of homeopathy.

HAI Abbreviation for **H**em-**a**gglutination **I**nhibition test.

Hailey-Hailey disease This refers to Benign Familial Pemphigus described by Hailey and Hailey.

hair This is appendage of the skin consist of keratin. Shaft, hair bulb and hair papilla are the parts of the structure of hair.

hairball Chronic accumulation of hair in the stomach to form a bundle called Trichobezoar, which needs surgical intervention.

Hakim's syndrome This refers to Normal Pressure Hydrocephalus described by Hakim.

Haldane chamber It is called Haldane chamber where animals are confined for metabolic studies and the chamber is air tight chamber.

half-life In case of elementary particle or in case of radionuclide half like is the time required for the decay of half of a sample of particles. It is also denoted by decay constant with symbol $t_{1/2}$ or $T_{1/2}$. which is also called half like of an element.

half-time In case of administered substance in the body, the time required for one half of a quantity of a substance to be eliminated from the system

half-value It is HVL called Half Value Thickness which describe the thickness of a given substance that will reduce the intensity of a beam of radiation to one half of its initial value.

halitosis Latin word meaning bad and offensive breath commonly by liver pathology called fetor hepaticus.

Hall's sign It is a shock called Tracheal diastolic shock felt in anaeurysm of the aorta.

Hallermann-Streiff syndrome This is referred to Oculo Mandubular Syndrome described by Hallermann and Streiff.

hallucination Latin word meaning a perception without any external source for that. We have visual hallucination, auditory hallucination, gustatory hallucination, Olfactory hallucination,

hallucinogen A drug, a chemical or a substance which produces hallucinations.

hallux This refers to Great Toe which is the first digit of the food. In clinical practice, we come across Hallux valgus, Hallux Varus

Hallwachs effect This refers to Photo Electric Effect described by Hallwachs in his physiology experiment.

halogen They are salt like chemical compound with sodium. The halogens in chemical table are Fluorine, chlorine, iodine

haloperidol Anti Psychotic drug used in Psychoses.

halothane An anesthetic agent used in General anesthesia which has proved good induction and good recovery.

Halsted's mastectomy This refers to Radical Mastectomy described by Halsted.

hamartoma Overgrowth of mature cells which show disorganized in histopathological examination. It is benign tumour like nodule which is common in pulmonary tissue and epithelial tissue.

Hamilton's, test It is useful to detect the luxation of shoulder joint. When a ruler is applied to humerus can be made to touch the outer condyle and the acromion at the same time.

hamster Rodent family animals used in laboratory for research purpose.

hamstring Muscle tendon that come in the popliteal fossa. Inner hamstring is by tendons of gracilis, sartorius and two other muscles. Outer hamstring is by tendon of biceps flexor femoris.

hamycin Antibiotic used in Trichomonal infection and in Fungal infections which is derived by Streptomyces pimprina.

Hand Distal end of upper limb which has five fingers and palm

H and E stain This refers to Hematoxylin and Eosin stains.

handedness This is commonly referable to Right handedness where person gives preference to use all voluntary motor acts in right hand. Quite opposite is left handedness which show low proportion of people.

handicap If a person is incapacitated to work and cannot have normal life because of physical defect or mental defect.

handle To help in grasping a big item, a part is provided to hold the item.

Hannover's canal A space which is potential in nature is available just in front and in back of suspensory ligament of the lens.

Hansen's bacillus Leprosy causing Mycobacterium leprae discovered by Hansen.

Hantavirus The word origin is name of river Hantaan in Korea where Epidemic hemorrhagic Fever or Pneumonia occurred caused by this virus.

haploid Gamete cell containing one of each pair of homologous chromosomes. Single set chromosome cell in reproductive cell division or meiosis.

hapten It is a micro molecule that can conjugate with a protein to form a carrier. Antibody production involves activation of B lymphocytes by the haptens and helper T lymphocytes by the carrier.

Harada syndrome This is found significantly associated with trauma during birth of a child and is characterized by the following manifestations:

- Both side athetosis
- Inabilities to walk
- Outburst of crying
- Disrupted speech
- Marbled appearance
- Mental retardation

It is also called Vogt Koyanagi Harada Syndrome.

harara Post sand fly bite syndrome with skin reactions. It is called Epidemic Urticaria.

Harden-Young ester This refers to Fructose 1,6 Biphosphate described by Harden and Young.

hardening This refers to induration and sclerosis of an area. In case of tissue preparation by process of rendering tissue firm for microscopic examination, where hardening help to cut the tissue.

hardness This refers to hardness of water which can be temporary or permanent in nature that can be due to bicarbonates in temporary hardness and due to sulphate, chlorides in permanent hardness. The unit of expression is PPM or mEq per litre.

Hardy-Weinberg law This refers to an equilibrium in Population gene tics described by Hardy and Weinberg. The law states that Alleles (say Tall=A and Dwarf =a) determine the proportions of genotypes in nature (say AA, Aa and aa) This follows the equation as under;

$(a+b)^2 = a^2+2ab+b^2$

That can be as .... aa + 2a b + bb

Or AA, Aa and aa

Which can describe AA=Tall, Aa= middle aa= dwarf

The law states that this equilibrium can be altered by many factors which are described as under:

- Mutation
- Selection
- Non random mating,
- Migration
- Genetic drift

Etc., in the community.

harelip Other name for Cleft lip which is a birth defect.

harmony Smooth working of organs in the body.

harpoon Surgical instrument used for removal of tissues for biopsy.

Harrison's groove This groove becomes prominent in children in rickets. The Harrison's groove is the depression along the lower border of the thorax corresponding to the costal insertion of the diaphragm.

Hartline American physician and physiologist who won Nobel Prize in 1967 for his work on chemical and physiological visual processes in the eye.

Harvey William Harvey (1578–1657). English physician who discovered Blood circulation in the body. His discovery gave fantastic report of heart function such as:

- Heart contraction and pulse coincide
- Pulse is an indication of filling up of arteries with blood
- Cardiac septum do not allow percolation
- Blood circulates from right ventricle to arteries of lung to pulmonary veins to left ventricle and thence through arteries to the body
- Comes back through veins to right ventricle.

Hashimoto's disease Thyroiditis described by Hashimoto which is an auto immune disease.

hashish Arabic word meaning herb. This is from female help plant called Cannabis sativa that has the intoxicating effect on the body. Marijuana is it's equivalent colloquial word.

Hassall's corpuscles They are spherical bodies present in thymus that contain epithelial cells with cytoplasmic filaments.

hatchet Dental instrument to break down tooth structure undermined by caries.

HAV Abbreviation for **H**epatitis **A** **v**irus.

haversian canal This is the nutrient canal of bone

HB_s Abbreviation for **H**epatitis **B** **s**urface antigen. Also denoted as **HBsAg**

Hb Abbreviation for **H**aemoglo**b**in.

HbO_2 Refer to Oxyhaemoglobin.

HCG Abbreviation for **H**uman **C**horionic **G**onadotropin.

HDCV Abbreviation for **H**uman **D**iploid **C**ell Rabies **V**accine.

HDL Abbreviation for **H**igh **D**ensity **L**ipoprotien

head Upper most part of human body that contain vital nervous system and special senses. This is referred to as Caput.

headache Pain in the head neurological or otherwise that are found to be due to anaemia, migraine, congestion, dynamite sound, exertion, emotional upset, histaminic reaction in the body, intra cranial pathology, post traumatic, high fever, nasal diseases, poisoning,

Heaf test This refers to Tuberculin test described by Heaf.

heal Refers to healing process which is restoration of wounded parts by repair through granulation or without granulation process.

health According to World Health Organisation it is a state of optimal physical, mental, and social well-being, and not merely the absence of disease and infirmity. Common terms used or Occupation health, public health, holistic health.

hearing Latin word meaning to hear a special sense to perceive sound. Hearing loss is called deafness which is a disability.

heart Main organ of blood circulation that contains two atria and two ventricles. Left atrium received pure blood from lungs. Through left ventricle and aorta blood goes to all parts of the body. The right atrium received impure blood which passes through right ventricle to lung where it gets oxygenated. Mitral valve, Tricuspid valve, Aortic valve land Pulmonary valves help in the process of physiological circulation.

heartbeat This denotes one complete cardiac cycle helped through electrical impulses.

heart block This refers to impairment of conduction of an impulse in heart excitation commonly referable to A.V. block.

heartburn Hotness and discomfort in food pipe area due to gastroesophageal reflux. This is retrosternal sensation of warmth due to acidity.

heart failure Heart when fails to function normally in cardiac pathology.

heatstroke Due to exposure to excessive heat, body is reacted with dryness of skin, vertigo, headache, thirst, nausea and muscle cramps.

hebephrenia Disorganised schizophrenia and the person with this manifestation is called hebephrenic.

Heberden's disease Rheumatism of distal interphalangeal joints which also show nodule formation.

hebetic Greek word which denote youthful or puberty. Hence the word is used for the event that occur at the time of puberty.

hedonism Main aspect of human behavior which avoids pain and always wants pleasure seeking behavior.

Hegar dilator Hegar dilators are widely used in gynecology **to open up the cervix**

height Vertical measurement of body.

HeLa cells He La was a cancer patient from whom cervical cancer cells were isolated in 1951. First cultured carcinoma cells used for research purpose.

Helicobacter Gram negative bacteria which cause gastritis, colitis which were formerly called as campylobacter.

Heller's plexus This refers to arterial network in intestinal submucosa described by Heller.

Heller-Döhle disease This refers to Syphilitic aortitis described by Heller and Dohle.

helminth They are parasites belonging cestoda, trematoda and nematode group.

helminthology Scientific study of parasitic worms.

Helweg's bundle This refers to Olivospinal Tract described by Helweg.

hemacytometer This is a blood count instrument used in haematology.

hemagglutination Clumping together of RBC due to haemagglutinins, influenza virus, mumps virus, lectins.

hemangioma Common but benign tumour of blood vessels which can be capillary haemangioma or cavernous haemangioma. They are due to malformation of angioblastic tissues in embryo stage.

Hematemesis Vomiting of blood

hematin Haeme is oxidized to form haematin which stimulates the formation of globin.

hematocele Effusion of blood into the tunica vaginalis testis.

hematocolpometra Accumulation of menstrual blood in the vagina and uterus.

hematocolpos Accumulation of menstrual blood in the vagina.

hematocrit This refers to Wintrobe Haematocrit tube used for packed RBC count.

Hematoid That which is related with blood

hematology Area of medical science that deals with the blood and blood-forming tissues.

hematoma Localised blood clot inside muscle or other tissues.

hematomanometer B.P. apparatus of sphygmomanometer which can be a) Mercury type, b) Anaeroid type and c) digital type.

hematometra Accumulation of blood in the uterus.

hematopoiesis Formation and development of blood cells.

hematoxylin An indicator of pH (5 to 6) and is used in stain preparation.

hematuria Presence of blood in the urine.

heme Combines with globin to form haemoglobin. It is pyrrole group of porphyrin

hemianopia Blindness in half of the visual field of one or both eyes

hemiparesis Partial paralysis affecting one side of the body.

hemiparesthesia Perverted sensation on one side of the body.

hemiplegia Paralysis of one side of the body. Common types are:

- Flaccid hemiplegia
- Contralateral hemiplegia
- Cerebral hemiplegia
- Infantile hemiplegia
- Crossed hemiplegia

Hemiptera insect with piercing or sucking apparatus such as Reduvid bug which has public health importance.

Hemiscotosis Other name for Hemianopia.

hemisphere One half of any spherical anatomical structure such as:

- Cerebral hemisphere

hemithorax It is one side of the chest.

hemlock Refers to poisonous herbal plant which produce fatal muscle paralysis and respiratory failure. Dried fruit portion has shown sedative, anodyne and antispasmodic effects on the body.

haemochromatosis Haemosiderin deposit in organs produces damage of liver, pancreas, heart and pituitary gland. Bronze pigmentation of skin and cirrhosis are common manifestations of haemochromatosis.

haemoconcentration Concentration of blood due to the decrease of fluid content of the blood

haemocyte It is the Blood Cell.

haemodiagnosis Diagnosis by examination of the blood.

haemodialysis With the help of haemodialysis blood is allowed to pass through semipermeable membrane to remove harmful elements of the blood, which otherwise would have been cleared by the kidney.

haemodialyzer It is an equipment used in Haemodialysis.

haemodilution Hypervolemia due to decrease in RBC count and blood will show an increase of fluid content.

Haemofil Available preparation of Coagulation Factor VIII.

haemoflagellate flagellate parasites in the blood, especially suborder Trypanosomatidae.

haemoglobin Blood pigment of RBC which carry oxygen which is a haemoprotein that contains Haeme and Globin. Existing available types are:

- Hb A normal adult type and common
  Bb A_2 normal adult but rare
- HB Bart's in Hydrops foetalis
- Hb C molecular abnormality
- HB D, E, G, H, I, M, and S(sickle cell trait) are abnormal
- DeOxy Hb
- Hb F foetal
- HB Muscle Myoglobin
- Hb Portland, foetal, normal later disappears

haemoglobinometer Instrument for measuring the hemoglobin of the blood.

haemoglobinopathy Inherited abnormalities of Hb such as Sickle cell anaemia, Haemolytic anaemia, Thalassemia etc.,

haemogram Blood picture a common investigation by blood examination.

haemolysis Breaking up and release of Hb from RBC caused by haemolysins, by antibodies.

haemolytic That which is related haemolysis.

haemopericardium Blood within the pericardium.

Haemoperitoneum Blood in the peritoneal cavity.

haemophil Pathogens that thrive in blood. .

haemophilia Royal disease carried by females and men get the disease. It is manifested by the bleeding in subcutaneous tissue, intramuscular bleeding, bleeding from mouth gum lip tongue and joints. It is sex linked disorder. Common types are:

a) Haemophilia A due to deficiency of Coagulation Factor VIII
b) Haemophilia B due to deficiency of Coagulation Factor IX

haemophiliac Patient exhibiting hemophilia.

haemophilic Affinity for blood by bacteria like Haemophilus and Bordetella. It also means that a person is having haemophilia.

haemoprotein Protein containing Haem such as Citochrome, Myoglobin, Haemoglobin and Catalase.

haemoptysis Sputum of Phlegm containing blood. Common clinical conditions for coughing out blood are;

- Telangiectasis of tracheobronchial tree
- Cardiac
- Parasitic by Paragonimus westermani

haemorrhage Bleeding which can internal or external by origin. In case of external it can be very small called petechiae, about 1 cm called purpura and very large called ecchymosis. In tissue the bleeding becomes haematoma.

- Sub arachnoid haemorrhage
- Sub dural haemorrhage
- Post partum haemorrhage
- Petechial haemorrhage
- Brain haemorrhage
- Venous haemorrhage
- Arterial haemorrhage
- Capillary haemorrhage

- External haemorrhage
- Internal haemorrhage
- Cerebral haemorrhage
- Extra dural haemorrhage
- Massive haemorrhage
- Nasal haemorrhage
- Pulmonary haemorrhage
- Renal haemorrhage
- Splinter haemorrhage

haemorrhoid Distension dilatation and tortuosity of rectal vein which is colloquially called piles. Hemorrhoidal plexus, resulting from a persistent increase in venous pressure. The types of haemorrhoid are:

- Sentinel piles
- External piles
- Internal piles
- Prolapsed piles
- Thrombosed piles

haemorrhoidectomy Surgical excision of haemorrhoids.

haemosiderin Iron pigment in intracellular space

haemosiderosis Raised tissue iron store in the body without any tissue damage. Common tissues involved are liver and lung.

haemospermia Presence of blood in the semen.

haemostasis Bleeding is stopped by coagulation or by vasoconstriction.

haemostatic Process of arrest of blood flow or haemostasis.

haemozoin Pigment produced by malarial parasites

Hench American physician who won Nobel Prize in 1950 for his work on Rheumatoid arthritis.

Henke's triangle This is also called Henke's space which is triangle space formed by descending portion of the inguinal fold, lateral portion of the inguinal fold and lateral border of the rectus muscle.

Henle's loop This is 'U' shaped part of renal tubule from proximal convoluted tubule to distal convoluted tubule. It has descending limb, thin tubule and an ascending limb.

Henry's law One of the chemistry law postulated by Henry which states "the solubility of a gas in a liquid solution at constant temperature is proportional to the partial pressure of the gas above the solution." .

heparin It is present in liver and lungs and is produced by mast cells and basophils of blood. It has powerful anticoagulant property.

hepatic That which is related to liver.

hepatitis Infection and inflammation of the liver. Common types seen in clinical practice are:

- Hepatitis A
- Hepatitis B
- Hepatitis C
- Hepatitis D
- Hepatitis E
- Hepatitis G
- Delta hepatitis
- Fulminant hepatitis
- Alcoholic hepatitis
- Chronic active hepatitis
- Non A and non B hepatitis
- Neonatal hepatitis

hepatobiliary Related to the liver and the bile

hepatocarcinoma Liver cancer and is called Hepatocellular Carcinoma.

hepatocirrhosis cirrhosis of the liver.

hepatojugular Related with liver and jugular vein such as hepatojugular reflux.

hepatologist a specialist in liver disorders.

hepatomegaly Liver enlargement

hepatosis functional disorder of the liver.

hepatotoxic Substance which is toxic to liver cells.

hepatotoxin Toxin that destroys liver cells.

heptadactyly Seven digits on one hand or foot.

herb Plant leaves which are used medicinally or as a flavoring.

herbal Related with herbs.

Herbert's operation Surgery treatment for glaucoma.

herbivorous Animals which live on plant food.

hereditary Diseases transmitted from parent to offspring which are genetic in nature.

heredity Genetic constitution. It also means the genetic transmission of a particular quality or trait from parent to offspring. This can be autosomal or X linked.

Hering-Breuer reflex It is nervous mechanism which limits expiratory process. In ordinary breathing inspiration and expiration are lowered by sensory nerve endings in the lung. .

hermaphroditism Both male and female organs and sex characteristics are present in an individual.

hernia Through abnormal opening loop of an organ is protruded. Common surgical hernias are:

- Inguinal hernia
- Hiatal hernia
- Epigastric hernia
- Scrotal hernia
- Congenital inguinal hernia
- Cerebral hernia
- Diaphragmatic hernia
- Abdominal hernia
- Femoral hernia
- Umbilical hernia

herniorrhaphy Surgical repair of a hernia.

herniotomy Surgical operation for the repair of hernia

heroin A narcotic drug which contain Diacetyl Morphine.

herpes Infection and inflammation by Herpes virus which can be herpes simplex or herpes zoster.

herpesvirus Virus belonging to Herpesvirdae that cause herpes infection.

Hers' disease This refers to Glycogen Storage Disease described by Hers.

Herter's disease This is infantile form of celiac disease described by Herter.

hertz A unit of frequency equal to one cycle per second usually written in the form of abbreviation Hz.

Herxheimer's reaction This is short term immunological response of the body due to released endotoxin like substances. This is following the antibiotic treatment for syphilis, borreliosis, brucellosis, typhoid, trichinella infection. It is also called Jarisch Herxheimer reaction which has the following manifestations:

- Fever
- Chills
- Headache
- Myalgia
- Skin rashes

Hess Swiss physiologist who won Nobel prize in 1949 on his work 'brain functions'

Hess capillary test This refers to Tourniquet test described by Hess.

Hesselbach's triangle Inguinal triangle. It is situated in anteroinferior abdominal wall bounded by the rectus abdominis muscle, the inguinal ligament and inferior epigastric vessels. The site is common site for inguinal hernia.

heterochromosome The name given to a sex chromosome.

heterogamy Meiosis or reproduction resulting from the union of two gametes that differ in size and structure

heterogeneous Not uniform in physical appearance. In genetics the term denotes a trait that can be produced by different genes

heterometropia There are differences in degree of refraction in the two eyes.

Heterophyes Trematodes found in the middle third of the small intestine of humans an helminthic infestation.

heterosexual Related to opposite sex. Non homosexual.

Hetrazan Preparations of Diethyl Carbamazine Citrate used in Eosinophilia and in Filarial treatment.

hexadactyly Six digits on one hand or foot.

Hexapoda Six foot insects.

hexavalent Having a valence of six.

hexavitamin Common preparation containing 6 vitamins viz., vitamin A, vitamin D, ascorbic acid, thiamine hydrochloride, riboflavin and niacinamide.

hexokinase Enzyme of the transferase class that catalyzes the phosphorylation of hexose in the cellular l'utilisation of hexoses.

hexylresorcinol Used as mouthwash, skin wound cleaner, anthelminthic. This is a substituted phenol with bactericidal properties

HF Abbreviation for **H**ageman **F**actor (Factor XII) under blood coagulation.

Hg Symbol for Mercury.

HI Abbreviation for **H**emagglutination **I**nhibition

hiatus It denotes a gap, cleft, or opening. E.g.,

- Hiatus for lesser petrosal nerve
- Oesophageal hiatus
- Hiatus femoralis
- Vena Caval hiatus

Hibbs' operation It is spinal surgery to fuse vertebrae by fracturing the spinous processes and pressing the tip downward.

hibernation Dormant state in which certain animal species pass the winter through reduced metabolism and reduced body temperature.

hiccup Sudden inspiration is checked by glottis closure that cause a sound. This is also coincided by spasmodic contraction of the diaphragm.

Hickman catheter This is a central venous catheter.

Hicks' syndrome This refers to Sensory Radicular Neuropathy that is significantly a hereditary disorder.

Hicks version This is also called as Braxton Hicks version. In case non viable fetus, internal podalic version is done through partially dilated cervix.

hidradenocarcinoma Carcinoma of the sweat glands.

hidradenoma Benign tumor originating in sweat gland

Highmore's antrum This refers to Maxillary sinus described by Highmore.

Hilton's line Not visible but palpable wavy zone at internal sphincter in the anus. Also called Anal Intersphincteric Groove.

hilum A depression or pit at that part of an organ where the vessels and nerves enter. E.g., Hilum of suprarenal gland, Hilum of the kidney, Hilum of the lung etc.,

Hind Meaning posterior such as the posterior organs like rhombencephalon, hindfoot, hindgut, hind kidney etc.,

hindfoot the posterior portion of the foot, comprising the region of the talus and calcaneus.

hip Area of the body lateral to and including the hip joint.

hippocampus Curved elevation of gray matter at the floor of the temporal horn of the lateral ventricle.

Hippocrates A physician in the history of Medicine Who is known for his Oath popularly called Hippocratic Oath. His observation of fever, skin , tongue, eyes, sweat, urine and faces are descried with vague anatomy. His treat was to restore the humoral therapy.

Hippocratic Oath This is the oath of professional behavior sworn by physicians as they embark upon their medical careers which is as under:

"I swear by Apollo the physician, by Aesculapius, Hygeia, and Panacea, and I take to witness all the gods, all the goddesses, to keep according to my ability and my judgment the following Oath: To consider dear to me as my parents him who taught me this art; to live in common with him and if necessary to share my goods with him; to look upon his children as my own brothers, to teach them this art if they so desire without fee or written promise; to impart to my sons and the sons of the master who taught me and the disciples who have enrolled themselves and have agreed to the rules of the profession, but to these alone, the precepts and the instruction. I will prescribe regimen for the good of my patients according to my ability and my judgment and never do harm to anyone. To please no one will I prescribe a deadly drug, nor give advice which may cause his death. Nor will I give a woman a pessary to procure abortion. But I will preserve the purity of my life and my art. I will not cut for stone, even for patients in whom the disease is manifest; I will leave this operation to be performed by practitioners (specialists in this art). In every house where I come I will enter only for the good of my patients, keeping myself far from all intentional ill-doing and all seduction, and especially from the pleasures of love with women or with men, be they free or slaves. All that may come to my knowledge in the exercise of my profession or outside of my profession or in daily commerce with men, whom ought not to be spread abroad, I will keep secret and will never reveal. If I keep this oath faithfully, may I enjoy my life and practice my art, respected by all men and in all times; but if I swerve from it or violate it, may the reverse be my lot."

hippuric acid An acid with the formula as $C_6H_5 \cdot CO \cdot NH \cdot CH_2 \cdot COOH$ (Urobenzoic acid) Present in the urine of animals and not in normal urine of man.

Hirschfeld's canals This refers to Interdental Canals described by Hirschfeld.

Hirschsprung's disease This refers to Congenital Megacolon described by Hirschsprung.

hirsutism Adult male pattern of hair distribution in women.

His' bundle Bundle or small band of atypical cardiac muscle fibers that originates in A V node in interatrial septum. This propagates atrial contraction rhythm to ventricles.

His-Purkinje system It is called Purkinje network which is portion of the conducting system of the heart.

His-Werner disease his refers to Trench Fever described by His and Werner.

histamine Present in body tissues, lung and mast cells. Chemically it is decarboxylation product of histidine with the formula $C_5H_9N_3$ Main functions are:

- Pupillary dilatation
- Smooth muscle contraction
- Secretion of gastric secretion
- Tachycardia
- Triple response

histidine This is an essential amino acid

histogram Graphic display of a frequency distribution, represented by a series of rectangles dividing the data into classes

histoid Weblike appearance or that which looks like a cell.

histology Human Anatomy which deals with the minute structure, composition, and function of the tissues. Normal histology is taught in Anatomy and abnormal histology is taught in Pathology.

histone Histone is a simple protein such as globin of Haemoglobin. Histone is present in the urine of patient suffering from Leukaemia and High fever.

HIV Abbreviation for **H**uman **I**mmuno deficiency **V**irus

Hodge's pessary This pessary is used in retro displacement of the uterus.

Hodgkin British physiologist who won Nobel prize for Medicine in 1963 for his Discovery and work on nerve cell membrane.

Hodgkin's disease This refers to Malignant Lymphoma described by Hodgkin.

Hodgkin cycle Circular sequence of events between depolarisation and permeability to sodium occurring in excitable cells. The cycle is as under:

Depolarisation

Increased permeability to sodium

Increased entry of sodium to cell (Na^+)

Increased concentration of sodium (Na^+)

Increased permeability to sodium

Further depolarization of cell membrane

Fig: Hodgkin cycle

Hoffmann's atrophy This refers to spinal muscular atrophy described by Hoffmann.

Hoffmann's duct This refers to Pancreatic duct described by Hoffmann.

hole An opening or perforation.

Holger Nielsen method Non mechanical method of emergency artificial respiration described by Holger Nielsen.

holistic This considers the man as a functioning whole or relating to the conception of man as a functioning whole. Under health it is called Holistic approach.

Holmes Noted American physician, anatomist, and writer, whose work on Puerperal fever in 1843 is ascribed to antecedent to the work of Semmelweis in its appeal for surgical cleanliness to combat this disease.

holography Recording of images in three-dimensional form on photographic film

Homans' operation Surgery for elephantiasis. The procedure included excision of subcutaneous tissue and redundant skin on lateral and medial aspects.

homatropine Anticholinergic effects similar to but weaker than those of atropine.

Homén's syndrome This refers to Post Concession Syndrome.

homeopathy Treatment founded by Samuel Hahnemann (1755–1843), in which diseases are treated by drugs which are capable of producing in healthy persons symptoms like those of the disease to be treated, the drug being administered in minute doses.

homeostasis The internal environment of an organism which has always has the tendency to stabilize the normal body status.

homicide Latin word meaning 'to murder', taking the life of another person.

homocysteine Sulfur-containing amino acid

homocystinuria Excretion of homocysteine in the urine, a biochemical abnormality with a variety of autosomal recessive genetic disorder.

homoeroticism Sexual feeling directed toward the same sex.

homogamy This is colloquially called Inbreeding.

homogeneous That contains similar elements or ingredients and which is clear.

homogenous Similarity of structure. Descent from a common ancestor.

homogentisic acid an aromatic hydrocarbon formed as an intermediate in the catabolism of *tyrosine* and *phenylalanine.* In case of Alkaptonuria it is accumulated abnormally and excreted in the urine

homologous In Greek it means corresponding. This correspondence is in with reference to structure, position and origin of an organ or a tissue.

homonymous It pertains to the corresponding vertical halves of the visual fields of both eyes. Viz.,
Nasal half of left eye and temporal half of right eye.
Temporal half of left eye and nasal of right eye.

homosexual One who is sexually attracted to persons of the same sex.

homosexuality Refers to sexual orientation in case of homosexuals.

homozygous That which possess a pair of identical alleles at a given locus

hookworm Nematode of the family Ancylostomatidae Common hookworm in India are:
- Ancylostoma duodenale
- Necator americanus

Hoover's sign In case of genuine paralysis and in normal condition, if the patient lying on a flat surface is directed to press the whole lower limb against the surface, there will be a lifting movement in the opposite limb. This phenomenon is absent in hysteria and malingering.

HOP Abbreviation for the regimen in the treatment of cancer which contain **H**ydroxydaunomycin, **O**ncovin and **P**rednisone.

Hope's sign Double heart beat in Aortic Aneurysm.

Hopkins British biologist who won Nobel Prize in 1929 for his discovery of the growth-stimulating vitamins.

hordeolum Localized, purulent, inflammatory staphylococcal infection of one or more sebaceous glands,

hormone In Greek it means 'to set in motion' Definition as per old concept was "substance secreted by Endocrine glands and transported in blood to distant target organ". But present concept is different and it defines the hormone as "Various substances having similar actions but not produced by special glands. Major hormones of the body are:
- Adrenocortical hormone
- Growth hormone
- Follicle stimulating hormone
- Luteinizing hormone
- Antidiuretic hormone
- Progesterone
- Oestrogen
- Gastrin
- Secretin
- Cholecystokinin hormone
- Gonadotropin hormone
- Prolactin
- Parathormone
- Chorionic gonadotropin
- Vasopressin
- Testosterone
- Thyroid stimulating hormone

Horner's law It is related to the transmission of colour blindness. Ordinary colour blindness is transmitted from males to males through normal females.

Horner's sign If positive it indicates death of fetus in X-ray. In the X-ray film of the fetus in uterus, overriding of the bones of the vault of the skill is present in positive sign.

hospice Facility provided directly or indirectly to palliative and supportive care for terminally ill patients and their families

hospital An Institution or an organization meant for the treatment of the sick and ill. Latin word meaning hospes, host or guest. The base hospital, the Camp hospital and the Teaching hospital are common ones seen in the society. The hospital is defined as:
"An institution suitably located, constructed, organized, managed and personneled, to supply, scientifically,

economically, efficiently and unhindered, all or any recognized part of the complex requirements for the prevention, diagnosis, and treatment of physical, mental, and the medical aspect of social ills; with functioning facilities for training new workers in the many special professional, technical and economic fields essential to the discharge of its proper functions; and with adequate contacts with physicians, other hospitals, medical schools and all accredited health agencies engaged in the better health program."

hospitalization Confinement of a patient in a hospital for the purpose of treatment

host Animal or man who harbors another organism (parasite). Definite host and intermediate host are common types of hosts.

hot line Phone assistance for crisis intervention to prevent suicide and mental patients to back up their lives.

Hounsfield British research scientist winner of Nobel Prize for his discovery of computerized axial tomography in 1979.

Houssay Argentine physiologist who won Nobel Prize in 1947 for his discovery of Pituitary gland work and diabetes.

Hoverbed Bed used for Burn patients in their treatment.

Howell's bodies This is present in patient after removal of spleen, in megaloblastic anaemia and in haemolytic anaemia. It is also called Howell-Jolly bodies.

HRIG Abbreviation for Human Rabies Immune Globulin.

HTLV Abbreviation for Human T Lymphotropic virus I, II and III types.

Hueck's ligament This refers to Trabecular ligament described by Hueck.

hum Indistinct, low, prolonged sound such as venous hum.

humerus The humerus is **the largest bone of the upper extremity** and defines the human brachium (arm). It articulates proximally with the glenoid via the glenohumeral (GH) joint and distally with the radius and ulna at the elbow joint.

humidity Water content in the air or the degree of moisture. Usual description of Absolute and relative humidity is seen in meteorological environment.

humoral Related to elements dissolved in the blood or body fluids

hump This denotes to a rounded eminence.

humpback This refers to Kyphosis.

Humphry's ligament This refers to anterior femoral ligament described by Humphry.

Hunter's canal This refers to Adductor canal which is an intramuscular interval on the medial aspect of the middle third of the thing, which contains the femoral vessels and the saphenous nerve.

Hunter's ligament This refers to Ligamentum teres uteri. Described by Hunter.

Huntington's chorea Autosomal dominant disorder which show progressive chorea and mental deterioration. .

hyaline glassy and transparent such as Hyaline membrane.

hyaluronic acid This is present in cartilage, vitreous fluid, synovial fluid and chemically glycosaminoglycan.

hyaluronidase This enzyme helps in breakdown of hyaluronic acid. They are hyaluronate lyase, hyaluronoglucosaminidase, and hyaluronoglucuronidase

hybrid Animal or plant produced from parents different in kind

hybridization Cross breeding.

Hydatid Referred to cyst like structure such as Hydatid cyst.

hydramnios Excess of amniotic fluid.

hydrocarbon Organic compound that contains carbon and hydrogen only. According to atom arrangement they may be Alicyclic or Aromatic.

hydrocele Collection of fluid in the tunica vaginalis of the testicle or along the spermatic cord.

hydrocephalus Clinical condition occurring secondarily to obstruction of the cerebrospinal fluid pathways that produces enlargement of the head, prominent forehead, brain atrophy and other neurological manifestations.

hydrochloric acid Aqueous solutions of hydrogen chloride

hydrocortisone Drug used in inflammations, allergies, pruritus, collagen diseases. Both natural and synthetic hydrocortisone are available.

hydrogen Element present in water and all organic compound.

hydrolase Enzymes that catalyze the cleavage of a chemical bond with the addition of water Common hydrolases are esterases, glycosidases, lipases, nucleotidases, peptidases, and phosphatases.

hydrometer Instrument for determining the specific gravity of a fluid.

hydrophobia Irrational fear of water. This is colloquial term for rabies.

hydrops Latin word meaning oedema such as Hydrops amnii, foetal hydrops,

hydrotherapy Water is used for externally in illness.

hydrothorax Pleurisy with effusion.

hydroxide When hydroxyl radical (OH) is present

Hygeia Goddess of health daughter of Aesculapius.

hygiene Science of health and of its preservation.

hygroma cyst or bursa distended with a fluid.

hygrometer This device is used to measure humidity.

hygroscopic Retaining moisture readily.

hymen Fold which occludes the external orifice of the vagina.

Hymenolepis Tapeworms of the family Hymenolepididae.

hyoscyamine Anticholinergic alkaloid

hyperacidity Excessive degree of acidity.

hyperbilirubinemia Excessive concentrations of bilirubin in the blood
hypercalcemia Excess of calcium in the blood
hypercapnia Excess of carbon dioxide in the blood.
hypercholesteremia High content of cholesterol in the blood.
hyperchromatic Staining more intensely than is normal.
hypercupremia Excess of copper in the blood.
hyperemic marked redness.
hyperextension Excessive extension of a limb or part.
hypergammaglobulinemia Excess of gamma globulins in the blood seen frequently in chronic infectious diseases.
hyperglycemia High blood sugar as in diabetes.
hyperhidrosis Excessive perspiration.
hyperkalemia High potassium concentration in the blood
hyperkeratosis Hypertrophy of the stratum corneum of the skin
hyperlipidemia a general term for elevated concentrations of triglycerides cholesterol
hypermetropia Refractory error called hyperopia.
hypernephroma This refers to Renal Cell Carcinoma.
hyperopia Error of refraction in which rays of light entering the eye parallel to the optic axis are brought to a focus behind the retina
hyperosmolality an increase in the osmolality of the body fluids.
hyperparathyroidism Because of high level of parathyroid hormone, calcium deposits in kidney and decalcification of bone occurs.
hyperpituitarism Excessive secretion of pituitary hormones.
hyperpnea Increase in the depth and rate of breathing;
hyperreflexia Exaggeration of reflexes.
hypersaline Addition of large doses of sodium chloride.
hypertension High arterial blood pressure
hyperthyroidism Condition caused by excessive production of iodinated thyroid hormones producing goiter, tachycardia or atrial fibrillation, widened pulse pressure, palpitations, fatigability, nervousness and tremor, heat intolerance and excessive sweating, warm, smooth, moist skin, weight loss, muscular weakness
hypertrichosis Excessive growth of the hair.
hypertrophy Overgrowth of an organ due to an increase in size of its constituent cells.
hyperventilation State in which there is an increased amount of air entering the pulmonary alveoli
hypervitaminosis clinical condition due to ingestion of an excess vitamins;
hypnosis Artificially induced altered consciousness which makes a person to respond involuntarily.
hypoalimentation Lowered nourishment.
hypobaric Low pressure and low weight of gases which determines specific gravity.
hypochlorite Dilute sodium hypochlorite which is antiviral and disinfectant.
hypochondriasis Meaning - disturbed function of the organs of the upper abdomen; such as heart problems, intestinal peristaltic movement which is producing discomfort.
hypofunction Diminished function.
hypogastric An area below the stomach.
hypoglossal Below the tongue
hypoglycemia Reduced blood sugar level .
hypokalemia Low potassium concentration in the blood which produces clinical manifestations.
hypomenorrhea Uterine bleeding of less than the normal amount occurring at regular intervals
hyponatremia Deficiency of sodium in the blood.
hyponitremia Low level of nitrogen in the blood
hypoparathyroidism Lowered function of parathyroidism producing clinical manifestations.
hypophysis The pituitary gland an epithelial body located at the base of the brain attached by a stalk to the Hypothalamus which secretes hormones.
hypopituitarism Diminution of function of the Pituitary gland producing clinical manifestations.
hypoplasia Underdevelopment of an organ or tissue
hypopraxia Diminished activity.
hypoproteinemia Decrease in the amount of protein in the blood resulting in edema and fluid accumulation in serous cavities.
hypoprothrombinemia Deficiency of Coagulation factor II or Prothrombin in the blood.
hypopyon Accumulation of pus in the anterior chamber of the eye.
hypospadias Developmental anomaly in the male in which the urethra opens on the underside of the penis or on the perineum.
hypostasis Stagnant circulation in a dependent part of the body
hypotension Low blood pressure seen in shock
hypothalamus It includes the preoptic area, optic tract, optic chiasm, mammillary bodies, tuber cinereum, infundibulum, and neurohypophysis which is also called Neurohypophysis.
hypothenar Eminence on the palm along the ulnar margin
hypothermia Lowering of core body temperature to 32°C (89°F) as that due to exposure in cold.
hypothesis Proposition that is subject to proof or to an experimental or statistical test.
hypothyroidism Deficiency of Thyroid gland giving rise to rise in basal metabolic rate, fatigue, and lethargy. Clinically it leads to Myxedema. It produces Cretinism in infants.

hypotonia Diminished tone of the skeletal muscles

hypotrichiasis This refers to Congenital Alopecia.

hypoventilation Clinical condition where reduced amount of air entering the pulmonary alveoli

hypovolemia Decreased volume of circulating blood in the body. The most common cause is hemorrhage.

Hypoxia Reduction of oxygen supply to tissue below physiological levels despite adequate perfusion of the tissue by blood.

hysterectomy Operation of excising the entire uterus, performed either through the abdominal wall or through the vagina

hysteria Colloquially it is mental disturbances. The types are Somatisation disorder, Conversion disorder, Dissociative disorder and Anxiety hysteria.

hysteromyomectomy This denotes Uterine Myomectomy.

hysteropexy Procedure of fixation of a displaced uterus by a surgical operation.

hysterosalpingectomy Excision of the uterus and uterine tubes.

I

IAEA Abbreviation for **I**nternational **A**tomic **E**nergy **A**gency.

iatraliptic Related to or concerned with the external application by massage of drug.

iatraliptics Treatment by inunction

iatro Related to the Physician.

iatrogenesis Complications resulting from treatment by a physician or surgeon. When complications occur during the course of treatment, it is called Iatrogenic.

ibuprofen a nonsteroidal analgesic, antipyretic, and anti-inflammatory agent

ICD Abbreviation for **I**nternational **C**lassification of **D**iseases (W.H.O.)

ice Solid form of water which melt at 0°C at 1 atmosphere.

Iceland disease Refers to Chronic Fatigue Syndrome seen at Atlantic.

ichthammol A chemical brownish in colour with strong odor obtained from the neutralization of ammoniacal substances. It is used as local antiseptic.

ichthyoid That which resembles a fish.

ichthyophthiriasis Skin manifestations with white spots.

ichthyosis Skin manifestations with keratinisation, scaling that are significant in genetic disorders. Dermatologists call this as Ichthyosis vulgaris.

ICN Abbreviation for **I**nternational **C**ouncil of **N**urses.

icon An image in computer science, specifically on monitor. Picture image in the mind often a person gets the perception of.

ICP Abbreviation for **I**ntra **C**ranial **P**ressure.

ICRP Abbreviation for **I**nternational **C**ommission on **R**adiological **P**rotection.

ICSH Abbreviation for **I**nterstitial **C**ell **S**timulating **H**ormone.

icteric Related to jaundice.

icterus Yellowish discoloration of skin, mucous membrane, nail bed and conjunctiva

ictus Refers to sudden attach of illness such as Epileptic attach (status epilepticus), Paralytic attach (ictus paralyticus), sun stroke (ictus solis) etc.,

ICU Abbreviation for **I**ntensive **C**are **U**nit.

id Psycho analytic position in which person harbors instinctive impulses and gets immediate pleasure of satisfaction.

idae It denotes the family in animal kingdom.

IDD Abbreviation for Insulin Dependent Diabetes.

idea This refers to thought or an impression of mind. Fixed idea, referential idea are examples.

ideal This speaks of a standard of any perfection.

identification A reflex process of defense mechanism wherein a person patterns himself with another person or in his society.

identity This refers to Man's aggregate characteristics.

ideology Scientific study of ideas which are characteristic of a person or of a society.

idiocy Mental retardation with very less I.Q. Mongolism, Familial disorders and Cretinism are common causes of idiocy.

idiopathic Refers to disease where cause cannot be ascertained.

idiosyncrasy This points out as to how a man behaves in the given circumstances. This can depict the quality of mind and the body. If a person is showing adverse reaction to consumed drug or protein.

idiot Person with very low I.Q. with mental retardation.

idiotype Used in the field of Immunology, in Immunoglobulin and in antigen binding situations.

idioventricular When condition is affecting only Ventricles of the heart such as Idiomas Ventricular Rhythm.

idoxuridine Substance which inhibit viral DNA synthesis and hence used in the treatment of herpes simplex keratitis.

IDU Abbreviation for **ID**ox **U**ridine

IFA Abbreviation for **I**mmuno **F**luorescence **A**ssay

Ig Abbreviation for Immunoglobulin. Main classes of Immunoglobulins are IgM, IgG, IgA, IgD, IgE. Subclasses are represented as IgG1, IgG2 and so on.

ignipuncture Traditional method of treatment by puncture with hot needles.

ignisation Producing hotness by artificial heat.

IGT Abbreviation for **I**mpaired **G**lucose **T**olerance.

IH Abbreviation for **I**nfectious **H**epatitis.

IHD Abbreviation for **I**schaemic **H**eart **D**isease.

ileac That which is related with ileum.
ileectomy Surgical removal of the ileum.
ileitis Infection and inflammation of the ileum.
ileocecal That which is related with ileum and caecum.
ileocolitis Infection and inflammation of the ileum and colon.
ileocolostomy Connection or an opening is created between ileum and colon for surgical therapy.
ileocolotomy Incision of the ileum and colon.
ileorectal Connection established between ileum and rectum such as ileorectal fistula.
ileorrhaphy Operative repair of the ileum.
ileum Portion of the small intestine from jejunum to cecum
ileus Intestinal obstruction.
iliac Which is pertaining to the ilium.
iliococcygeal Which is pertaining to the ilium and coccyx.
iliocostal Which is pertaining to the ilium and ribs.
iliofemoral Connected with Iliac and femoral such as iliofemoral artery.
ilioinguinal Which pertains to the iliac and inguinal regions.
iliolumbar Related to the flank and loin.
iliopagus Conjoined twins united in the iliac region which are symmetrical
iliopectineal That is related to the ilium and pubic bone.
iliosacral That which is related to the ilium and the sacrum.
iliospinal That which is related to the ilium and the spinal column.
iliothoracopagus Twins fused from the pelvis to the thorax.
iliotibial That which is extending from the ilium to tibia.
iliotrochanteric pertaining to the ilium and a trochanter.
ilioxiphopagus Twins fused from the pelvis to the xiphoid process.
ill Opposite of wellbeing. A disease an illness.
illinition External application of an ointment or liniment with rubbing.
illness This refers to the Disease status.
illumination To put the light to a cavity or organ for examination. In Lighting one of the physical environment it is expressed in Foot Candles.
illuminator Equipment for the source of light (for viewing an object).
illusion When a person get false image rather than a real image it is called illusion or misinterpreted impression of sensation.
IM Abbreviation for Intra Muscular referable to injection.
image A visual picture conceived which is far from objective reality.
imaging Radiological and Ultra sound images that are clear, detailedly and good contrast.
Types of such images are:
- Echo planar imaging
- Colour Doppler imaging
- Cardiac imaging
- Hot spot imaging
- Electrostatic imaging
- MRI i.e., Magnetic Resonance Imaging
- Thallium imaging

imago It can be adult stage of an insect or an unconscious mental image.
imbalance This refers to Autonomic imbalance, Vasomotor imbalance, Muscular imbalance or Postural imbalance.
imbecile Refers to a stage of Mental Retardation where I Q is very low.
imbricated overlapping of illness or of a surface.
Imferon Preparation of Iron Dextran injection for Therapy.
imipramine An antidepressant drug which contains Dibenzazepine.
immature That which is not fully developed.
immediate To occur without delay..
immedicable Illness which has very poor prognosis
immersion To plunge a structure into a liquid. In Medical vocabulary we commonly come across Oil immersion and Water immersion in day to day practice.
immobilization By using available sapling or cast the parts are made immobile for a cure in cases of fracture or injury.
immortalization When a thing overcomes the limitations on growth or life span.
immune Having body resistance that one cannot get diseases is said to be immune.
immunity Body protective mechanism is developed either by vaccine administration or by acquiring a disease.
immunization Producing body immunity by giving active immunisating agents or by giving passive immunizing agents.
immunize To give immunizing agents to render immune.
immunoassay Quantitative analysis of immunological aspect of a substance which are referable to Immunoassay for Radioactivity, for Enzyme activity, for Fluorescence activity.
immunoblast Other name for Lymphoblast.
immunocomplex This refers to Antigen Antibody Complex
immunocompromised When a person has immuno-deficient status by known causes such as Drug, Radiation, Malnutrition or by Disease.
immunodeficiency Deficient immune response which may be Antibody Type, Cellular type or Combined type in nature. Common Known Immunodeficiency diseases are as follows:
i. X linked Agammaglobulinemia
ii. Hypogammaglobulinemia of infancy
iii. Thymic Hypoplasia
iv. AIDS

v. Reticular dysgenesis
vi. Lazy Leucocyte Syndrome
vii. Alkaline Phosphate Deficiency
viii. Glucose 6 Phosphate Dehydrogenase Deficiency

immunodiagnosis Diagnosis based on blood serum reactions

immunofluorescence This is an immunohistochemical method using antibody labeled with a fluorescent dye

immunoglobulin They are Glycoproteins which function as antibodies which are 5 in numbers. (IgM, IgG, IgA, IgD, and IgE). Basic unit of Ig is made of 2 heavy 'H' chains and 2 'L' light chains which is Y shaped molecule.

immunologist Person who is specialist in immunology.

immunology The scientific study of organism to Antigenic property and to Antigen Antibody response. Different areas of interest are developed which are:

- Basic Immunology which highlights immune system.
- Clinical Immunology which highlights vaccination, Organ transplantation, Blood transfusion.
- Laboratory Immunology which highlights testing for humoral and cellular immunity
- Serology which highlights laboratory testing of antigen antibody reactions.

immunoregulation Through Lymphocytes and Immunoglobulins Immune response is controlled in the body.

impact Collision which is sudden and forceful.

impacted Firmly driver such as impacted tooth.

impalpable Unable to feel by palpation which indicates that it is small.

imperforate Referred to imperforate anus which is a birth defect.

impervious Hard layer which do not permit the movement of or passage of fluid.

impetigo Skin infection by bacteria belonging to either staphylococci or streptococci which is a contagious pyoderma.

implant Insertion of a material containing drug, chemical, hormone to body tissue.

implantation Fertilised ovum getting attachment to or embedding to endometrium. This is a preparatory approach for the attachment to the endometrium to develop into the state of fetus.

impotence No copulating power on the part of male in sex act which may be lack of erection.

impregnate To allow semen into vagina for fertilization through ejaculation.

impression Indentation on a structure or an effect on the mind.

impulse Sudden act by a person which cannot be controllable by him. Usually referred to nerve impulse.

inactivation To take away the activity of and pathogenicity of bacteria, virus or an enzyme by available means of chemical and physical agents.

inanition Weight loss and decreased metabolism due starvation.

inarticulate Do not have joints or do not utter normal speech.

inborn Something which is acquired in intra uterine life such as inborn error of metabolism.

inbreeding Close circle marriage leading to the mating of closely related individuals

incandescent That which gives light on heating.

incest Sexual activity between persons who are closely related that marriage between them is legally and culturally prohibited.

inch Unit of linear measure which is equivalent to 2.54 cms.

incidence It signify the rate of occurrence of events. It is expressed as number of new cases that occurred in a year for a disease or for an event.

incineration Act of burning hospital waste material to ashes

incipient That which comes to an existence.

incised That which is cut or made to cut.

incision To made a cut with a sharp instrument like knife. Always it is referred to a surgical incision.

incisor This refers to the tooth which is moulded to cut before mastigation.

incisura A notch or an indentation particularly for a depression in an anatomical structure.

inclination To lean vertically or horizontally, a sloppy position, It can also be an inclination for learning.

incoagulability Which cannot get clotted or the state of being incoagulable.

incoherent Specifically referable to speech which is without proper sequence or incongruous.

incompatibility Not adjustable or not compatible. In specific it refers to blood matching at blood transfusion.

incompetence One who cannot maintain himself, Anything that is inadequate or insufficient. Common medical terminologies are; Aortic incompetence, Mitral incompetence, Ileocaecal incompetence etc.,

incontinence Person when he cannot control urination or defecation

incoordination No harmonious working of organs in the body.

incrustation kin manifestations such as scale, scab or a crust.

incubation Time in which the entered pathogen produce pathology and clinical features start appearing.

- It can also be the development of embryo in the egg.
- In laboratory procedures maintenance of room temperature or required standard physical

environment in terms of Temperature, Humidity, and oxygen content.

- To culture organisms for better growth in laboratory.

incubator Instrument used or equipment used for Incubation.

incurable Prognosis of a disease in not at all good.

incus This is the middle small bone of middle ear which help in conduction of vibration and noise. Incus along with stapes and malleus form three ossicles of the ear. The middle of the three ossicles of the ear, which, with the stapes and malleus, serves to conduct vibrations from the tympanic membrane to the inner ear.

indapamide Pharmacological agent which has the property of antihypertensive and diuretic actions

indentation Depression, pit or notch in an organ.

Inderal Pharmacologically it contains Propranolol Hydrochloride.

Inderide Pharmacologically it contains Propranolol Hydrochloride and Hydrochlorthiazide.

index Index finger indicate index finger. This can be ratio of two measurable quantities. When there is collection of objects index is done for their sequence

indication Which serves as a guide in treatment of given disease. The mode of treatment is indicated by signs and symptoms which serve for line of management.

indicator Denotes to a chemical which can serve to show the concentration of a substance. This also can refer to Index Finger.

indigenous Refers to native which means it is of ones own country's material or substance.

indigestion Eaten food is not digested or not made to simpler substances which is ready for absorption.

indinavir sulfate Drug used in HIV/AIDS which belong to protease inhibitor group.

indiscriminate To affect all parts or all organs without any specificity to any one part or organ.

indisposition Unable to attend to his routine when a person is ill.

indole This is responsible for the odour of stool that is produced by the decomposition of tryptophan in the intestine.

indolent Means little pain, also means slow growing.

indomethacin Drug acting as anti inflammatory that is not a steroid. It is mainly used in the treatment of a) Gout b) Ankylosing spondylitis c) Osteoarthritis and d) Rheumatoid arthritis.

induced Artificially produced or induced such as Induced abortion.

induction This is referable to starting of drug regimen for a disease. This also can mean induction of anaesthesia in surgical operation.

indurated That which is hardened such as induration after a skin test.

indwelling Refers to leaving a catheter or a tube for Therapeutic purpose or for diagnostic purpose. Examples are urinary catheter, Ryles tube etc.,

inebriation When alcohol content goes beyond a certain level in the blood, person gets the toxic effect of alcohol which is called alcohol intoxication. Colloquially it is called Drunkenness.

inert It refers to inert gases or that which has no action .

inertia No activity found or which do not move at all.

infancy 0 to 1 year age group which is the early period of life

infant This include Neonate and Post Neonate period in early life which comes to the period of 0 to 1 year of age.

infanticide Killing infant of 0 to 1 year age with or without intension.

infantile That which is related to infancy

infantilism Usual term for Dwarfism which is Hypothyroid condition. Otherwise it denotes to mental retardation and no development of secondary sexual characters.

infarct Loss of local blood supply that causes necrosis of tissue. This is due to blocking by a blood clot called thrombus. Common infarct is coronary artery infarct causing heart attack.

infarctectomy Removal of thrombus through a surgical approach.

infarction Clot blocking a vessel or formation of an infarct such as Acute Myocardial Infarction, Cerebral Infarction etc.

infaust Not unfavorable.

infection Entry of pathogen in to human body causing inflammatory changes and later clinical manifestations of signs and symptoms that result in cure, defect or death if not treated. Types of infection are local and systemic and based on the nature of infection it can be acute, sub acute or chronic. Common terminology used are as under (depending on way of transmission)

- Air borne infection
- Water borne infection
- Vector borne infection
- Droplet infection
- Milk borne infection
- Food borne infection
- Faecal borne infection
- Soil borne infection
- Cross infection
- Ascending infection
- Descending infection
- Endogenous infection
- Exogenous infection
- Blood borne infection
- Iatrogenic infection

- Latent infection
- Mixed infection
- Nosocomial infection
- Opportunistic infection
- Perinatal infection
- Puerperal infection
- Transplacental infection

infectiosity The degree infection

infectious Disease caused by pathogens which are capable of spreading from one person to another.

infective Pathogens which are capable of producing infection in man.

infecundity This refers to person who is not capable of producing offspring.

inferior This anatomical terminology indicate that a structure is lower, directed downward or situated below etc.,

infertile One who cannot produce offspring or not fertile; Exhibiting infertility.

infertility Not capable of producing offspring in relative sense as compared to absolute term sterility. Common clinical types are Primary and Secondary.

infestation Infection with ticks, mites insects which produce lesion on the skin. Present concept has extended to parasites of intestine to depict Intestinal Parasitism.

infibulation Ancient custom of putting clasps to male organ or female organ to see that intercourse is not possible from any outside person. They used to use buckles to fasten labia or penis.

infiltrate To penetrate to surrounding tissues by a material or by a solution.

infiltration Tissue or material getting accumulation into tissues in excess. Different types of infiltration are:

- Fatty infiltration
- Cellular infiltration
- Lymphocytic infiltration
- Tubercular infiltration
- Serous infiltration

infirmary Space or building to attend to people for their need such as a hospital for the sick, a church for prayer etc.,

infirmity Weak state of Mind.

inflammation Local protective phenomenon seen in case of infection. Major protective responses are a) Pain b) Redness c) Raised temperature d) swelling and may be associated with loss of function. In pathological descriptions it shows the following:

- Dilatation of vessels
- Increased tissue permeability
- Fluid exudation
- Increased protein content
- White cells migration to inflammatory site.

Common types of inflammations are:

- Acute inflammation
- Atrophic inflammation
- Catarrhal inflammation
- Chronic inflammation
- Disseminated inflammation
- Diffuse inflammation
- Focal inflammation
- Interstitial inflammation
- Necrotic inflammation
- Pseudomembranous inflammation
- Purulent inflammation
- Sclerosing inflammation
- Suppurative inflammation
- Toxic inflammation
- Ulcerative inflammation

inflammatory Related to inflammation.

inflation Pushing the air or gas to make the container distended.

inflorescence The arrangement of the flowers in a plant.

influenza This is a viral infection of Respiratory tract which is an acute infection. Influenza epidemics are known in the history of medicine.

infolding It is the act of folding inward of a layer of tissue.

infra- Meaning below, beneath or inferior to other structure.

infra-axillary Below the axilla or inferior to the axilla.

inframammary Below the breast or submammary position.

Infra-mammillary Below the nipple or inferior to the nipple.

infrared These rays are the basis of thermography in medical profession. In the light spectrum, waves having wavelength of 0.75 and 1000 μm. are called infra red rays.

infundibulum Anatomical structure which is funnel-shaped

infusion Intra venous infusion or introduction of fluid or blood to the body for the purpose of treatment.

ingestion Consumption of food or medicine through oral route.

ingrowth Refers to ingrowth of epithelia, stroma or nail which grow inwards.

inguen Junction between the abdomen and thigh.

inguinal Related to groin.

inguinoscrotal Related to the groin and the scrotum.

INH Abbreviation for **I**so **N**icotine **H**ydrazine a drug in the treatment of Tuberculosis.

inhalation Biological process of inhalation which allow air taken in to the lungs.

inherent Present since birth which is also called as intrinsic or innate.

inheritance Qualities inherited from parents which is called genetic in disposition.

inion Prominent point of the external occipital protuberance.

iniopagus Birth defect with twins fused at occiput region.

initial It denotes first or first stage of any biological process.

injectable Drug introduced through injections through any one of the tested routes such as intra muscular, intra venous, sub cutaneous or intra dermal.

injection Injection given for treatment through Parenteral route (other than oral route.)

injury Damage by external force usually by trauma or accident. Common terms are Birth injury, Traumatic injury, Accidental injury.

inlay Putting bone or skin into other bone or other tissue to cover a defect. It also mean dental restoration.

innate Physical or biological change present since birth or congenital in nature.

innervation Describes the nerve supply to a part or to a structure.

innocuous That which is harmless.

innominate In Anatomy it refers to Hip bone and to Brachiocephalic artery which are not named. Any structure which do not have a name.

innoxious Not hurtful.

inoculation Viral or Bacterial portions which are not virulent are introduced to human body to produce mild illness followed by immunity.

inoperable A surgical problem which is not suitable for operation.

inorganic When a chemical is not derived from Hydrocarbons. Opposite to organic.

inosine It is a nucleoside which is responsible in Purine metabolism.

inositol Inositol, or more precisely myo-inositol, is a carbocyclic sugar that is abundant in the brain and other mammalian tissues; it mediates cell signal transduction in response to a variety of hormones, neurotransmitters, and growth factors and participates in osmoregulation..

inpatient With admission to a hospital a patient gets the investigation and treatment.

inquest Legal enquiry on the cause of death before a coroner or a Medical Examiner.

Insall-Salvati ratio In the normal knee it should be **One**.

$$\text{Insall Salvati Ratio} = \frac{\text{Length of the ligamentum patellae}}{\text{Height of the patellae}}$$

insalubrious Opposite of salubrious which means that it is not conducive to health.

insane Not behaving normally or that which is related to insanity.

insanitary Refers to a thing which is not in a good sanitary condition

insanity A person cannot take the responsibility for a crime and legally denoting that he is having mental derangement

inscription To write the name and quantity of ingredient in medical prescription.

insect They are vectors in the transmission of diseases such as Mosquito, Fly, Ticks, Mites, Cyclops and so on.

Insecta Belong to Arthropoda (jointed legs) which have cutting mouth parts mentioned under insect.

insecticide Substances which kill insects which may be chemicals, which may be natural or synthetic in origin.

insemination Depositing semen within vagina or cervix by natural means (intercourse) or by artificial means (A.I.H or A.I.D)

insert Refers to putting inside of Copper T or an Implant.

insertion This is the place of attachment of a muscle.

insidious Slow development of a disease.

insight Appropriate solution to a problem by forethought. Person understands of attitude, feeling, behaviour.

in situ Confined to the site of origin without invasion of neighboring tissues.

insomnia Loss of sleep or abnormal wakefulness.

inspiration Taking the air inwards or inhalation

inspissated Thick, Dry or a thing with less fluid.

instillation Administration of a liquid drop by drop.

instinct Unlearned responses that is characteristic of a species. E.g., Aggressive instinct, Sex instinct, Ego instinct etc.,

institutionalization Admission of a patient for a longer time for a course of long time treatment.

instrument Medical tool, Medical appliance or Medical apparatus.

insufficiency The condition of being inadequate to the performance of the allotted function.

insufflation Blowing a medicament into the body cavity.

insulin A hormone secreted by Beta cells of the Pancreas which is responsible for the regulation of Blood Sugar. It's deficiency causes Diabetes mellitus.

intake This refers to the intake of calorie or fluid by a person which is normal or sick.

integument This refers to a covering or an investment of an organ.

intelligence The ability to understand

intensive Good and continuous approach as in Intensive Care Unit Therapy.

interaction The process of acting on each other. Human interaction, Drug interaction are common terms.

interatrial Between the atria of the heart.

intercerebral Between the two cerebral hemispheres.

intercostal Between the ribs.

intercourse Mutual exchange of ideas. Coitus involving introduction of male organ into female vagina in sexual act.

interdigital Between two adjacent fingers or toes.

interferon A glycoprotein found to have immunoregulatory function. It exert specific antiviral activity by inhibiting the synthesis of viral RNA.

interior Inner part of an anatomical structure.

interlobar Between lobes.

interlobular Between lobules.

interlocking Complication of labor in twin births

intermammary Between the breasts.

intermammillary Between the nipples.

intermarriage To wed within ones own group may be ethnical, social or religious .

intermenstrual Between the menstrual periods.

intermittent That which occurs at separated intervals

intern Clerkship of a Medical graduate or Dental graduate to make him eligible to receive final degree in Medicine or Dentistry.

internal Situated within the Body.

internist Specialist in Internal Medicine.

internship One year clerkship for intern in a hospital.

interosseal Situated between bones.

interosseous Between Bones.

interphase Resting phase in Cell division.

interscapular Between the scapulae.

intersection Site where one structure cuts across another.

intersex Not male or female but a Hermaphrodite which can be True, Male or Female1.

interstitial Situated between parts or in the interstices of a tissue.

intertrigo Intertrigo is **a common inflammatory skin condition that is caused by skin-to-skin friction (rubbing) that is intensified by heat and moisture**. It usually looks like a reddish rash. Trapped moisture, which is usually due to sweating, causes the surfaces of your skin to stick together in your skin folds.

intervention Measures to improve health or to alter the course of illness.

Level could be a) Primary b) Secondary c) Tertiary. Stages could be a) Health Promotion, b) Specific Protection c) Early Diagnosis and Treatment d) Disability Limitation e) Rehabilitation.

intestinum G.I. tract from Pyloric opening of stomach to Anus. Colloquially called Bowel or Gut.

intolerance Unable to withstand a drug or a food by a sensitive person.

intoxication This refers to Chemical poisoning or Drug poisoning.

intra It is a prefix meaning within such as intra abdominal, intra arterial, intra articular etc.

intradermal Method of injection in medicamentation.

intragastric Occurring within the stomach.

intrahepatic Within the liver.

intramammary Within the breast.

intramedullary That which is within the bone marrow of the bone, within in the medulla Oblongata or within the spinal cord.

intramural That which is within the wall of an organ.

intramuscular Injection given to the substance of a muscle for medicamentation.

intraocular Refer to a structure or for a pathology within the eye.

intraosseous Anything that occur within a bone.

intraperitoneal Refer to an organ or pathology within the peritoneal cavity.

intravaginal Referable to organ pathology or surgery within the vagina.

intravenous Drug or fluid given to a vein

intrinsic Factors that are within.

introitus This term is used to denote vaginal entrance or pelvic entrance.

introjection To control the aggression on hated person by one self internally.

intromission Referred to the insertion of penis into vagina in sex act.

introspection Analysis of one's own thoughts and feelings which is called self analysis

introversion Lack of interest in outside world by a person. Opposite of Extroversion.

introvert Person who do not show any reaction outwardly.

intubation Insertion of tube into trachea, into urethra, into nose, into the mouth, for the purpose of or part of treatment.

intumescence An organ or a gland getting swollen may be normal or pathological.

intussusception Intestinal lumen of one part getting prolapsed into adjoining part. Surgically there are 4 types:

1) Enteric intussusception
2) Colic intussusception
3) Ileocolic intussusception
4) Ileocaecal intussusception.

intussusceptum The invaginated portion of intestine in intussusception.

intussuscipiens Portion of intestine into which another portion has invaginated in intussusception.

inunction To apply ointment with friction on the skin.

invagination To get invaginated as in intussusception.

invalid Disabled by illness or injury.

invasion This gives the meaning of pathogen invasion into human body or invasion of cancerous tissues.

invasive Investigations or surgery which involve incision, cut, introduction of instrument for diagnostic purpose or for therapeutic purpose.

inventory Taking into stock of material, making a comprehensive list of personality traits, aptitudes, and interests.

inversion Reversal of a part, Homosexuality, Chromosomal aberration

Invertebrata All animal kingdom which do not have backbone or spinal cord.

in vitro Biological event undertaken in laboratory environment say in a glass tube .

in vivo Biological event undertaken in living body or experimental animal.

involucrum Refers to sequestrum of a necrosed bone in a case of osteomyelitis.

involuntary Action, movement etc. are performed independently of the will such as heart contraction, respiration etc.,

involution Going back to its normal structure and function as in the case of involution of uterus after delivery. Body changes as age advances as in senility.

iodide One of the required mineral Iodine in the form of iodide for normal body function particularly for the physiological function of Thyroid gland.

iodine Essential in nutrition. It is required for Thyroid hormone regulation.

iodixanol Contrast medium used in angiography, computed tomography, and excretory urography.

iododerma Skin lesion resulting from iodism.

iodolography Visualization of an organ or part after the injection of Iodised oil in Radiodiagnosis.

iodoquinol Drug used in the treatment of intestinal amebiasis and in Vaginitis due to Trichomonas vaginalis.

iodotyrosine Iodinated derivative of tyrosine.

iodoxamic acid Radiopaque medium used in cholecystography.

ion An atom having a charge of positive (cation) or negative (anion) electricity by gain or loss of electrons.

ionization Radioactive particles getting entry and stored in the tissues. Passage of radioactive particles in to living tissue.

ionize Radioactive particles get separated into ions.

ionotherapy Ultra Violet Ray therapy.

IOP Abbreviation for **I**ntra **O**cular **P**ressure.

iopromide Used in C.T scan for enhancing contrast.

ioseric acid This is a radiopaque medium and has the formula $C_{15}H_{16}I_3N_3O_7$.

iota This is a Greek alphabet.

ioversol A Contrast Media used in C.T. Scan.

ioxaglate Salt of ioxaglic acid used as radio opaque medium.

ioxaglic acid Radiopaque medium of low osmolality.

ipecac An emetic used in poisoning.

ipsilateral Situated on same side as against contralateral.

IQ Abbreviation for **I**ntelligence **Q**uotient.

iridectomy Surgical excision of the iris

iridencleisis Surgical operation for Glaucoma or increased Ocular Pressure wherein a drain is created by a corneal incision as a wick through which aqueous is filtered to subconjunctival tissues.

iridocele Iris prolapse through cornea.

iridocoloboma Coloboma or congenital fissure of the iris.

iridocyclitis Infection and inflammation of the iris and ciliary body.

iridoplegia Paralysis of the sphincter of the iris

iris Circular pigmented membrane behind the cornea which is perforated by the pupil

iritis Infection and inflammation of the iris characterized by pain, congestion, photophobia and contraction of pupil and change in the colour of the iris.

iron Essential mineral for human body for Haemoglobin formation to transport oxygen to tissues. Iron deficiency anaemia is common in developing countries.

irradiate Means Radiotherapy where ionizing radiation is used for diagnosis and Treatment. Tissues are irradiated by the process of irradiation. Following are the types of irradiation;-

- Beam irradiation
- Interstitial irradiation
- Inverted Y field irradiation
- Radical irradiation
- Whole body irradiation
- Lymphoid tissue irradiation in toto.

irreducible That which cannot be reduced such as irreducible hernia, irreducible fracture, irreducible dislocation or irreducible chemical.

irreversible One cannot reverse or that which is incapable of being reversed.

irrigate Wash given to a wound. The process is called irrigation. Common solutions are ;-

- o Sodium chloride for wound irrigation and colon irrigation
- o Glycine or acetic acid for bladder irrigation

irritability Abnormal stimuli for stimuli. Muscle, Bowel and Intestine irritability are known in medical practice.

irritant Substance which produce irritation.

Isaacs' syndrome Muscular illness similar to neuromyotonia. This is characterstised by:

- Muscle stiffness which is progressive
- Muscle spasm which is progressive

ischemia Because of constriction of artery deficiency of blood supply to a part occurs.

ischiofemoral Related to the ischium and femur.

ischiopagus Twins fused at the ischia

ISGE Abbreviation for **I**nternational **S**ociety of **G**astro-Enterology.

ISH Abbreviation for **I**nternational **S**ociety of **H**ematology.

Ishihara's test By using pseudoisochromatic plates test for colour vision is made in eye examination for detecting colour blindness.

ISO Abbreviation for **I**nternational **S**tandards **O**rganization.

iso It is a prefix used in words such as Isomer, Isograft, Isoantigen etc.,

isoagglutination Cell agglutination by agglutinins of same species.

isoantigen In tissue graft or in blood transfusion an antigen that induces an immune response in the same species .

isocarboxazid An anti depressant which is a monoamine oxidase inhibitor

isochromosome Abnormal chromosome having a median centromere and two identical arms

isocitrate Fully ionized salt of isocitric acid.

isocitric acid Isomer of citric acid found in the citric acid cycle

isoconazole Antifungal and antibacterial used in the treatment of vaginal candidiasis and in dermatophytes

isocoria Both the pupils are equal in size.

isogamete Union of gametes by same size gametes.

isogamy In case unicellular organism reproduction resulting from the union of two gametes that are identical in size and structure

isohemagglutination RBC agglutination by haemagglutinin from other person of same species.

isohemagglutinin Hemagglutinin that agglutinates R B C of other individuals of the same species.

isoimmunization Antibodies are produced by antigen from genetically dissimilar individual of same species. Clinically Rh Isoimmunisation is important to prevent erythroblastosis foetalis.

isolate Refers to isolation of pathogen from culture for sub culture. Isolation for preventing interbreeding as a social barrier.

isolation Refers to chemical isolation, Bacteriological isolation, Human isolation for Quarantine.

isoleucine This is an essential amino acid produced by the hydrolysis of proteins

isomer That which is capable of showing isomerism.

isomerase An enzyme that catalyze a molecule to form a single product.

isomerization Under required special temperature pressure and catalyst an isomer is converted into another.

isometric Maintaining the same dimensions. Isometric contraction and isometric exercises are known terminologies in this regard.

isometropia Both the eyes have the same refractive errors.

isoniazid INH it is called is an antibacterial, used as a tuberculostatic, administered orally and intra-muscularly.

Isordil Isosorbide dinitrate a coronary vasodilator.

Isospora This is a genus of coccidian protozoa characterized by the presence of two sporocyst in each oocyst and four sporozoites in each sporocyst

isotonic A solution in which movement of solvent is not possible. Maintaining same tonicity in mixture such as blood serum and salt solution. Maintaining isotonic contraction or isotonic exercise.

isotope An element having the same atomic number as another which can radioactive or stable in nature.

isotropic Substance with same refraction as one piece which show the property of similarity in all direction. E.g., cubic crystal.

isozyme Enzymes with different chemical physical or immunological characters but are structurally related. This is also called Isoenzymes.

isthmus Narrow connection between two larger bodies such as isthmus of auditory meatus or Eustachian tube isthmus.

ITA Abbreviation for **I**nternational **T**uberculosis **A**ssociation.

itch Skin sensation marked by pruritus. Refers to Itch mite infestation called Scabies.

itching Skin sensation called Pruritus.

itis Word termination denoting inflammation of the part indicated by the word stem to which it is attached.

ITP Abbreviation for **I**diopathic **T**hrombocytopenic **P**urpura.

itraconazole Antifungal agent belonging to triazole compound that inhibits the synthesis of ergosterol

IU Abbreviation for **I**nternational **U**nit.

IUCD Abbreviation for **I**ntra **U**terine (**C**ontraceptive) **D**evice. Now it is called IUD without mentioning Contraceptive word.

IV Abbreviation for **I**ntra **V**enous a route of administration or a route of investigation in therapy and diagnosis.

Ivemark's syndrome It is called asplenia which is manifested with the following:

- Congenital splenic agenesis
- Cardiac malformations
- Visceral situs inverses

IVF Abbreviation for **I**n **V**itro **F**ertilisation. A mode of treatment of infertility.

IVIC syndrome It is also called Oculo Oto Radial Syndrome which is having following clinical manifestations;-

- Ophthalmoplegia
- Hearing loss
- Long slender thumb
- Deformity of upper limb

It is a rare autosomal syndrome.

IVP Abbreviation for **I**ntra **V**enous **P**yelography.

Ivy loop wiring Wiring of two adjacent teeth to provide attachment to intermaxillary elastics. It is a Fascio Maxillary surgical procedure.

Ivy's test A test to find out bleeding time in a patient. First incisions are made on the forearm along with a sphygmomanometer inflated around the upper arm.

Time taken for the control of bleeding is noted in seconds.

Ixodes Ticks of the family Ixodidae parasites on humans

Ixodidae They are hard ticks belonging to Dermacentor or Haemaphysalis.

J

Jaboulay's operation This refers to Hemipelvectomy described by Dr. Jaboulay.

Jaccoud's syndrome Chronic Arthritis occurring after Rheumatic Fever.

jackscrew For the approximation of teeth, orthodontic appliances which has threads to fix

Jackson's law The law of Jackson states '*The nerve functions that are latest developed are the first to be lost when the brain is damaged by disease*'

Jackson's membrane Thin sheet of peritoneum that extends from lateral abdominal wall to the caecum. This membrane can also produce intestinal obstruction at the level of caecum.

Jackson's safety triangle This triangle allows safety area to incise trachea in case of emergency tracheostomy. The boundaries are as under:

- Suprasternal notch is apex of triangle
- Lower end of thyroid cartilage is base of triangle
- Inner edges of sternocleidomastoid muscle are the sides of the triangle.

jacksonian epilepsy Fits starts as focal epilepsy in one group of muscle showing clonic movements which is followed by other group of muscles. Jackson described this type of epilepsy as March of the epileptic activity through the motor cortex.

Jacob François. French biologist, born 1920; co-winner, with André Michael Lwoff and Jacques Lucien Monod, of the Nobel prize in medicine and physiology for 1965, for discoveries concerning the genetic control of enzymes and virus synthesis.

Jacob's membrane Layer of Rods and Cones described by Jacob.

Jacobson's retinitis Syphilitic Retinitis described by Jacobson.

Jacob's triad This is clinically known as petrosphenoidal syndrome characterized the following triad:

1) Trigeminal neuralgia
2) Ophthalmoplegia
3) Unilateral Blindness

Jacquet's dermatitis Dermatitis caused by Diaper among children described by Jacquet.

jactitation Making unnecessary movement of patient from one place to the other or from one doctor to another who actually is in need of emergency treatment.

Jaffe's test This is a qualitative test for the detection of creatinine. Sample of liquid (urine) is tested with addition of trinitrophenol and sodium hydroxide give red colour if creatinine is present.

Jakob's disease Spongiform degeneration of neurons which is found fatal in few years of onset identified as autosomal dominant disease.

Janet's test The test is done to find out whether loss of touch sensation is by organic lesion or just functional.

janiceps Conjoined twins with one head and two opposite faces.

Jansen's disease Metaphyseal Dysostosis described by Jansen.

jar Wide-mouthed glass container.

jargon Words pronounced in an incoherent manner

Jarisch-Herxheimer reaction This is short period side reaction for an antibiotic treatment that can be attributed to liberation of endotoxin like substances from killed microorganisms of antibiotics. Headache, chills, fever and skin changes are common.

jaundice Clinically yellow bile pigment is found deposited in skin, mucous membrane, sclera which results in yellow colour on these parts. This is associated with hyperbilirubinemia.

jaw Lower jaw is made of mandible bone and upper jaw is made of maxillary bone which have teeth that have the function of seizing the food, biting the food and chewing the food for nutrition.

Jectofer Commercial preparation of iron tonic.

Jefferson's fracture Fracture of First Vertebra i.e., # of Atlas Vertebra.

jejunocolostomy Joining or anastomosis of jejunum and colon.

jejunoileostomy Joining or anastomosis of proximal jejunum and the terminal ileum.

jejunum This refers to the portion of intestine from Duodenum to the Ileum.

jelly This is a soft substance which is colloidal mass. e.g., are contraceptive jelly, Petroleum jelly etc.,

Jenner He discovered the vaccination to prevent smallpox by inoculating cowpox vaccinia vaccine.

Jensen's disease This refers to Retinochoroiditis described by Jenson.

jerk This is a sudden involuntary or produced movement to elicit reflex which may be superficial reflex or deep reflex. e.g., are Biceps jerk, Knee jerk etc., a sudden reflex or involuntary movement.

jet Describes the projection of a fluid with high pressure and high velocity such as water jet, steam jet. etc.,

Jeune's syndrome The syndrome consists of Thoracic Dystrophy which gives rise to Asphyxia

jigger Skin burrowing flea Tunga Penetrans which cause intense irritation and ulceration.

Jimson weed Source of scopolamine and hyoscyamine. When contaminated with feeds it can cause saturnism.

Joffroy's reflex In cases of spastic paralysis any pressure on buttocks produces twitching of gluteal muscles.

Johne's bacillus Mycobacterium para tuberculosis described by Johne.

Johnson-Stevens disease Severe mucocutaneous lesion which is called Fatal Erythema Multiforme with the development of pseudomembrane and Haemorrhagic crusts that are oronasal and anogenital in distribution. Ocular complications like blindness and opacities are common.

joint Junction between two or more bones that are called Articulations.

Jolly's bodies They are remnants of nuclear chromatic present in RBC in the following conditions:

- Haymolytic anemia
- Megaloblastic anaemia
- After splenectomy operation

Jolly's reaction When Faradic stimulation is given to a muscle it fails to respond to that stimuli even when Galvanic response to stimulation is present and there is voluntary contraction of that muscle.

Jones fracture This is the # of diaphysis of 5th Metatarsal bone.

Jonnesco's fold This refers to Parieto peritoneal fold described by Jonnesco.

Jordans' anomaly Granulocytes and Monocytes contain lipid vacuoles which are seen associated with the development of Muscular Dystrophy and Ichthyosis.

joule This is the unit of energy and heat which give an account of work done by a force.

jugular That which is related with neck or Jugular vein.

juice Fluid from an animal such as Gastric juice, intestinal juice etc.,

junction Point where two tissue or two organ meet.

junctional This pertains to a junction.

Jung Swiss psychiatrist and philosopher, 1875–1961 is the founder of Analytic Psychology who gave an account of Introvert, Extrovert, Libido and Ego.

jurisprudence the scientific study of the application of the principles of law and justice. It refers to Medical Jurisprudence or Forensic Medicine.

juvenile That which is related with childhood or immature stage.

juxta- That which is situated near or adjoining.

juxta-articular It denotes Periarticular.

juxtaglomerular Near the glomerulus of the kidney such as juxtaglomerular cells.

juxtaposition Meaning organs in Apposition.

juxtapyloric Meaning prepyloric

juxtaspinal Meaning Para Vertebral

juxtavesical Meaning near the bladder

K

K Chemical symbol for Potassium element.

κ This is Greek Alphabet Kappa.

Kader's operation Gastrostomy for introducing feeding tube. A special valve like flap is put which closes on withdrawal of the feeding tube.

Kahler's law This law states 'Ascending branches of the posterior roots of spinal nerves pas within the cord in succession from the root zone toward the mesial plane.

kala-azar This is a protozoal infection of man causing Visceral Leishmaniasis.

kalemia When potassium is present in the blood.

kallikrein They are proteinases that go to form Bradykinin, kallidin in the body. They can be tissue kallikrein or plasma kallikrein.

Kallmann's syndrome Hypogonadotropic Eunuchoidism described by Kallmann.

Kambin's triangular working zone This is a safe space for orthopaedic operation on Lumbar Disc surgery. The boundary of this triangle is as under:

A. Spinal nerve in anterior
B. Lateral edge of the superior articular process posteriorly
C. Upper rim of lower vertebra inferiorly

Kammerer-Battle incision This incision is Vertical Abdominal Incision through the skin and superficial fascia for abdominal operations.

kanamycin Clinically there are three known component called Kanamycin A, Kanmycin B and Kanamycin C. They are derived from Aminoglycoside derived from Streptomyces kanamyceticus. Because of resistance it's sparingly used.

Kanavel's sign In case of tendon sheath infection maximum tenderness is elicited 1" proximal to the base of little finger of that palm.

Kanner's syndrome Autistic disorder described by Kanner.

Kantor's sign A string like configuration of contrast material through a filling defect is seen in Radiography of colon.

kaolin This is colloquially called as China Clay which contain Hydrated Aluminium Silicate which has the medicinal value in day to day clinical practice. In pharmacy common preparation of Kaolin are Kaolin Mixture and Kaolin with Pectin mixture.

Kaplan-Meier survival curve This is called "Product Limit Estimate in Statistics. This refers to the conditional probability of survival during the interval since the last death is calculated as the number of patient observed to survice beyond that point divided by the number at risk.

No. of patient observed to survive beyond a given point of time

$$\text{Kaplan Meier Survival curve} = \frac{}{\text{Number of people at risk}}$$

for all the intervals upto that point of consideration to get **the value of survival curve.**

Kaposi's sarcoma This is described as Multiple Idiopathic Pigmented Haemorrhagic sarcoma which is malignant tumour of proliferates in vessels producing red cutaneous nodules in lower limbs. Human Herpes Virus is found to be significantly related in this sarcoma.

kappa A Greek Alphabet. This signified in statistics the extent of difference between observe value and expected value.

Karnofsky scale This is a Performance Scale by assigning scores.

0 Scale = Dead patient (Non functional)

100 Scale = Fully normal (Functional)

Karplus' sign This sign is observed in case of Pleural Effusion where on auscultation spoken letter U is heard as A over the effusion area.

Kartagener's triad This seems to be Autosomal Recessive Trait which contains the following manifestations:-

1) Situs Inversus or Dextrocardia
2) Bronchiectasis
3) Sinusitis

karyo That which is related with Nucleus.

karyocyte This refers to a nucleated cell.

karyogenic Which forms the nucleus of a cell

karyokinesis This refers to Mitosis wherein we observe the process of cell division.

karyolymph In the nucleus of the cell excluding the solid structures like chromatin and linin, the remaining liquid part is termed karyolymph.

karyolysis The nucleus of the cell swells up and looses the chromatin. This biological process is called Necrobiosis.

karyoplasm The Protoplasm present within the nucleus of cell.

karyosome Inside the cell there lies the irregular condensed clump of chromatin.

karyotype At the time of arrested cell division, the chromosomes are taken and arranged according to the specified classification.

Kasai operation Portoenterostomy described by Kasai.

Kashin-Bek disease This is chronic degenerative disease of joints and spine among children caused by ingestion of cereals adulterated with Fusarium.

katathermometer This is a materialogic instrument which is used to find out cooling power of the air. Dry kata and wet kata are two types known. In practice Standard kata, High temperature kata and very high temperature kata are differentiated with colour in the alcohol used.

katharometer This is used to find out B.M.R.

Kauffmann-White classification In Widal test use of O, H and Vi antigenic tirtre is observed for their classification of reactions.

Kawasaki disease This refers to Mucocutaneous Lymph Node Syndrome described by Kawasaki.

Kayser-Fleischer ring This ring is seen in Descemet's membrane of cornea in Liver diseases and in Wilson's disease. This is greenish discolouration in limbic region of the cornea.

Kazanjian forceps This is a cutting forceps which is used for resection of the nasal dorsal hump. This is used in surgery for increasing height of buccal vestibular sulcus of edentulous ridges that give denture retention. This is also used in Maxillofacial surgery for zygomaticomaxillary fractures..

kcal This denotes **Kilocal**orie.

kCi This denotes **Kilo**Curie.

kcps This denotes **K**ilo **C**ycles **P**er **S**econd.

Keen's sign In case of Pott's fracture of Fibula, there will be increased diameter at the level of Malleoli in lower limb.

Kehr's sign Rupture of spleen produce severe pain in left shoulder.

Kehrer's reflex Thermal stimulation of external auditory meatus produces closure of eyes.

Keith-Wagener-Barker classification They have given a type of classification of hypertension and arteriosclerosis which is based on retinal changes which is as under:

- Moderate arteriolar attenuation on retina – Group I.
- More arteriolar attenuation and localised vascular constriction – Group II.
- Cotton wool exudates and haemorrhage on retina — Group III.
- Papilloedema — Group IV

kelectome Kelectome is used to take the specimen from a tumour.

Keller operation This is surgical correction technique devised by Keller for Hallux Valgus. Base of the proximal phalanx of the great toe and head of first metatarsal bone is resected at medial prominence.

Kellock's sign Positive sign of Pleural Effusion. Sharp percussion by one hand when other hand is placed on thorax under nipple produce more vibrations.

Kelly's operation Surgical operation for stress incontinence in women. Wide shelf is produced for support by suturing connective tissue between vagina and urethra

keloid Keloid are produced when connective tissue repair occurs by the formation of excessive collagen in the corium which is a type of scar which goes on enlarging.

Kelvin scale This is the unit of measurement of temperature called "Kelvin" which is also called absolute temperature scale.

0 degree Centigrade = 273.15 kelvins

100 degree Centigrade = 373.15 kelvins

kelvin This is the SI unit of thermodynamic temperature equal to 1/273.15 of the absolute temperature

Kenalog Trade name for Triamciolone Acetonide preparation.

Kendall Edward Calvin. American biochemist, 1886–1972 who discovery on hormones of adrenal cortex.

Kendall's rank correlation coefficient When graded variables are present which are represented in ordinal data such as mild, moderate and severe, use of multiple grading is done so that multiple samples can be assigned to each grade.

Kennedy classification In case of partial toothing, classification is done based on location of the edentulous spaces in relation to other teeth.

Kennedy's syndrome Tumour of frontal lobe producing following symptoms in a patient;-

- Papilloedema on opposite side of tumour
- Central Scotoma on lesion side
- Optic neuritis on lesion side
- Optic atrophy on the lesion side

Kenny's treatment This is a rehabilitative treatment for poliomyelitis patients followed by Kenny, which consists of:

1. Wrapping of back with hot clothes
2. Wrapping of limb with hot cloths
3. Passive exercise when pain subsides
4. Advising exercises for muscles

keno Meaning 'emptiness.

kenotoxin This toxin generated in muscle during contraction causes muscular fatigue.

Kent-His bundle Atypical cardiac muscle fibre which arises in the node in interatrial septum. This propagates the contraction rhythm.

keratalgia Pain in the cornea.

keratectasia Cornea which is scarred and thinned out is seen protruded outside the eyeball which is also called corneal ectasia.

keratectomy Surgical exclusion for treating anterior staphyloma where the affected portion of cornea is excised.

keratin Keratin is present in skin, hair, nail and horns. Keratin is not soluble in gastric juice and hence it is used in coating tablets.

keratitis Infection and inflammation of the cornea.

keratoacanthoma An epithelial tumor resembling squamous cell carcinoma.

keratocele Inner layer of cornea, the Descemet's membrane gets protruded and is called Hernia of Descemet's membrane.

keratoconjunctivitis Infection and inflammation of the cornea and conjunctiva.

keratoconus This is called Conical Cornea which is the protrusion of the cornea which is bilateral and is seen as hereditary disorder.

keratoid That which resembles either horn or cornea.

keratoiridocyclitis Infection and inflammation of the cornea, iris, and ciliary body.

keratolysis The Horney layer of epidermis gets softened and peeled off.

keratomalacia Clinical manifestation of Vitamin A deficiency. This is the stage of softening and necrosis of cornea in severe Vitamin A deficiency.

keratome An Ophthalmic instrument viz., a knife for incising the cornea.

keratometry With the help of this Ophthalmometery, measurement of the anterior curvature of the cornea is done.

keratomileusis keratoplasty in which a slice of the patient's cornea is removed, shaped to the desired curvature on a lathe after freezing, and then sutured back on the remaining cornea to correct optical error.

keratomycosis Fungal infection and inflammation of the cornea

keratopathy Diseases of the cornea which are non inflammatory in origin.

keratophakia Cornea which is donated by a donor is sliced to suit to a recipient which is also called Keratoplasty.

keratoplasty Corneal grafting.

keratosis This refers to a wart or horny layer growth of skin.

Kergaradec's sign This refers to Uterine Soufflé described by Kergaradec.

Kerley's lines In Chest X-ray Linear densities of about 1 inch which is seen horizontally. It is seen stepladder fashion and could be due to interlobular septa secondary to Mitral stenosis or Silicosis.

kernicterus Clinically it is called Bilirubin Encephalopathy which involves yellow discolouration of Basal nuclei, Globus Pallidus, Putamen, Caudate nucleus, Cerebellar nuclei bulbar nuclei and Gray matter of cerebrum. Since commonly seen in neonates it is called Icterus Gravis Neonatorum.

Kernig's sign It is a sign of Meningitis. Patient cannot extend the lower limb in sitting posture or when lying with thigh flexed upon the abdomen.

Kesling appliance This is an occlusion splint which is used in Bruxism. It is made of latex rubber to fit over the occlusal and incisal surfaces of teeth.

keto In chemical structure for the chemical to contain carbonyl groups such as **C[dbond]O**

ketoacidemia Clinical condition containing the presence of keto acids in the blood.

ketoacidosis Accumulation of Ketone bodies to give rise to the following conditions:
- ✓ Starvation Acidosis
- ✓ Diabetic Acidosis.

ketoconazole This is a broad spectrum antifungal agent used for systemic and local infections.

α-ketoglutaric acid This is an intermediate product in Tri Carboxylic Acid Cycle.

ketone An organic compound containing the carbonyl group **C[dbond]O**

ketonuria Presence of ketone bodies in urine as seen in Diabetes mellitus.

ketose A Monosaccharide containing nonterminal keto group.

ketosis After total fat metabolism, increased level of ketone bodies in tissues and fluids. Diabetes, alcoholism and starvation has ketosis manifestation.

ketosteroid They are urinary metabolites of androgens from adrenal cortex and gonads.

ketosuria Presence of ketose in the urine.

kg Abbreviation for Kilogram.

Khorana Har Gobind Khorana an Indian. Along with Robert William Holley and Marshall Warren Nirenberg won Nobel prize for medicine and physiology in 1968 for the discovery of the process by which enzymes determine the function of a cell in a genetic environment.

kHz Symbol for Kilohertz.

kidney Main excretory organ of human body. It excretes the end products of body metabolism. It regulates the ion concentrations of Hydrogen, Sodium, Potassium and phosphate. Each kidney has outer cortex and inner medulla and about one million renal tubules called nephrons.

Kiel classification Morphological and cryptologic criteria based classification of Non Hodgkin's Lymphoma.

Kielland's forceps It is an Obstetrical forceps which does not possess the pelvic curve.

Kienböck disease Clinical condition of Osteochondrosis of the Semilunar Bone.

Kiernan's spaces A triangular space between liver lobes which contain larger interlobular branches of the portal vein, hepatic artery and hepatic duct.

Kilian's line On the promontory of the sacrum it is a prominent line.

Killian's operation To produce permanent communication with the nose, and to remove the diseased tissue, excision of the anterior wall of the frontal sinus is done.

Killian-Freer operation Surgical operation which include submucous resection of the nasal septum , septal cartilage, vomer and perpendicular plate of the ethmoid bone.

kilocalorie This refers to Large Calories.

kilocurie Radioactivity unit which explains that the quantity of radioactive material in which the number of nuclear disintegrations is 3.7×10^{13} per second is present.

kilogram Mass by weight is expressed in S.I. Unit being 1000 grams or one cubic decimetre of water. It is defined as the mass equivalent to 2.2 pounds avoirdupois.

kilohertz 1000 cycles per second or one thousand (10^3) hertz

Kiloh-Nevin syndrome This is Ocular Myopathy. Clinically we observe Ptosis and severe external ophthalmoplegia.

kilometer A unit of linear measurement of the metric system which is equivalent to 1000 meters or 3280.83 feet or 1/5th of a mile.

kilovolt Unit of electromotive force which is equivalent to 1000 volts.

Kimmelstiel-Wilson lesion This refers to Intercapillary Glomerulosclerosis described by Kimmelstiel and Wilson.

Kimura's disease Angiolymphoid hyperplasia described by Kimura.

Kimura cartilage graft This graft is used in tracheal stenosis where split thickness costal cartilage graft is used.

kinesics Organised study of body movement for communication.

kinesiology This refers to Bio-mechanisms where motion of human body is studied in a scientific manner.

kinesthesia Human awareness of position, movement, weight and tension of different parts of the body.

kinetic That which produce motion .

kinetics The expression of rate at which a thing occur such as Erythrokinetics, Leuko kinetics Ferrokinetics etc.,

kinetogenic When a movement is produced.

kinetoplasm Refers to the cytoplasm of the cell which has contractile action.

King syndrome Malignant Hyperthermia associated with physical deformities and congenital defects.

King unit In certain clinical conditions alkaline phosphatase under alkaline conditions and acid phosphatase under acidic conditions are measured which expresses the amount of phosphatase that liberates one mg. of phenol from an excess of disodium phenyl phosphate.

kingdom Refers to Animal Kingdom or Plant Kingdom.

Kingsley appliance This is colloquially called Jumping the Bite Plate because the biting plate is inclined anter4iorly to move the mandible forward by jumping the bite.

kinin This is responsible for vascular permeability causing vasodilation of vessels except pulmonary vessel.

kinship Relationship is maintained with the sign of descent which can be traced from a common ancestor.

Kirchner's diverticulum This diverticulum is present in Eustachian tube.

Kirk's amputation Amputation of leg is done above the femoral condyles. This amputation is called Tenoplasty Transfemoral Amputation.

Kirschner wire It is steel wire used for skeletal traction and skeletal fracture of bones. The insertion is done through soft tissues and bone.

Kirstein's method Direct Laryngoscope described by Kirstein.

Kisch's reflex Tactile sensation of Tympanum causes closure of the eye.

Klapp's creeping treatment Exaggerated movement of spine is advocated in the treatment of Scoliosis. This looks as though the patient is creeping on the floor.

Klatskin's tumor Cholangiocarcinoma described by Klatskin.

Klebs-Löffler bacillus Diphtheria bacillus discovered by Klebs and Loffler which is well known as Corynebacterium diphtheriae.

Klebsiella This is Gram negative Facultatively anaerobic bacteria which belongs to the family Entero-bacteriaceae. This causes Urinary and Pulmonary infections. They are isolated very commonly in wounds.

Klein-Waardenburg syndrome Genetic disorder which an Autosomal Dominant disorder characterised by the following manifestations:

- Acrocephaly
- Orbital deformity
- Brachydactyly
- Cleft palate
- Hydrophthalmos
- Cardiac malformations
- Elbows and Knees are contracted by contractures.

Kleine-Levin syndrome Among Adolescents Sleep, overeating and Amnesia are seen for which no cause is attributed.

Kleist's sign It is positive in Frontal lesions and Thalamic lesions. When fingers of the patient is is gently elevated by the fingers of examiner, patient's fingers will hook into the examiner's fingers.

Klemm's sign This is a Radiographic sign in Chronic appendicitis. Indication of Tympanites in right lower quadrant is a positive sign of chronic appendicitis.

klepto Anything that is related to stealing.

kleptolagnia In a person sexual gratification produced by stealing.

kleptomania Urge to steal objects that do not serve any purpose. Here at no cost there will not be any vengeance.

Klinefelter's syndrome This is called XXY syndrome with the clinical manifestations of a) Small testes b) Azoospermia c) Gynaecomastia. This is justifiably called male syndrome.

Klippel-Feil syndrome Because of reduced number of cervical vertebrae and due to fusion of a few vertebrae to one osseous mass, patient will have low hair line, limited neck movement and short neck.

Klippel-Trénaunay syndrome Usually lower limb showing the manifestations of Haemangioma, Hypertrophy of bone and soft tissues and Nevus flammeus along with skin varices.

Klippel-Weil sign This is seen in Pyramidal tract lesion . When patient's flexed fingers are quickly extended by doctor, flexion and adduction of thumb occurs. .

Klumpke's paralysis Due to Birth injury so common in breech deliveries, new-born gets brachial plexus paralysis

Klüver-Bucy syndrome Bizarre behaviour disturbances following head injury, probably damage to limbic structures.

km Abbreviation for Kilo Meter.

Knapp's operation Cataract surgery without Iridectomy. Through peripheral opening in the capsule behind the iris.

kneading Muscle massage with pressure and kneading.

knee Bent Mid leg potion which is major flexible joint .

kneippism System of Hydrotherapy introduced by Rev. Sebastian *Kneipp*

Knies' sign In Graves' disease, unequal dilation of the pupils is present apart from other symptoms.

knife This is a cutting instrument that can be any size or any shape.

Knight brace One of the oldest type of brace developed by Knight called chair back brace wherein the upper and lower bands are made of metal. Upright bars also are made of metal. Common metal used is aluminium.

knock Commonly refers to Pericardial Knock which is a sound as of a blow against a firm surface.

knock-knee This condition is called Genu Valgum.

knuckle Four prominence on the dorsal aspect of palm at the site of phalangeal joints

Koch Robert Koch a German physician and bacteriologist, 1843–1910 who discovered Tuberculosis bacteria. He was awarded Nobel prize for medicine or physiology in 1905

Koch's node Atrioventricular Node described by Koch.

Koch's postulate Koch postulated the statement of experimental evidence required to establish the cause and relationship disease producing microorganisms and the disease. Following are the known postulate:

- Microorganisms must be observed in a disease
- Isolation of such organisms and culture

➢ The cultured organism when inoculated should produce illness

In addition to the above it also postulates that the pathogens must be recovered from diseased animal or man.

Koch-Weeks bacillus Haemophilus bacilli is called Koch Weeks bacillus which was discovered by Koch and Weeks.

Kocher Swiss surgeon is known for his work on Thyroid.

Kocher's forceps Forceps used to hold tissues and for compressing bleeding tissue. Tips of forceps are with sharp points and has transverse serrations along the full length for holding tissues.

Koeberlé's forceps They are Haemostatic forceps.

Koebner's phenomenon In case of Psoriasis, Lichen Planus skin manifestations are seen on uninvolved skin at the site of injury which is called *Isomorphic effect.*

Köhler He discovered Monoclonal antibodies.

koilo This refers to a hollow or concave area such as spooning on nail.

koilonychia Sign of Anaemia which is caused by dystrophy of the fingernails

Kolmer test It is a complementation test used in earlier times for test for syphilis which is a modified Wassermann test.

König's syndrome Syndrome of constipation and diarrhoea which is associated with following symptoms;-

- Gurgling sounds on auscultation in right lower abdominal area
- Meteorism
- Abdominal pain

konimeter Instrument used for air analysis in Occupational Health centres . It measures dust in air.

Koplik's spots One of the sign of Measles. They are small irregular bright red spots on buccal and lingual mucosa with a white speck in centre of spot.

Kornberg He discovered the biologically synthesised DNA and RNA.

koroscopy It is the other name for Retinoscopy.

Korotkoff's sounds This is heard in auscultation for B.P recording with sphygmomanometer. Pneumatic cuff tied produces the distention of artery which produces the sound.

Kossel's test This is a qualitative test for the detection of Hypoxanthine. The material containing Hypoxanthine when combines with Zinc and HCl in presence of NaOH in excess, produces ruby red colour.

Kostmann's neutropenia This refers to Infantine Genetic Agranulocytosis described by Kostmann.

Krameria A herb whose extract is used as Astringent which was discovered by Kramer.

kraurosis Clinical condition in which vulva is brittle and dry.

Krause-Wolfe graft It is Full thickness graft described by Krause and Wolfe.

Krebs Described the action of protein kinases in cell metabolism. Discovered Krebs cycle (citric acid cycle)

Krebs cycle This refers to Tricarboxylic Acid Cycle.

kreotoxicon Toxin present in putrefied meat which cause meat poisoning. It is also called Crotoxin under food poisoning.

Kretschmann's space A depressed area in Tympanic membrane.

Kretz's granules This is seen in Cirrhosis of Liver.

Kreyszig's sign It is a sign of Adherent Pericarditis. Clinically there is depression of intercostal space.

Kromayer's lamp This is high pressure mercury arc lamp used in the treatment of skin disorders.

Kronecker's center Cardio Inhibitory Center described by Kronecker.

Krönlein's hernia Inguino Peritoneal hernia described by Kronlein.

Krukenberg's veins Central Hepatic Veins described by Krukenberg.

krypton (krip′ton) Element present in atmosphere which is inert.

Kufs' disease Progressive neurological degeneration of CNS.

Kuhlmann's test Used for demining mental age of children which is a modification of Binet's test.

Kunkel's syndrome This is Lupoid Hepatitis described by Kunkel.

Küntscher nail It is an Orthopaedic nail used for fixing in intramedullary fractures. By shape it is tubular metal nail.

Kupffer's cells Pyramidal cells with oval nucleus in liver which are part of R.E. system.

kurtosis This describes the degree of peakedness of a curve of normal distribution.

Kussmaul's disease Poly Arteritis Nodosa described by Kussmaul.

Kussmaul-Kien respiration Deep and Rapid respiration in Metabolic Acidosis.

Kussmaul-Landry paralysis Acute Idiopathic Polyneuritis described by Kussmaul.

Kussmaul-Maier disease Poly Arteritis Nodosa described by Kussmaul and Maier.

Kveim test is a skin test used to detect sarcoidosis, where part of a spleen from a patient with known sarcoidosis is injected into the skin of a patient suspected to have the disease. If non caseating granulomas are found, the test is positive.

kW Abbreviation for kilowatt.

kwashiorkor Protein malnutrition, or kwashiorkor, is mostly found in people living in geographical areas that have limited food resources. It's most commonly seen in children whose diets are low in protein and calories.

Kyasanur Forest disease Kyasanur Forest disease (KFD) is **caused by Kyasanur Forest disease virus (KFDV), a member of the virus family Flaviviridae**. KFDV was identified in 1957 when it was isolated from a sick monkey from the Kyasanur Forest in Karnataka (formerly Mysore) State, India.

kyllosis Deformity of the foot including Clubfoot.

kynocephalus Dog headed foetus which is a birth defect.

kyphos The visible prominence of Kyphosis.

kyphoscoliosis This is common clinical manifestation of Osteochondrosis where spinal column is bent backward and lateral wards.

kyphosis Increased convexity in the Thoracic curvature of spine which is called Humpback appearance.

Kyrle's disease A chronic disorder of Keratinisation in the body.

L

Labarraque's solution Sodium Hypochlorite solution and water in 1:1 ratio.

Labbé's triangle an area bounded below by a horizontal line touching the lower edge of the cartilage of the left ninth rib, laterally by the line of the false ribs, and to the right side by the liver; here the stomach is normally in contact with the abdominal wall.

label To identify an object a tag used is called label.

labial That which is related to lip.

labile That which fluctuate or that which is unstable.

labium Any lip like structure in anatomical description. Labia which is pleural form is reserved for parts of external genitalia in females viz., Labia majora and Labia minora.

labour This is referred to stages of delivery of child in woman. This is colloquially called as child birth or delivery. The stages of labour are:

I stage : Dilatation of cervix (from the start of uterine contraction till Os dilated.

II stage : Expulsion of foetus (Os dilation to child expulsion)

III stage : Delivery of placenta (Child expulsion to placenta expulsion)

IV stage : Uterine tone establishment (Placenta expulsion till uterine tone)

laboratory This is the place or area where chemicals are produced, drugs are prepared, experiment done, research done. When examination of excreta or secrete of man is done it is called clinical laboratory.

Laborde's method In cases of asphyxiation Laborde method is adopted to stimulate the respiratory centres. This is done through rhythmic traction movement on tongue.

labrum This mean the brim of a structure and even a lip like structure.

labyrinth System of intercommunicating canals. Common terms that are in use are:

- Membranous labyrinth
- Bone labyrinth
- Vestibular labyrinth
- Cochlear labyrinth.

labyrinthectomy Surgical treatment for severe hearing loss due to vestibular dysfunction. Excision of the labyrinth of the ear, done for implacable vestibular dysfunction when severe hearing loss is already present.

lac Latin word meaning milk particular reference to human milk and cows milk.

laceration a deep cut or tear in skin or flesh.

lacrimal Related to the tears.

lacrimation Physiological or pathological secretion of tears.

lactagogue That which produces milk called galactogogues.

lactalbumin It is milk protein present in why of human milk.

lactase This enzyme is present in intestinal mucosa that is responsible for the convention of Lactose to galactose and glucose. Absence of lactase is responsible for the clinical condition lactose intolerance.

lactase deficiency This is an inherited deficiency of enzyme lactase among patients of lactose intolerance that manifests in the form of diarrhoea, flatulence and abdominal pain . Failure to thrive among children is called congenital lactose intolerance

L-lactate dehydrogenase Commonly called LDH has five different entities like M_4, M_3H, M_2H_2, MH_3, and H_4. This is the catalyst in reduction of pyruvate to lactate in biological situations like glucose conversion in liver, combustion of lactate of red fibres and glycolysis of white fibers.

lactation From Latin word meaning to suckle babies. Lactation denotes the period of milk secretion during which time baby is fed with breast milk by mother.

lactic acid Lactic acid is the end product of glycolysis. This provides energy to skeletal muscles. In liver lactic acid is converted back to glucose by gluconeogenesis process. Lactic acidosis by elevation of lactic acid in blood is seen in Diabetes.

lactiferous That which produces milk.

lactifuge That which inhibits the production of milk.

Lactobacillus Gram positive and rod l shaped bacteria that are anaerobic present in oral cavity, intestinal and female reproductive system. One type of lactobacillus produces only lactic acid and other type produces the end products of fermentation.

lactogen That which enhances milk production such as Prolactin. Human placental lactogen 'hPL' is a placental hormone present during pregnancy disappears after delivery that is known to increase the glucose supply to foetus .

lactogenesis The production of milk by the mammary glands.

lactogenic Substance that stimulates the production of milk.

lactometer Instrument used to find out the specific gravity of milk.

lactose Main ingredient of breast milk in human beings. In infant's intestine with the help of intestinal lactase, lactose is converted into galactose and glucose. It is a disaccharide.

lacuna A hollow cavity in bone or blood such as bone lacuna or blood lacuna.

Ladd's bands Peritoneal bands that connects the caecum to the right lateral abdominal wall.

Ladd's procedure In case of intestinal malrotation and intestinal obstruction, Ladd's band is cut and the correction is effected.

Ladd's syndrome Malrotated caecum produce obstruction of duodenum by peritoneal bands which is invariably congenital in origin.

Ladd-Franklin theory This theory explains the evolution of colour vision. The Evolution is as under;-

i. White light sensation is produced in visual cells by the stimulation of light
ii. Reactive products are produced namely blue and yellow
iii. From yellow becomes two more products for red and green.

Incomeplete recapitulations of this evolutionary development causes either dichromacy or trichromacy.

Laënnec's cirrhosis Laennec was French Physician who invented stethoscope. This type of liver cirrhosis was described by Laennec is due to chronic alcohol ingestion.. Initially there is fatty infiltration of liver cells followed by necrosis and inflammation. Later progressive fibrosis occurs.

lag It is the interval between stimuli and result such as Nitrogen lag.

lagophthalmos a condition in which the eye is protruded or which cannot be completely closed.

Lagrange's operation A combined iridectomy and sclerectomy that is performed in glaucoma for the purpose of forming a filtering cicatrix.

laiose This is present in the urine of Diabetes patient which is that do no ferment on its own.

lallation Uttered speech by infant which is called babbling,

Lamarck's theory This natural theory of transmission of acquired characteristics in man states that acquired characteristics may be transmitted in man.

Lamaze method This refers to the method adopted in a pregnant woman for preparing her for natural delivery. Health education on physiology of pregnancy and delivery, breathing exercise that can help for bearing down at delivery.

lambda Greek alphabet written as Λ or λ. Lambda refers to posterior fontanel where lambdoid and sagittal suture meet that is used as a landmark in craniometrics analysis.

lambdoid That which looks like lambda.

lambert A unit of expression to express the lighting in a given area may be in one square foot or in a square cm.

lame One who limbs and cannot have normal locomotion as in the case of polio lameness.

lamella Denotes thin plate like part of a bone such as basic lamella or articular lamella.

lameness This is lame condition of a person.

lamina This plate like projection of a vertebrae.

laminaplasty Orthopaedic surgery performed for relieving compression of spinal cord.

laminar laminar flow, also called streamline flow, **type of fluid (gas or liquid) flow in which the fluid travels smoothly or in regular paths**, in contrast to turbulent flow, in which the fluid undergoes irregular fluctuations and mixing.

Laminaria This is sea weed that is used as Laminaria tent in cervical dilatation for abortion.

Lancefield classification Group A Haemolytic, Group B haemolytic etc from group A to O are classified by this method of serological classification based on specific carbohydrate antigen in the cell.

lanceolate That which is shaped like a lance.

Lancereaux-Mathieu disease This refers to Spirochetal jaundice that is manifested with following manifestations:

- Haemorrhage
- Anaemia
- Fever
- Azotaemia Disturbance of consciousness.

landmark The point for any measurement and for referring other structures in anatomical descriptions.

Landolt's operation Done in the lower eyelid formation by using skin of upper eye lid through bridge flap.

Landry's paralysis This refers to Acute Idiopathic Polyneuritis described by Landry.

Landsteiner Austrian pathologist and immunologist who won Nobel Prize for his discovery of Blood Group in the year 1901.

Langerhans' cells The precursor cells in bone marrow that has indented nucleus and inclusion granules in cytoplasm. The cells have been identified in spleen, thymus and lung. They are called antigen presenting cells in lymph nodes.

lanolin Common pharmaceutical preparation as water in oil ointment base.

lanugo Fine hair on the body of the fetus

Lanz's point The location of vermiform appendix at a point on a line connecting the two anterior superior iliac spines one third of the distance from the right spine.

Laparo That which is related to flank. Loosely referred to abdomen in recent days.

laparorrhaphy Surgical repair of abdominal wall.

laparoscope An endoscope that is introduced to inspect peritoneal cavity for the purpose of diagnosis.

laparoscopic That which is related to laparoscope.

laparotomy Surgical intervention through incision on abdomen or flank .

lard Fat taken out from abdomen of hog which is cleaned.

larva It is second stage in the life cycle of insects . Larva is from egg. Larva changes to pupa in succeeding stage.

larvicide Insecticide that is used to kill the larval stage of insect.

larvivorous This refers to certain fishes like Gambusia or Lebistes which feed on larvae.

laryngectomy Removal of the larynx for treatment.

laryngitis Infection and inflammation of the larynx which is manifested with cough, dysphagia, dryness in throat.

laryngoscope For direct endoscope visual examination of larynx this instrument is used.

laryngoscopy Through laryngoscope examination of larynx is done. Two types of laryngoscopy are Direct laryngoscopy and Indirect laryngoscopy

laryngospasm Larynx is closed because of spasm which is called spasm of glottis.

larynx This structure connects trachea and pharynx. Larynx is made up of nine cartilages which are connected with muscles and ligaments

laser When light is converted into monochromatic radiation in visible region is called laser.

LASER stands for **L**ight **A**mplification by **S**timulated **E**mission of **R**adiation.

Lassa fever This is a viral fever first identified in Lass a town in Nigeria in the year 1959.

lassitude It is a state of exhaustion or weakness in some of the clinical conditions.

latent It means hidden disease or dormant disease.

lateral That which is away from median plane or midline of the body.

latex Plant secretion in the form of white viscid fluid that has the commercial value.

lathyrism A kind of poisoning in man by consumption of contaminated seeds of Lathyrus sativus. Lathyrism produces spastic paraplegia.

latissimus Meaning very wide such as latissimus dorsi muscle.

latus That which is wide.

Lauber's disease This refers to Fundus Albi Punctatus described by Lauber.

laudable That which is commendable and healthy.

laughter A condition of merriment in the form of series of spasmodic involuntary expirations that may or may not be associated with articulations.

Laugier's hernia This is Femoral Hernia which is perforated to Gimbernat ligament described by Laugier.

Laumonier's ganglion This refers to Carotid Ganglion described y Laumonier.

Laurence-Moon syndrome This is an autosomal recessive disorder. Common manifestations are:

- Hypogonadism
- Retinopathy (Pigmentary type)
- Mental Retardation
- Spastic paraplegia

laureth Popularly called laureth 9 which is used as sclerosing agent in the treatment of varicose veins. This has shown other actions like spermicidal and surfactant.

lavage French word meaning washing out of an organ like stomach lavage, Peritoneal lavage.

law This refers to facts and principles such as All or none law, Boyle's law, Law of conservation of energy etc.,

laxative Drugs that help in evacuation of bowel. They are called purgatives. Types of laxatives are:

- ➢ Bulk laxatives
- ➢ Saline laxatives
- ➢ Contact laxatives
- ➢ Lubricant laxatives

lb Abbreviation for pound.

LBW Abbreviation for **L**ow **B**irth **W**eight

LD Abbreviation for **L**ethal **D**ose

LD_{50} Abbreviation for Median **L**ethal **D**ose

LDL Abbreviation for **L**ow **D**ensity **L**ipoproteins.

lead They are ECG conductors and we have three common lead which are lead I , lead II and lead III.

leaf Refers to plant leaf which are responsible for photosynthesis.

leaflet Small leaf in plant kingdom.

learning Permanent adaption of behaviour by day to day experience. Common types of learning are a) Observational learning b) Insight learning and c) latent learning.

Leboyer method Gentle and controlled delivery without any painful stimuli that help in good personality in new-born life.

lechopyra Other name for Puerperal Fever.

Le Dentu's suture Suture used to tie the divided tendon by three suture method described by Le Dentu.

Lederberg American biochemist who won Nobel Prize for his discovery on Genetic Recombnation in 1958.

LeDuc technique This is Uretero Intestinal anastomosis described by LeDuc

Lee's ganglion This refers to Cervical Ganglion of the Uterus described by Lee.

leech They are blood sucking annelids used in leeching in earlier centuries. Medicinal leech is called Hirudo medicinalis.

leg Anatomical portion between knee and ankle.

legume Leguminosae plant seeds.

Leigh disease (le) [Archibald Denis *Leigh,* British neuropathologist, born 1915] This refers to Sub Acute necrotising Encephalo Myelopathy. Described by Leigh.

Leishman's stain This is common stain to stain a) blood cells and b) parasites. This stain contains mixture of Methylene Blue and Eosin.

Leishmania This is flagellate protozoa that cause disease in man. Common species are L. donovani and L. tropica.

leishmaniasis Infection caused by L.donovani and L.tropica.

Lembert's suture Suture used in G I surgery.

lemon Citrus fruit that contain citric acid, ascorbic acid and lemon oil.

Lenègre's disease Due to degeneration of conductive system acquired complete heart block in a patient.

length This refers to the measurement between the two ends.

Lennert's classification Lymphoma which do not respond to chemotherapy and is non Hodgkin's type. On pathological examination plenty of epithelioid histiocytes are present and bone marrow involvement is present.

Lennhoff's index This is found out by:

$$= \frac{\text{(Sternal notch to symphysis pubis) X (100)}}{\text{Greater circumference of abdomen}}$$

lens This refers to convex or concave glass which transparent to help in convergence of light for visual acuity. Types of lenses are: Acrylic lens, Achromatic lens, Contact lens, Bi convex lens, Biconcave lens, Bifocal lens, Bi spherical lens, Compound lens,

lentiform That which is shaped like a lens

lentigo Melanosis which is not raised above the surface of the skin.

Lentivirus They belong retroviruses that produce HIV infections that lead to AIDS. They also known to cause anaemia, encephalitis and arthritis

Lenz's syndrome This is Sex linked inherited disorder which show following clinical manifestations:-

- Small eye ball or absence of eye ball
- Abnormal fingers including 2 thumbs
- Very narrow shoulders,
- Teeth defects
- Heart defects
- Genital defects
- Kidney defect

Leo's test This is a lab test for free acidity. Addition of calcium carbonate produces neutral status in the test solution.

leper A leprosy patient. This is not a socially acceptable term for the patient suffering from leprosy.

lepra Greek word meaning scaly skin as in case of leprosy. Skin test in leprosy is called lepra reaction.

leprologist A Dermatologist who is experienced in the study and treatment of leprosy.

lepromatous Related with a type of leprosy called lepromotour leprosy.

lepromin Heat killed leprosy bacteria that is used as antigen in lepra reaction.

leprosarium Place for the treatment of leprosy patients. After domiciliary care the role of leprosarium is not significant.

leprosy A chronic bacterial infection caused by leprosy bacteria. It is also called Hansen's disease after the scientist who discovered the pathogen. Types of leprosy are

- o Tuberculoid leprosy
- o Lepromotous leprosy
- o Borderline leprosy
- o Indeterminate leprosy

Leptomonas Elongate flagellar stage of a protozoan parasite

Leptospira One of the spirochaetales that produce jaundice and bleeding (Leptospira Icterohaemorrhagiae)

leptospirosis Leptospira infection which produces fever, jaundice. The illness is transmitted by infected urine of rats, pigs and dogs.

leptotene One of the stages in meiosis in which chromosomes are seen as threads.

Lerch's percussion This refers to Drop Percussion described by Lerch.

Léri's sign In case of hemiplegia, normal flexion at the elbow is lost on the affected side when passive flexion of the hand is done.

Leriche's disease This refers to Post Traumatic Osteoporosis described by Leriche.

lesbian They are female homosexuals.

lesion Lesion is defined as a pathological discontinuity of tissue. This also refers to traumatic discontinuity of tissue. When there is loss of function of an organ or of a part it is also called lesion.

let-down This denotes to milk yield by lactating woman.

lethal That which is fatal in nature.

lethargy Person who show indifference or apathy.

leucine This is one of the essential amino acid that is necessary for the growth and development and nitrogen equilibrium in the body.

leukemia Blood cancer which show distorted WBC in blood and bone marrow. Types of leukaemia are:
- Acute leukaemia
- Chronic leukaemia
- Myelogenous leukaemia
- Lymphocytic leukaemia.

leukocidin A toxic substance produced by staphylococci and streptococcus bacteria that is lethal to white cells.

leukocyte WBC in blood which can be a) Basophils b) Eosinophil c) Neutrophils d) Lymphocytes and e) Monocytes.

leukocytolysis Destruction of white cells due to various reasons.

leukocytosis A high WBC count seen in infection and inflammation

leukoderma White depigmented patches on the skin that are acquired in later life. Which is called vitiligo.

leukoma Dense white opacity of the cornea.

leukonychia Whitish discoloration of the nails

leukopenia Low WBC count which can of any type like Agranulocytosis, Neutropenia or Pancytopenia.

leukorrhea White discharge from vagina which is always pathological

leukotriene Three double bonds containing compound that is formed from Arachidonic acid in the presence of Lipoxygenase. They are responsible for the regulation of allergy and inflammation

Lev's disease Complete heart block due to sclerosis of heart skeleton.

levamisole An anthelmintic used in the treatment of round worm and hook worm infections.

levator Refers to muscle which help to elevate an organ or a structure such levator ani levator anguli oris.

Lévi-Lorain infantilism This refers to Pituitary Dwarfism described by Levi and Lorain.

Levin's tube This is a Nasogastric Tube.

levocardia Left sided heart which is normal .

levorotatory Plane of polarisation is turned to left.

Levret's forceps Forceps which has the curvature corresponding to the curve of the birth canal devised by Levre

levulose Other name for Fructose.

Lewis blood group This type of classification done on the basis of plasma glycolipids. (depending on Le antigen). We have three types of grouping:
- Double negative Le (a- b-)
- Le without H Le (a+ b-)
- Le with H Le (a- b+)

lewisite American chemist discovered a lethal gas which was named after him as Lewisite.

Lewy bodies Lewy body dementia, also known as dementia with Lewy bodies, is the second most common type of progressive dementia after Alzheimer's disease.

Leyden's disease Periodic vomiting which is idiopathic in nature.

Leyden-Möbius muscular dystrophy syndrome This refers to Limb Girdle Muscular Dystrophy described by Leyden and Mobius.

LH Abbreviation for Luteinising hormone.

libido They are major expressions of love and pleasure which are described as sexual desire.

license Legal permission to perform any act to make that act as legal.

licentiate Licence to practice a profession..

Lich technique Ureter is dissected and reattached to bladder to submucosal tunnel created within the bladder which is called ureterocystostomy.

lichen Skin manifestations which ae raised above the surface of the skin. Lichen planus is common variety of lichen.

lidocaine A local anaesthetic applied topically to the skin and mucous membranes.

lie Refers to Transverse lie and Oblique lie of foetus in the womb in relation to uterus.

Lieberkühn's crypts Simple tubular intestinal glands called Crypts of Lieberkuhn present in mucous membrane of small intestine.

life The total of vital events of an organisms such as growth, movement, reproduction and adaptation.

ligament Modified connective tissue which connects bone and surrounding viscera or surrounding tissue.

ligation Ligature application such as Tubal ligation Rubber band ligation etc.,

ligature Substance used to ligate such as silk, wire, cat gut etc.,

light Light is required for subjective sensation of sight in man and animals. Light is the electromagnetic radiation having a velocity of 186,284 miles per second

lightening An obstetrical term which denotes the descent of uterus into pelvic cavity 3 to 4 weeks before the labour

limb Referred to arms and legs for grasping and for locomotion.

lime Common calcium oxide used for white wash is disinfectant. Second meaning is the citric acid fruit containing vitamin C.

lincomycin Antibiotic used against Gram positive organisms.

lindane is used to treat lice and scabies, but it may cause serious side effects. Safer medications are available to treat these conditions.

Lindau's tumor This refers to Hemangioblastoma described by Lindau.

linear That which looks like a line.

lingua Latin word meaning the tongue a muscular organ in the mouth which aid in tasting, masticating, deglutition and articulation of words.

lingual That which is related with tongue.

lingula Anatomical structure which looks like a small tongue such as Cerebellar lingual or mandibular lingual etc.,

liniment Oily liquid preparation used for applying on the skin. Common liniments are Turpentine liniment, camphor liniment etc.,

linnaean Named after Botanist from Sweden who developed the system of taxonomic classification of living organisms.

linoleic acid Unsaturated 18-carbon fatty acid present in vegetable oils which is an essential fatty acid

linolenic acid Unsaturated 18-carbon fatty acid present in fish oils and seed oils which is an essential fatty acid.

lint This is an absorbent surgical dressing material

lip The margin of the mouth which are fleshy and flexible called labia oris or oral folds. This can mean margin of any structure which is lip like in its appearance.

lipase An enzyme that hydrolyse Triglyceride or Phospholipid.

lipid They are Fat, Fatty acids, Neutral fats , waxes and steroids that are made of aliphatic hydrocarbons. Fat is major source of energy since they yield 9 calories per Gram of fat.

lipidemia High level cholesterol in the blood called hypercholesterolemia. Since they are in the form of lipoprotein the word Hyperlipidemia is used.

lipochrome Fat soluble pigments like carotene, lycopene, lutein, xanthophylls.

lipodystrophy Absence of fat in sub cutaneous tissue which may be congenital or acquired .

lipogranuloma Foreign body reaction in fat tissue leading to granulation and cysts.

lipoma Tumour which is containing fat tissue and is benign usually occur in isolated areas.

lipopolysaccharide This is the combination of lipid and polysaccharide that is found in cell wall of Gram negative bacteria.

lipoprotein They are triglycerides or cholesteryl esters . Types of Lipoprotein are:

- Chylomicrons
- Very Low Density Lipoproteins
- Low density lipoproteins
- High density lipoproteins

lipoproteinemia Presence of excessive lipoproteins in the blood.

liposuction With the help of high pressure vacuum fat deposits are removed for reverting to normal shape of an organ.

liquefaction When a substance is converted into liquid.

liquid Physical status of a substance which will be in a position to flow readily.

liquor Name of fluids in the body such as liquor amnii or liquor chorii.

Lissauer's paralysis An apoplexy with paralysis of Posterolateral Tract.

Lister English surgeon who used carbolic acid along with heat sterilised instrument did surgeries which showed remarkable reduction in post operative infection. This is documented in 1865.

Lister's tubercle This refers to Dorsal Radial Tubercle described by Lister.

lithiasis Calculi or concretions formed in urinary bladder, kidney or gall bladder.

lithocystotomy Bladder stone is removed through incision through bladder through abdominal route.

lithotomy For removal of bladder stone, incision of bladder through abdominal route.

lithotripsy Non invasive procedure for crushing the bladder stone and washing it off.

litmus This is from lichens as pigment prepared used in pH tests which hs the range of pH of 4.5 to 8.3

Little's area This is common site for Nose Bleeding since it is richly vascularised. It is the area of anterior part of nasal septum above intermaxillary zone.

Little's disease Cerebral palsy occurring in new-born due to trauma or foetal anoxia. This produces spastic stiffness of limbs producing difficulty in walking.

livedo Discoloured spot on the skin due to passive congestion

liver (liv'[schwa]r) Part of G I system liver in upper right part of abdomen has the functions of blood filtration, bile secretion, bilirubin excretion glycogen formation from sugar .

liver phosphorylase Isozyme of glycogen phosphorylase present in the liver. It's deficiency causes glycogen storage disease type VI.

liver phosphorylase kinase is a serine/threonine-specific protein kinase which activates glycogen phosphorylase to release glucose-1-phosphate from glycogen.

livid Discolouration due to contusion.

Livingston's triangle This area is important in eliciting hypersensitive area on palpation on a triangular area bounded by lines from umbilicus to iliac crest, from here to right public spine and are there to umbilicus.

LMP Abbreviation for **L**ast **M**enstrual **P**eriod

LOA Abbreviation for **L**eft **O**ccipito **A**nterior the position of the foetus.

lobar That which is related with a lobe

lobe Well defined portion of lung, liver or any organ that are demarcated by sulci, fissures or by shape.

lobectomy Excision and removal of a lobe of any organ say that of lung, brain, thyroid or liver.

Lobo's disease This refers to Blastomycosis with Keloid described by Lobo.

Lobstein's disease This refers to Osteogenesis Imperfecta described by Lobstein.

lobule This denotes to a small lobe

local That which is not generalised and is only localised that means restricted to one spot.

lochia Vaginal discharge during the first week. Lochia rubra, Lochia alba and Lochia serosa are three common types of lochia.

Locke's solution Used in Physiology experiments of mammalian heart. This contains the following:-

- ✓ NaCl
- ✓ KCl
- ✓ $NaHCO_3$
- ✓ Dextrose

lockjaw This is one the symptoms of Tetanus which is called Trismus.

Lockwood's ligament Thick ligament which extends from Tenon's capsule and the sheaths of inferior rectus and inferior oblique muscles.

locomotion One of the property of living organisms which allow the function of movement from one place to another.

locus This is the position of the gene on a chromosome

Loewi German-born American physiologist and pharmacologist who won Nobel Prize for Medicine in 1936 for his work on chemical transmission of nerve impulses..

Löffler's methylene blue Stain used to demonstrate Diphtheria bacteria. Stain contains Methylene blue made alkaline and potassium hydroxide, which is applied to the slide for a few minutes and the slide, is washed. Granules appear deep blue in lighter blue cells.

logarithm From a base number we get a second number which is computed in natural base 'e'. this is denoted by:

$e = \log_e$

$\log_e (y) = x$

$e^x = y$

logopedics This refers to speech pathology and speech therapy i.e., the study and treatment of speech defects.

longevity Good health condition which allow a man to live longer.

longissimus The word mean 'any long anatomical structure' such as longissimus muscle.

longitudinal This denote that any thing in reference is parallel to the long axis of the body or an organ.

longsightedness This refers to Hypermetropia, a refractive error.

loop When there is a curve in thick cord like anatomical structure. Common terms in use are:

i. Henle's loop
ii. Spinal nerve loop
iii. Ventricular loop
iv. Capillary loop
v. Subclavian loop
vi. Cervical loop

loopful Thin layer of fluid in a loop of wire used in transferring pathogens in culture media.

LOP Abbreviation for **L**eft **O**ccipito **P**osterior position of foetus in the womb.

loperamide hydrochloride Oral antiperistaltic drug used in inflammatory bowel syndromes.

Lorain-Lévi dwarfism This referred to Pituitary gland hypo function called hypophysial infantilism described by Lorain and Levi.

lordosis Increased anterior curvature of back bone producing hollow back or saddle back

Lorenz Austrian zoologist who got Nobel Prize for his work on Ethology in 1973

Lorenz's operation Orthopaedic correction for developmental dysplasia of hip joint.

losartan potassium This is an angiotensin II receptor antagonist used in the treatment of high blood pressure.

loss Functional loosing such as hearing loss, visual loss etc.,

Lossen's rule In case of Royal disease Haemophilia, Men gets disease or inherits disease where as women only carry or transmits the disease.

LOT Abbreviation for **L**eft **O**ccipito **T**ransverse position of the foetus in the womb.

lotion An external application of liquid suspension of medication . Common lotions are:

- Calamine lotion
- Benzyl benzoate lotion
- Lindane lotion

Lou Gehrig disease Lou *Gehrig was an* American baseball player who succumbed to this disease and hence the name Lou Gehrig disease which is Amyotrophic Lateral Sclerosis.

Louis's angle It is called sternal angle or Ludwig's angle which is formed on the anterior surface of the sternum at the junction of its body and manubrium.

Louis-Bar's syndrome This is referred to Ataxia associated with Telangiectasia described by Louis Bar.

loupe This is a magnifying glass or convex lens put to spectacles.

louse Referable to head louse, body louse and pubic louse which are of medical importance in Medical Entomology . Head and body louse transmit Typhus, Trench fever and Relapsing fevers.

lovastatin Drug used in Hypercholesterolaemia

Löwe's ring Ring observed in the visual field which is due to macula.

Lowe's syndrome This is referred to combination of diseases of the eye, of the brain and kidney diseases called Oculocerebrorenal Syndrome. It is also called Lowe Terrey Mac Lachlan syndrome.

Löwenberg's canal It is called cochlear canal which lye between the Scala tympani below and the Scala vestibule above.

loxotomy Type of limb amputation called oval amputation.

lozenge Chewable or suckable tablet with medication , In case of plastic surgery this denote to an area marked on the skin for its for removal.

LSD Abbreviation for **L**y**S**ergic Acid **D**iethylamide a hallucinogen.

lubb This is referable to first heart sound described in auscultation.

lubb-dupp Term used to explain normal first and second heart sound in auscultation.

lubricant Oily non toxic substance used as surface applicator to reduce friction in moving parts or joints.

Luc's operation Antrostomy operation through supradental fossa opposite premolar teeth.

Lucas' sign This is a sign of Rickets where we observe the distension of abdomen. This is supposed to be early sign of rickets.

lucid Latin word meaning that which is clear such s Lucid interval.

lucidity Clarity of mind in a person.

Lucio's leprosy Diffuse lepromatous infiltration of skin . In severe cases it is called Lucio's phenomenon where dermal necrosis is seen.

Ludwig's angina Severe cellulites of submaxillary space by infection or injury which is manifested by fever, tachypnoea, oedema of glottis and difficulty for swallowing or eating.

Ludwig's angle This refers to Sternal Angle described by Ludwig.

Luer's syringe This is named after Luer a German instrument maker in France who developed the Luer Lock syringe in 19th century. This is a glass syringe for I V, I M and Hypodermic injections

Lugol's caustic This refers to Strong Iodine Solution identified by Logol which is still a best antiseptic in medical practice.

lumbago Latin word denoting the loin region where pain is perceived.

lumbar This refers to loin which is sides of the back between pelvis and thorax.

lumbosacral Related to loins and sacrum.

lumbricoid Referred to round worm which resembles earthworm.

lumen Inside a tubular structure it is a cavity.

luminescence Which emits light without production of heat.

Lumsden's center This refers to Pneumotaxic Center described by Lumsden.

lunacy In Latin this means the moon and name is given to a personality which is not normal or insane.

lunatic Mentally ill person.

Lung A pair of organ in thorax for respiration which are separated by mediastinal structures. Lung help in exchange of gases that is vital to the existence.

lungworm Longest nematode parasite called Paragonimus westermani which produce lung lesion.

lunula Any anatomical structure which is moon shaped such as lunula of nail, lunula of aortic valve etc.,

lupus Refers to Lupus erythematosus or Lupus Vulgaris. Latin word means destruction of skin.

Lust's phenomenon In case of presence of muscular spasm of leg muscle, tapping peroneal nerve just below the head of the fibula produces abduction with dorsal flexion of the foot.

luteinization Development of corpus luteum and lipid accumulation gives the luteinisation a sort of yellow colouration.

luteotropin Other name for Prolactin.

lux Unit of illumination called foot candle.

LVH Abbreviation for **L**eft **V**entricular **H**ypertrophy

Lyell's disease This refers to Toxic Epidermal Necrolysis described by Lyell.

lying-in Post delivery period of women called puerperium.

lymph Liquid present in Lymphatic vessels that contains liquid portion of and lymphocytes.

lymphadenitis Infection and inflammation of one or more lymph nodes

lymphadenopathy This is referred to as the disease of the lymph nodes.

lymphangiectasis Dilatation of the lymphatic vessels.

lymphangioma This is referred to as Cavernous lymphangioma unless otherwise mentioned. This is a benign tumor representing a congenital malformation of the lymphatic system

lymphangiosarcoma This is a malignant tumor of vascular endothelial cells from lymphatic vessels

lymphangitis Infection and inflammation of a lymphatic vessels.

lymphatic That which is related with lymph vessels.

lymphedema Chronic oedema of lower limbs or upper limbs due to interstitial fluid accumulation by stasis of lymph.

lymphoblast Immature lymphocyte that are due to antigenic stimulation.

lymphocyte They are mononuclear white cells present in blood, lymph and lymphoid tissues that are responsible for body immunity.

lymphocytosis Increased number of lymphocytes in the blood which reveals the presence of an infection which could be acute in nature.

lympholytic Substance that cause destruction of lymphocytes.

lymphoma Cancerous disorder of the lymphoid tissue

Lynch's incision In case of tumours of sinus, pyocele and mucocele removal that content is made by incision of the frontal sinus to remove the floor and contents.

Lynen German biochemist who received Nobel prize for his work in biosynthesis of fatty acids and cholesterol in the year 1964.

lynestrenol It is the component of oral contraceptives which has the action of progestational activity.

lyophilization Rapid freezing and dehydrating blood plasma or serum to get a stable preparation. This is also called Freeze Drying.

lysergic acid Present in natural alkaloid ergot and is obtained by hydrolysis. Same synthetic ergot alkaloid with psychotomimetic properties is called LSD.

lysin Substance which help to dissolve in biological science.

lysine This is an essential amino acid required for growth of infants and required for nitrogen equilibrium of adults. .

lysis Greek word meaning destruction or dissolution. This can be cellular, tissue, organ lysis. This can also mean gradual cure of an illness.

lysosome They are electron microscopic bodies that service the function of intracellular digestion. Their release causes tissue damage. There are two types namely Primary and Secondary lysosomes.

lysozyme This is an enzyme of the hydrolase class that catalyzes the hydrolysis of glycosides. This enzyme is present in saliva, tears and egg white

Lyssavirus Rhabdoviridae viruses which include Rabies virus which causes hydrophobia.

M

μ (μ) mu, Symbol for Micron and it is the twelfth letter of the Greek alphabet

Macaca Monkey species used in laboratory research.

McArdle's disease This refers to Glycogen Storage Disease described by McArdle.

McBurney's point This refers to a point about one 1/3rd the distance between the right anterior superior iliac spine and the umbilicus. This corresponds with the normal position of the base of the appendix and is a point of special tenderness in acute appendicitis.

MacConkey's agar This a culture medium used to differentiate coliforms (lactose fermenters) from non lactose fermenters (among enteric bacilli). The ingredients are:

- Peptone
- Lactose
- Bile salts
- Sodium chloride
- Neutral red
- Crystal violet

McDonald's maneuver Measurement of contour of abdomen to calculate the duration of pregnancy. This follows the rule which estimate gestational age of pregnant woman in her 3rd trimester. If a pregnant women showed the measurement as 30 cm from the fundus to the pubis, the gestational age can be estimated by using McDonald's Rule as under;

$$\frac{\text{Fundal height in cms.}}{3.5} = \frac{30}{3.5} = 8.5714 = 8.6 \text{ lunar months.}$$

maceration Degenerative changes with discolouration and softening of tissues.

Macleod Scottish physiologist during 1876–1935 won Nobel prize with Banting on their discovery of Insulin.

Macleod's syndrome This is also called Swyer James Syndrome which is characterised by the following manifestations

- Unilateral emphysema which is acquired
- Severe airway obstruction
- Oligemia
- Presence of a small hilum

McMurray's test This test is positive in case of tear in lateral or medial meniscus of the knee joint. Patient lies supine with knee fully flexed, the examiner rotates the patient's foot fully outward and the knee is slowly extended. Painful click indicates tear of the medical meniscus. With same procedure painful click when patient's foot fully rotated inwards the diagnosis is tear of the lateral meniscus.

macrogamete Larger less active female anisogamete.

macrogametocyte Larger less active macrogametocyte.

macrognathia Abnormally large jaws.

macrolide Antibacterial antibiotics containing a macrolide ring (large lactone ring containing multiple keto and hydroxyl groups) produced by species of streptomyces. Common available antibiotics are erythromycin, azithromycin and clarithromycin.

macronutrient Carbohydrates, fats, proteins, water, minerals like calcium, chloride, magnesium, phosphorus, potassium, sodium, and sulphur

macropathology Morbid (seen by naked eye) pathological changes of an organ or tissue.

macrophage Different forms of mononuclear phagocytes present in tissues.

macrophallus Abnormally large male organ.

macrophthalmous Abnormally large eyes.

macroscopic Visible to the naked eye.

macroscopy Examination with the naked eye.

macula Discoloured spot on the skin that is not elevated above the surface;

maculopapular An eruption consisting of both macules and papules

Madura foot Named after a place called Madurai in Tamil Nadu State of South India. It is mycetoma of the foot.

maggot Larva of an insects living in decaying flesh and wounds of live animals, including humans

Magnan's movement Forward and backward movement of the tongue when it is drawn out. This present in general paresis.

magnet Native iron oxide that attracts iron that has magnetic polarity.

magnification Increase in size as under the microscope.

Mahler's sign This is positive in thrombosis wherein a steady increase of pulse rate without corresponding elevaton of temperature.

maintenance Providing a stable state over a long period

mal Denotes disease or pathological state. Grand mal, Petit mal are common disease entities.

malabsorption Impaired intestinal absorption of nutrients

malacia Softness of a part or of tissue.

maladie Refers to a disease

malaise Vague feeling of bodily discomfort

malalignment Displacement out of line such as malocclusion of teeth or malalignment of teeth.

malar meaning buccal.

malaria It means bad air. An infectious disease caused by obligate intracellular protozoa of the genus Plasmodia, transmitted by the bite of infected Anopheles mosquito.

malathion An organophosphorus insecticide and veterinary topical parasiticide.

maldevelopment Abnormal development.

male Represents masculine sex and that produce spermatozoa.

malformation Morphological defect or anomaly.

malfunction This refers to dysfunction.

malignancy Cancerous that potentially cause death.

malignant This can be anaplasia, invasion, and metastasis; said of tumors.

malingering Wilful, deliberate, and fraudulent exaggeration of the symptoms of illness

malleable That can be beaten out into a thin plate.

Mallory's bodies This is seen in alcoholic cirrhosis and hepatic disorders. Mallory's bodies are hyaline cytoplasmic inclusions of cytokeratin in liver cells.

malnutrition Disorder of nutrition due to insufficient diet or defective assimilation

malocclusion Malposition of maxillary and mandibular teeth which come in the way of mastication. Depending on anteroposterior jaw relationship there are four major groups of malocclusion in dentistry management.

malpighian bodies bodies where the smaller veins enter into the larger veins of the spleen.

malpractice Unskilled improper practice

malpresentation Abnormal foetal presentation.

malrotation When organs fail to rotate at embryological development.

malt Barley soaked in water for germination, dried. The malt contains dextrin, maltose, and diastase.

maltase They are glycolytic enzymes.

malthusian law This postulates that over population is controlled by natural calamities like volcano, earthquake, floods, epidemic etc. Though it is not a scientific version it can only be an antithesis of population. The law states that population tends to outrun the means available to sustain it..

maltose A reducing disaccharide composed of two glucose residues

mamma Breast that secrete milk for nourishment of the young.

Manchester operation Named after the place where it was developed. Operation for prolapse of uterus. The steps include D & C, anterior repair, amputation of the vaginal portion of the cervix, shortening of the cardinal ligaments and posterior colpoperineorrhaphy.

mandelic acid Bacteriostatic used in urinary tract infections, usually as the ammonium salt.

mandible Bone of the lower jaw

maneuver Any dexterous procedure such as Adson's maneuver for thoracic outlet syndrome, Allen's maneuver for scalenus anterior syndrome, Brandt Andrews maneuver for expression of the placenta, Kocher maneuver as operative mobilisation of the duodenum, Ortolani maneuver to diagnose congenial hip dislocation, Valsalva maneuver for forcible exhalation effort against a closed glottis,

mania Greek word meaning madness. A psychiatric disorder with elation, agitation, hyperexcitability, flight of ideas called manic syndrome.

manikin Body model which is movable and removable used for teaching purpose.

manipulation Skilful treatment by the hand.

Mann-Whitney test Statistical Rank Sum Test described by Mann and Whitney.

mannerism Stereotyped movement or habit of an individual.

mannitol Reduction of mannose or fructose present in plants and fungi.

mannose This is produced in oligosaccharides like glycoproteins or glycolipids.

Manson's hemoptysis Schistosoma parasitic haemoptysis described by Manson.

Mansonia Mosquito that transmits filarial caused by Brugia malayi.

Mantoux test Tuberculin test using PPD to find out whether a person is exposed to infection with Mycobacterium tuberculosis.

manual Procedure performed by the hand

manubrium Handle like structure referable to Manubrium sterni.

MAO Abbreviation for **M**ono **A**mine **O**xidase.
map Graphic representation of a space which is two dimensional.
mapping Locating the relative position of genes on chromosomes.
marasmus Protein-Energy Malnutrition predominantly due to prolonged severe caloric deficit, chiefly occurring during the first year of life characterized by growth retardation and progressive wasting of subcutaneous fat and muscle. Appetite and mental alertness are retained.
Marfan's syndrome Congenital disorder of connective tissues. Clinical manifestations are:

- Lengthy fingers and toes
- Subluxation of the lens
- cardiovascular abnormalities

margin Referable to the edge,
marijuana Cannabis preparation which has euphoric effect.
Marion's disease Congenital malformation of urogenital system with stenosis of bladder neck producing obstruction of posterior urethra.
Marjolin's ulcer Ulcer seated on old cicatrix. This is associated with malignancy.
mark Spot on the skin or mucous membrane. E.g., Birth mark, Pock mark etc.,
marrow Bone marrow which is soft substance in the bone.
Marsh's disease This refers to Graves' disease described by Marsh.
Marsupialia Order of the class Mammalia which include Kangaroos
Marsupialization Surgical exteriorization of a cyst by resection of the anterior wall and suture of the cut edges of the remaining cyst to the adjacent edges of the skin.
masculine Presence of qualities the male sex.
Masochism Gaining pleasure from experiencing physical or psychological pain referable to sexual masochism.
mass A lump made up of cohering particles
massage Systematic therapeutic stroking, and kneading of the body.
massive Solid and bulky form
mastectomy Surgical excision of the breast called mammectomy. This can be total or partial mastectomy.
mastication The process of food chewing
mastitis Inflammation of the breast.
mastoid That which is breast shaped such as mastoid process of temporal bone.
mastoidectomy Excision of the mastoid cells or mastoid process of the temporal bone.
mastoiditis inflammation of the mastoid antrum due to otitis media or ear infection.
masturbation Self-stimulation of the genitals for sexual pleasure.
Masugi's nephritis This refers to Nephrotoxic Serum Nephritis described by Masugi.
matching Selection of objects having similar or identical characteristics as done in clinical trials or case control studies.
maternal Related with the word the mother.
maternity A lying in hospital for obstetric cause or gynaecological cause.
mating Pairing of individuals of the opposite sex for reproduction.
matrix Intracellular substance of a tissue from which a structure develops.
maturation Stage of becoming mature or fully developed.
maturity Period of attainment of maximal development.
Maurer's dots Irregular dots staining red with Leishman' stain seen in RBC from malaria patients infected with plasmodium falciparum.
maxilla Bone that form upper jaw and that possess orbit, nasal cavity , palate and upper teeth.
maximum Actual effect or quantity.
Mayo's operation Excision of pyloric end of stomach with G.J, Surgical method of treatment for umbilical hernia and also for formal method of operation for varicose veins.
Mazzoni's corpuscle Small encapsulated nerve ending in skin or mucous membrane or conjunctiva which act as thermoreceptors for cold.
MCH Abbreviation for Mean Corpuscular Haemoglobin.
MCHC Abbreviation for Mean Corpuscular Haemoglobin Concentration.
MCI Abbreviation for Medical Council of India.
MCV Abbreviation for Mean Corpuscular Volume
MD Abbreviation for Doctor of Medicine
MDT Abbreviation for **M**ulti **D**rug **T**reatment adopted in Leprosy.
meal Food taken at some particular and fixed time.
mean French work meaning middle. It refers to mathematics mean in statistics. Other types of mean are geometric mean, harmonic mean, population mean and sample mean.
measles Viral disease caused by a paramyxovirus, common among children is an acute communicable disease.
measure To determine the extent of a substance.
meatus It refers to an anatomical opening.
mebendazole An anthelmintic agent that irreversibly inhibits glucose uptake in the parasite used in the treatment round worm, thread worm, hookworm
meclizine hydrochloride Antihistamine used as an antiemetic in the management motion sickness.
meconium Dark green mucilaginous material in the intestine of the full-term fetus
medial nearer to midline of a body or structure.
median Median is the middle value of an odd number of values arranged in ascending order

mediastinum Tissues and organs separating the two pleural sacs, between the sternum anteriorly and the vertebral column posteriorly and from the thoracic inlet superiorly to the diaphragm inferiorly.

medical That which is related with medicine and treatment of illness.

medicament Medicinal substance

medication Administration of remedies. Common terminologies are conservative medication, sublingual medication, and parenteral medication.

medicine Drug which is used as remedy. This can also detail a discipline like aviation medicine, behavioural medicine, clinical medicine, comparative medicine, Emergency medicine,
Environmental medicine, Experimental medicine, family medicine, forensic medicine, geriatric medicine, and holistic medicine.

medicolegal Pertaining to medicine and law, or to forensic medicine.

medicosocial Discipline that has both medical and social aspects,

Medin's disease This refers to Poliomyelitis described by Medin.

medium Substance used in the culture of bacteria called culture medium.

MEDLARS Abbreviation for **MED**ical **L**iterature **A**nalysis and **R**etrieval system from which Index Medicus is produced. It is a computerised bibliographic system.

MEDLINE This is an on line segment of MEDLARS.

medroxyprogesterone acetate Progestin orally in the treatment of secondary amenorrhea and functional uterine bleeding. Progestin intramuscularly as an antineoplastic in the treatment of metastatic endometrial and renal carcinoma. Progestin as a contraceptive.

medulla Most interior portion of an organ or structure. Examples are adrenal medulla, renal medulla, and medulla oblongata.

mega- Large, enlarged, or of abnormally large size

megacolon An abnormally large or dilated colon

megaloblast Large, nucleated, immature progenitor of an abnormal red blood cell series seen in some types of anemia

meiosis Cell division, occurring in maturation of the sex cells, by means of which each daughter nucleus receives half the number of chromosomes characteristic of the somatic cells of the species.

melancholia Major depressive disorder called Melancholia.

melanin Dark amorphous pigment of the skin, hair, and various tumors, of the choroid coat of the eye and the substantia nigra of the brain.

melanoblastoma Malignant melanoma

melanocyte Dendritic clear cells of the epidermis that synthesize tyrosinase and, within their melanosomes, the pigment melanin

melanoma Tumor arising from the melanocyte of the skin and other organs.

melena Dark stools stained with altered blood.

membrane Layer of tissue which covers a surface or lines a cavity

memory Mental faculty by which sensations, impressions, and ideas are recalled.

menadione Provitamin that can be chemically converted in the body to active vitamin K

menarche Beginning of the menstrual function.

Mendel's laws It is called laws of inheritance which is the basis of genetics. Gregor Mendel described this in the year 1865. From experimental crosses of pea plants differing in one or more characteristics determined by single genes, and counting the types of progeny in successive generations, Mendel derived laws that are called LAW OF SEGREGATION and LAW OF INDEPENDENT ASSORTMENT.

Meniere's disease It is popularly called Endolymphatic Hydrops (nonsuppurative disease of the labyrinth with oedema) which has the following clinical manifestations:

- hearing loss
- tinnitus
- vertigo

meningioma Benign, slow-growing tumor of the meninges

meningism Symptoms and signs of meningeal irritation associated with acute febrile illness or dehydration without actual infection of the meninges.

meningitis Infection and inflammation of the meninges, usually by either a bacterium or a virus

meningocele Called Spina Bifida is hernial protrusion of the meninges through a bony defect

meniscus In chemistry basic term upper meniscus and lower meniscus represent a crescent-shaped structure appearing at the surface of a liquid column

menopause Cessation of menstruation in the human female occurring usually around the age of 45 years which is called Climacteric.

menses Refers to menstruation which is the monthly flow of blood from the genital tract of women

menstrual Related with menstruation

menstruation Cyclic, physiologic blood discharge through the vagina nonpregnant. Types of menstruation are:

- ❖ Vicarious menstruation
- ❖ Anovular menstruation
- ❖ Scanty menstruation.

mensuration Process of measuring.

mental Related with either mind or chin.

mercaptopurine Purine analogue used in the chemotherapy of cancer such as Leukaemias, Crohn's disease, ulcerative colitis, psoriatic arthritis, polycythemia vera.

merozoite One of the stage in the life cycle of certain sporozoan protozoa

mesencephalon Midbrain developed from middle of three primary brain vesicles of embryo.

mesenteritis Inflammation of the mesentery.

mesial This refers to nearer the center line of the dental arch.

mesmerism Named after Franz A Mesmer which means hypnotism.

mesocolon This contains ascending, transverse, descending, and sigmoid portions, according to the segment of the colon to which it gives attachment with peritoneum.

mesoderm Middle layer of the three primary germ layers of the embryo, from which connective tissue, bone, cartilage, muscle, blood vessels, lymphatics pleura, pericardium, peritoneum, kidney and gonads are derived.

mesosome Invagination of the cell membrane occurring in certain bacteria.

mesothelioma Tumor derived from mesothelial tissue like peritoneum, pleura, pericardium

mesothelium Flat cells, derived from the mesoderm, which lines the body cavity of the embryo.

meta-analysis Systematic method that uses statistical analysis to integrate the data from a number of independent studies.

metabolism This include Anabolism (produced and maintained) and Catabolism (available for use of organism) . Common entities are:

- Basal metabolism
- Energy metabolism
- Inborn error of metabolism

metabolite Substance produced by a metabolic process.

metacarpal Related with metacarpus.

metacarpus Part of the hand between the wrist and the fingers,

metacercaria The encysted resting stage of trematode parasite in the tissues molluscs or on vegetation.

metamorphosis Transition from one developmental stage to another such as from larva to adult form.

metaphase Second stage of cell division

metaphysis Wider part at the extremity of the shaft of a long bone,

metaplasia Changes that are not normal to a tissue such as Squamous, nephrogenic or myeloid.

metastasis Transfer of cells as in malignant tumors.

metatarsal Pertaining to the metatarsus.

metatarsus Part of the foot between the tarsus and the toes.

Metazoa Multicellular animals whose cells become differentiated to form tissues.

Metchnikoff Russian zoologist co-winner with Paul Ehrlich, of the Nobel prize for medicine or physiology in 1908 for his discovery of phagocytes and phagocytosis.

meter Basic unit of linear measure in the metric system

metformin Anti Hyperglycaemic agent used in the treatment of Type 2 Diabetes.

methanal Other name for Formaldehyde.

methane Methane CH_4, produced by decomposition of organic matter,

methaqualone A non-barbiturate compound used as a sedative and hypnotic

methemoglobin Brown pigment formed from Haemoglobin formed in injury or by toxic agents.

methemoglobinemia Presence of excessive methemoglobin in the blood, which can occur as congenital or as acquired condition.

methionine Naturally occurring essential amino acid necessary for normal metabolism.

methodology Principles of procedure in research and in scientific study.

methotrexate Drug used in cancer treatment which inhibits the synthesis of DNA, thymidylate and protein.

methylcellulose Methyl ether of cellulose used as a cathartic, and applied topically to the conjunctiva to protect and to lubricate the cornea.

methyltestosterone Synthetic androgen similar to testosterone used in replacement therapy and inoperable breast cancer.

metoprolol Hypotensive agent which is a cardioselective β_1-adrenergic blocking agent.

metra Greek word meaning uterus.

metritis Infection and inflammation of the uterus.

metronidazole Antiprotozoal and antibacterial effective against Trichomonas vaginalis infection, giardiasis, and amoebiasis.

Mg symbol for Magnesium

mg symbol for milligram.

µg symbol for microgram.

MI Abbreviation for Myocardial infarction.

miconazole Broad-spectrum antifungal agent

microbe Microorganism like bacteria, protozoa and fungi which cause diseases in man.

microbiology Science that deals with the study of microorganisms

microfauna Animal life visible only under the microscope

microfilaria Prelarval stage of Filaria worm which produce elephantiasis.

microfilm High-speed automatic machines for the photographic reproduction, in greatly reduced size, of books and documents

microgamete Smaller flagellated and actively motile male anisogamete.

microglia Supporting structure of the central nervous system.

micronutrient Essential dietary element required in small quantities such as trace elements.

microorganism These are microbes seen under microscope such as bacteria, fungi or protozoa.

microphone For amplification a device is used which can convert acoustic signal into an electric signal .

microscope Laboratory instrument used to obtain an enlarged image of small objects . Types of microscope in use are:

- Binocular microscope
- Compound microscope
- Dark field microscope
- Electron microscope
- Fluorescence microscope
- Operating microscope
- Simple microscope

microscopy Observation by means of the microscope.

microsurgery Surgery under microscope as in ENT, Eye etc.,

microtome Instrument for cutting thin slices of tissue for microscopical study.

microvilli Processes on the free surface of a cell specifically in intestine and renal tubule.

micturition The act of urination.

mid-diastolic Occurring in the middle third of diastole.

midwife One who practices midwifery

midwifery Clinical practice of assisting in childbirth.

migraine Periodic attacks of vascular headache,

Mikulicz'scells They are called foam cells that are seen in rhinoscleroma that contain the bacillus of the disease.

Miles' operation Operation done for cancer of sigmoid and rectum. This drastic operation for cancer includes removal of pelvic colon, mesocolon, adjacent lymph nodes, wide perineal excision of rectum, wide excision of anus and a permanent colostomy.

miliary That which resembles millet seed. Generally applicable to miliary tuberculosis.

milieu French word meaning environment which can be external or internal. Claude Bernard's internal environment is well known postulation.

milk Mammary gland secretion for the young.

milking Pressing out of the contents of a tubular part

Milkman's syndrome Generalised bone disease with transparent stripes of absorption in long and flat bones.

Miller-Abbott tube Inflammable balloon holding double channel intestinal tube used in the treatment of intestinal obstruction.

Mills' disease This is referred to Ascending Hemiplegia described by Mills.

Milroy's disease Congenital hereditary lymphedema of legs caused by chronic lymphatic obstruction.

Milton's disease This refers to angioedema described by Milton.

Minamata disease Named after Minamata bay in Japan where Minamata disease was caused by poisoned seafood.

mind Mind is the seat of consciousness where men experiences feelings, emotions, and desires, and is able to attend, to remember, to learn, to reason, and to decide.

mineral Nonorganic solid substance from the earth's crust.

mineralocorticoid This is involved in the regulation of electrolyte and water balance . Principally it refers to aldosterone which is stimulated by angiotensin II.

Minerva jacket This is **used to immobilise the various levels of the cervical and thoracic spine**. A minerva cast is generally made of fibreglass casting material and remains in place for approximately four to 12 weeks. The cast can only be removed by a cast technician or orthopaedic doctor.

minilaparotomy Short incision laparotomy.

miosis Greek word meaning diminished referable to papillary contraction

mirror Concave or convex mirror which reflect light to yield images of objects in front of it.

miscarriage Spontaneous abortion before the fetus is viable;

miscible That can be mixed.

misogamy Aversion to marriage.

misogyny Aversion to women.

mite Trombiculid mite and Itch mite are of public health importance. They produce skin irritations called acariasis since they belong to order Acarina.

mitochondria (mi″to-kon′dre-[schwa]a) Small spherical to rod-shaped components in the cytoplasm of cells, they are the principal sites of the generation of energy

mitosis Indirect cell division. In different stages like prophase, metaphase, anaphase and telophase. Daughter cells receive identical complements of number of chromosomes characteristics of somatic cells of given species.

mitotic pertaining to mitosis.

mitral Related to mitral valve.

Mitsuda reaction It is called Lepromin reaction. It is a skin test to differentiate tuberculoid and lepromatous leprosy. It is negative in lepromatous and positive in tuberculoid leprosy.

mixture Combination of different drugs or ingredients in the form of fluid for administration orally during treatment. Common mixtures are:

- o Pectin Kaolin mixture
- o Sodasol mixture
- o Sedative expectorant mixture
- o Cough mixture

MLD Abbreviation for **M**inimum **L**ethal **D**ose

mm Symbol for Millimeter.

mm Hg Expression for millimeter of mercury, a unit of pressure equal to sea level 760 mm.Hg.

MMR Abbreviation for **M**aternal **M**ortality **R**ate and for **M**easles, **M**umps and **R**ubella vaccine.

mnemonic That which promotes recollection or memory.

mnemonics Improvement of memory by special methods

MO Abbreviation for **M**edical **O**fficer

mobilization This refers to mobilisation of finance, manpower or material in Health administration.

Möbius' disease This refers to Ophthalmoplegic Migraine described by Mobius.

modality Employment of any therapeutic agent in the management of a case.

mode Most frequently occurring value in a distribution

model A replica or a facsimile of the body

moiety One half of a portion.

mold Parasitic or saprobic fungi.

mole This refers to any one of the following:

- Atoms
- Ions
- Molecules
- Radicals
- Blemish spot of the skin

molecular That which composed of molecules.

Molecule Smallest amount of a substance in the nature. This can be aggregation of atoms.

Molisch's test Test for glucose in the urine sample. 2 ml. of urine + 2 drops of 15% thymol + equal volume of strong sulphuric acid. Deep red colour is positive for the presence of glucose in the sample of urine.

molluscum Soft rounded cutaneous tumours of skin such as Molluscum contagiosum.

Monge's disease This refers to chronic mountain sickness described by Monge.

mongolian Related to the resembles of Mongols and formerly it was applied to Down syndrome.

mongolism Down Syndrome because of facial characteristics typical of this condition.

monitor The procedure of checking constantly on a state of signs or symptoms in patients.

Moniz Portuguese neurosurgeon co-winner of the Nobel prize for medicine or physiology in 1949 for his development of cerebral angiography and the introduction of prefrontal lobotomy as a therapy for certain psychoses.

monkeypox Epidemic, exanthematous disease occurring in captive monkeys, which can be transmitted to humans, in whom it causes a disease clinically similar to smallpox.

monoamine oxidase Flavin containing amine oxidase abbreviated as MAO.

monocular One eye piece of microscope.

monocyte Mononuclear phagocytic leukocyte

monogamy Marriage to a single spouse.

monoiodotyrosine Intermediate in the thyroidal biosynthesis of thyroxine and triiodothyronine.

monoparesis Paresis of a single limb.

monorchism Condition of having only one testis in the scrotum.

monosaccharide Simple sugar that cannot be decomposed by hydrolysis.

monoxide An oxide containing one atom of oxygen such as carbon monoxide.

Monro's bursa Intra tendinous bursa of olecranon.

Mons An eminence such as Mons Pubis,

Montgomery's follicles Cyst like formation by occlusion of Lumina of glands in mucosa of uterine cervix.

mood Emotion that when extreme can affect behavior.

Mooren's ulcer Chronic ulceration of the marginal cornea having a serpiginous in old age, cause of which is not known.

morbid Disease condition of man.

morbidity State of disease condition in a community.

Mordant Refers to mordents like Alum, Aniline, Oil, Phenol etc., which are capable of intensifying the reaction of a specimen to a stain.

mores Traditions and habits which are generally regarded as conducive to social welfare.

morgue Place where dead bodies are temporarily kept

moribund Person or an animal in a dying state.

Morison's pouch Peritoneal pouch below the liver and to the right of the right kidney that extends inferiorly to the transverse mesocolon.

moron Low I Q leading to mild mental retardation.

morphine Opium alkaloid which is central stimulant and narcotic. Morphine dependence is known.

morphology Science which deals with structure and form of an organism.

morphosis Process of formation of an organ.

Morris syndrome This is referred to Complete Androgen Resistance described by Morris.

mors Latin word meaning Death. Mortal means destined to die; mortality is death rates.

mortuary Place where dead bodies are kept till the disposal of the dead body.

morula Cleavage of a zygote.

mosaic Pattern made up of small pieces fitted together.

mosquito Insects which are vectors of many diseases which are of following types:

- Anopheles
- Culex
- Aedes
- Mansonoides

mother Female parent.

motile That which has the appreciable movement.

motivation Activating behavior toward or achieving goals.

motor That which movement.

mottling Condition of patches of color.

mourning Processes that follow the loss of a loved one called grief.

mouse Small rodents

mouth Proximal opening of the Alimentary Tract.

mouthwash Rinsing the mouth with some of the preparations like Potassium bicarbonate, Amaranth solution, Glycerin or purified water.

MPH Abbreviation for **M**aster of **P**ublic **H**ealth.

MRCP Abbreviation for **M**ember of the **R**oyal **C**ollege of **P**hysicians.

MRDM Abbreviation for **M**alnutrition **R**elated **D**iabetes **M**ellitus.

MRI Abbreviation for **M**agnetic **R**esonance **I**maging.

mRNA Abbreviation for Messenger RNA.

mucin Protein-containing glycoconjugates with sulfated polysaccharide content

mucolytic Substance which dissolve mucin

mucopolysaccharide Polysaccharide with a high hexosamine content

mucopurulent Mucus and pus both are present.

mucormycosis Mycosis by Mucorales fungus which infects palate, pharynx or cerebrum.

mucosanguineous When blood and mucus are present.

Muller American biologist and geneticist Winner of Nobel Prize for his discovery on spontaneous genetic mutation

Müller Swiss chemist winner of the Nobel prize for his discovery of DDT.

multibacillary That which is made up of a number of bacilli.

multicellular Composed of many cells.

multifactorial Caused or precipitated by many factors. This is said of disease in man.

multigravida Woman who has been pregnant several times.

multipara Woman who has more pregnancies which resulted in viable fetuses

mummification Drying up of a dead body or fetus.

mumps (mumps) Acute infectious disease caused by a paramyxovirus seen in children under the age of 15, clinically called parotitis

Munro's point This point is used for performing abdominal puncture. This is situated midway between the umbilicus and the left anterior iliac spine.

murine Related to rats or mice.

murmur Sound heard by auscultation which may normal or abnormal.

- Pathological murmurs are Anaemic murmur, Aneurysmal murmur, Aortic murmur, Crescendo murmur.
- Early diastolic murmur, Early systolic murmur, Mid diastolic murmur, Pansystolic murmur, Pre systolic murmur.

Murphy American physician, winner of Nobel prize for his work on Anaemia.

Murray American plastic surgeon winner of Nobel Prize for his work on Kidney transplantation.

Murray Valley Fever Named after Murray Valley in Australia where Murray Valley Fever was first detected. It is a mosquito borne viral infection caused by flavivirus which produce encephalitis.

Musca Flies under Muscidae specifically house fly called Musca domestica.

muscarine Alkaloid from mushrooms which produce poisoning.

muscle Muscle is an organ which by contraction produces the movements of an animal or man.

mutant Gene or organism that has undergone genetic mutation.

mutation Permanent transmissible change in the genetic material, usually in a single gene.

mute One who cannot speak.

mutilation Severe disfigurement which can be depriving of an organ.

muzzle Region of the face of animals,

myalgia Muscular pain.

myasthenia Constitutional anomaly of muscle.

mycetoma Progressive, destructive infection of skin fascia, and bone caused by certain actinomycetes.

Mycobacterium Genus of bacteria of the family Mycobacteriaceae that causes Pulmonary tuberculosis, non pulmonary tuberculosis and leprosy in man.

mycolic acids Fatty acids found in the cell walls of Mycobacterium bacteria

mycology Scientific study of fungi.

Mycoplasma Genus of bacteria of the family Mycoplasmataceae, that are distributed in mucous membrane of human beings.

mycosis Disease caused by a fungus.

mydriasis Dilatation of the pupil.

myelin Referable to Myelin sheath which is the substance of the cell membrane of Schwann's cells

myelitis Infection and inflammation of the spinal cord. Common clinical entities are Acute myelitis, Bulbar myelitis, Chronic myelitis, Compression myelitis, Post vaccinal myelitis, Transverse myelitis, Viral myelitis.

myeloid That which resembles bone marrow.

myeloma Tumor composed of cells of the type normally found in the bone marrow

myiasis House fly larvae infestation. Creeping myiasis, cutaneous myiasis, and traumatic wound myiasis are common entities.

myocardial Related with muscular tissue of the heart

myocarditis Inflammation of the muscular walls of the heart.

myocardium Middle thick layer of the heart wall.

myoclonus Shock-like contractions of a portion of a muscle

myope Nearsighted person called myopia.

myopia Near sightedness where rays of light entering the eye parallel to the optic axis are brought to a focus in front of the retina

myopic Person with Myopia.

myosin It is a globin which is the most abundant protein in muscle is responsible for the contraction and relaxation of muscle.

myosin ATPase An enzyme activity of muscle that uses the energy derived from the hydrolysis of ATP to drive a cycle of muscular contraction and relaxation.

myxedema Primary hypothyroidism manifested with dry, waxy swelling of the skin,

myxoma Benign tumor of connective tissue cells and stroma

myxovirus RNA viruses characterized by special affinities for mucopolysaccharides and glycoproteins

N

N Abbreviation and symbol for Nitrogen. It also denotes the strength of solution as Normal.

ν One of the Greek alphabet

Na Symbol for Sodium.

Naboth's follicles Cysts due to occlusion of lumina of glands in uterine cervical mucosa which is also called as Montgomery's follicle.

NAD Abbreviation for Nicotinamide Adenine Dinucleotide.

Naegeli's leukemia This is Acute Myelomonocytic Leukaemia described by Naegeli.

Naffziger's syndrome This is Scalenus Syndrome described by Naffziger.

Nagel's test Colour vision test where the test is done by matching half standard yellow and matched yellow for patients who mixes red and green.

Nageotte bracelets, cell They are bands covered with circular spines on the axons.

nail Dead tissues of the skin in the form of nails in fingers and toes. This also denotes the metal rod that can be fixed to bones in fractures. Aberrant growth of nail is called ingrown nail. Kuntscher nail and Jewett nail are nails used in Orthopaedics.

nailing Always refer to intra medullary nailing, marrow nailing or medullary nailing in fractured bone fixation.

nalidixic acid Quinolone drug used orally in the treatment of urinary infections caused by gram-negative organisms like Proteus.

nalorphine An antagonist to Morphine and other narcotics.

NANBH Abbreviation used for Non A Non B Hepatitis.

nandrolone Non methylated anabolic steroid which is different from methylated testosterone.

nanogram A unit of weight in metric system which is equivalent to 10^{-9} gram

nanoliter A unit of volume which is equivalent to 10^{-9} of a liter

nape This refers to the back of the neck.

naphthalene Hydrocarbon from coal tar oil which is used as moth repellent, fungicide, and preservative

naproxen It is a nonsteroidal anti-inflammatory drug used in osteoarthritis and rheumatoid arthritis.

narcissism Showing interest and love in one's own body. The word came to existence from a Person called Narcissus in Greek who fell in love with his own image in water. There are two types described one is Primary infantile phase type and the other is Secondary adult type.

narcoanalysis Mind analysis by injecting Barbiturates drug which help in psychotherapy.

narcolepsy Paroxysmal sleep or Brief episodes of sleep which is uncontrollable in nature.

narcosis CNS depression by opioid drugs.

nares This refers to Nostrils. External orifices of nose.

nasal Related to nose such as nasal speech sound.

nascent Just liberated item such nascent oxygen.

nasogastric That which related with nose and stomach. E.G., Naso Gastric tube.

nasolacrimal That which is related with nose and lacrimal apparatus.

natal This refers to buttocks.

Nathans American microbiologist who won Nobel Prize in Medicine in 1978 for his work in molecular genetics.

natrium Latin word denoting Sodium.

natriuresis Sodium or salt losing in urine

naturopathy Treatment with physical material such as water therapy, heat therapy, massage, light therapy etc.,

nausea Sensation in epigastrium which is unpleasant that culminates in vomiting.

nauseant Substance which produce nausea.

navel Refers to Umbilical area.

navicular A structure which is boat shaped.

NBS Abbreviation for **N**ational **B**ureau of **S**tandards.

near-sight This sis called refractive error called Myopia.

nebula This is a corneal opacity that is not significant.

nebulizer Small device for creating and throwing an aerosol spray.

Necator Hookworm genus and is called Necator americanus.

neck Is a constricted part such as Neck of humerus, Neck of ankle, neck of bladder etc.,

necrolysis Destruction due to necrosis.

necrophilia Sexual contact with dead bodies.

necropsy Post death examination to ascertain cause of death which is also called autopsy.

necrosadism Sadistic mutilation of dead to get sexual pleasure.

necrosis Progressive degradation by enzymes after death that produce morphological changes to indicate death.

necrospermia Dead sperms in semen.

necrotoxin Toxins from Clostridium and Staphylococcus bacteria that kills tissue cells,

needle This can be puncturing needle or suturing needle which is made up of metal as sharp instrument. Common needles used in medical practice are:

- Fine needle
- Hagedorn needle
- Aspiration needle
- Veress needle
- Ligature needle
- Hypodermic needle
- Cataract needle
- Biopsy needle.

negativism resistance exerted by patients in clinical practice.

neglect Disregard to do or to perform a task or function.

Negri bodies Intra cytoplasmic inclusion bodies in Rabies diagnostic of Rabies infection.

Negro's phenomenon This refers to Cog Wheel Rigidity wherein passive stretch of muscle produce series of jerks.

Neher German biophysicist who won Nobel Prize for Medicine in 1991 for his work on ion channel communication in living cells.

Neill-Mooser reaction This is an animal inoculation test for Murine Typhus. When suspected material is inoculated to laboratory animal, it develops scrotal swelling that contains large mononuclear cells filled with rickettsia.

Neisser's diplococcus Gonococcus belonging to Neisseria gonorrhoeae described by Neisser.

Neisseria Gram negative bean shaped and paired bacteria that include Gonococcus, Meningococcus.

Nelson's syndrome Bilateral adrenalectomy produce a sequelae that produce aggressive growth of Adreno cortico Tropic hormone producing tumors and hyperpigmentation of skin.

nemathelminth Nematode parasites called nematodiasis.

Nematoda They are cylindrical or round Worms that cause illness. They are studied under Helminths .

neoantigen Tumors Associated Antigen is called Neoantigen.

neocerebellum They are Cerebellar hemisphere and middle portion of the vermis. This is attributed to be the Phylogenetically new part of cerebellum.

neocortex Evolution attained cerebral tissue with sex layered portions that is stratified and organized.

neo-hippocratism Bed side Medicine with Physician's observation for a human approach to illness.

neomorphism During evolution if an organ or tissue takes a new form it is called neomorphism.

neomycin Broad spectrum antibiotic used against Gram negative bacilli in clinical practice.

neon An inert gas discovered in 1898 and used in neon light.

neonatal Related to period from birth to 28 days of life in the new born.

neonate New born baby.

neonatologist Pediatrician who is trained in handling the health problems of neonates.

neonatology The art and science of diagnosis and treatment of disorders of the newborn

neoplasia Cancerous growth of a tissue where uncontrolled multiplication of cells occurs for which cause is not known.

neoplasm High degree anaplasia, invasion and metastasis in a given tissue which is called cancerous growth.

Neopsylla One of the genus of fleas.

Neospora One of the genus of protozoa.

neostigmine This is an anticholinesterase used in the treatment of following conditions:

- Myasthenia gravis,
- Post operative stasis,
- G I tract atony
- Atony of urinary bladder
- Post surgery recovery in tubocurarine injections.

neothalamus Neocortex region which phylogenetically a new part.

neovagina New vagina created after vaginectomy or in sex transformation surgery.

nephrectomy Removal of kidney in surgical treatment. Surgical techniques include a) Posterior nephrectomy b) Abdominal nephrectomy c) Para peritoneal nephrectomy d) Lumbar nephrectomy and e) Radical nephrectomy.

nephritic That which is related to kidney.

nephritis Infection and inflammation of the kidney which can be focal or diffuse involving glomerulus, tubule and interstitial tissue.

nephroblastoma Other name for Wilms' Tumors.

nephrologist Physician who is trained and an expert in nephrology.

nephrology Scientific study of the kidney which include pathology, diagnosis and treatment of diseases of kidney.

nephron Functional unit of the kidney consisting of the renal corpuscle, proximal convoluted tubule, descending and ascending limbs of Henle's loop, distal convoluted tubule and collecting tubule.

nephropathy Disease of the kidneys.

nephropexy Surgical fixation of a floating kidney.

nephrosis Diseases like Nephritis or Nephrotic syndrome that are degenerative disease of renal tubules. Clinical manifestations are a) Hypercholesterolaemia b) Oedema and c) Hypoalbuminemia.

nephrotomy Surgical incision into the kidney through abdominal or lumbar route.

nephrotoxic Substances that are toxic or destructive to kidney cells.

Neri's sign When leg is passively lifted spontaneous bending of that side knee occurs. This is positive is organic hemiplegia.

Nerium Flower is ornamental and bark is cardiac glycosides.

nerve Contain nerve fibres that is responsible for nerve conduction.

nervous Excitable and agitated conditions.

Nesokia Burrowing rodents found in India which are called Bandicoots.

Nessler's reagent This is used in qualitative and quantitative analysis of ammonia. The reagent contains:

- KI 5 percent
- $HgCl_2$ 2.5 percent
- KOH 16 percent in aqueous solution.

Nettleship-Falls type ocular albinism Albinism manifested by X linked genetic disorder which ws described by Nettleship and Falls.

Neufeld's reaction Capsular swelling in capsular organisms when they are mixed with specific immune serum due to the presence of capsular polysaccharide

Neumann's law This Physics law by Neumann states ' the molecular heat in compounds of analogous constituting is always the same'.

Neumann's sheath It is dentinal sheath which is an area of interface in dental structure.

neuralgia Pain extending along the course of nerves such as Trigeminal neuralgia, Occipital neuralgia, Intercostal neuralgia, Supra Orbital neuralgia, Sciatic neuralgia,

neurapraxia Injury and compression causing disturbance in nerve conduction.

neurasthenia Fatigue, mental weakness and Physical weakness which was attributed to exhaustion of nervous system. But the cause is now questionable.

neurilemma Spiral entrapment of myelin layers of peripheral nerves. It is called Sheath of Schwann or Neurolemma.

neuritis Infection and inflammation of a nerve which cause pain, paralysis and absence of reflexes. Common causes are Viral infections, alcohol, Amyotrophic sclerosis, Leprosy, Lead intoxication, Radiation,

neuroblastoma Malignant condition of Neuroblasts in Autonomic Nervous System.

neurocysticercosis Infection with larval forms of Tape worms causing convulsions, nervous dysfunctions.

neuroepithelium They are specialized cells in Cochlea, Vestibule, Nasal Mucosa and Tongue which receive sensations by external stimuli.

neurofibroma Benign tumors of peripheral nerves. The cause could be abnormal proliferation of Schwann cells.

neurofibromatosis Multiple pedunculated soft neurofibromatosis tumors which is a familial condition along with areas of pigmentation.

neurofibrosarcoma Malignant schwannoma which mimics Sarcoma of fibrous tissue.

neurogenetics Genetic basis of nervous disorders are studied in this discipline.

neuroglia Supporting structure of nervous tissue which is formed by astrocytes and oligodendrocytes.

neurohypophysis This considers posterior lobe of Pituitary gland which secretes Vasopressin, Oxytocin and Neurophysins.

neuroleptic Old generation of anti psychotic drugs which used to reduce emotion and agitation and normalizing psychomotor activity. But New generation of anti psychotic drugs have different mode of action and hence are called as ANTIPSYCHOTIC rather that NEUROLEPTIC.

neurologist Physician whose is trained in the field of Neurology.

neurology The Science that deals with the conditions that keeps the nervous system normal or pathological.

neuroma Usually a benign tumors formed from nerve cells and nerve fibres. Common neuromas are:

- Acoustic neuroma
- Ganglio neuroma
- Traumatic neuroma

neuron One of the main conducting cell of nerve system. This has a body, a nucleus, perikaryon, dendrites and axon. Afferent neurons are sensory nerves and Efferent neurons are motor nerves.

neuropeptide Chemicals found in nervous tissues which are mainly endorphins, enkephalins and vasopressin.

neurophysiology This is the study of physiology of the nervous system.

neuropsychiatrist Physician who specializes in neuropsychiatry.

neuropsychiatry This is the branch of medicine which includes both neurology and psychiatry.

neuropsychology An area which deals with neurology and psychology to study the relation between brain function and behavior.

neurorrhaphy Suturing of a cut nerve.

neurosarcocleisis Bone resection and transplanting nerve in soft tissue for the treatment of Neuralgia.

neurosarcoma Sarcoma with nerve elements.

neuroschistosomiasis Infection with Schistosoma japonicum causing CNS disorder.

neurosis This includes anxiety, dissociative disorder, mood changes, sexual disorders and psychosomatic disorders in man where actual organic cause cannot be demonstrated.

neurosurgeon A surgeon who specializes in neurosurgery.

neurosurgery Surgical treatment of nervous disorders.

neurosyphilis Syphilis involving nervous tissue which can be symptomatic or asymptomatic that are clinically seen as a) General Paralysis of Insane b) Paralysis c) Tabes dorsalis.

neurotendinous Related to both nerve and tendon

neurotensin It is found in brain and small intestine which has the function of vasodilation, hypotension and neurotransmitter in human body.

neurotic That which is related with Neurosis.

neurotome Nerve cutting knife which is needle like instrument.

neurotoxic Substance which is poisonous to nerve tissue.

neurotoxin Nerve toxin produced by Clostridium, Shigella and Corynebacterium bacteria.

neurotransmitter Some of the substances like Acetylcholine, Epinephrine, Endorphins and Serotonin travel across the synapsis to excite or to inhibit target cell.

neurovaccine Culture of virus in brain tissue of animals produce vaccine.

neutron Uncharged protons in the atoms of element is called neutron which are electrically neutral.

neutropenia Reduced number of neutrophils in the blood in conditions like Acute Lymphoblastic leukemia, Infiltrative disorders, severe bacterial infection.

neutrophil They are polymorphonuclear leukocytes which have the property of phagocytosis.

nevus Birth mark by a hamartoma which is circumscribed stable malformation of the skin.

newborn Just born baby

Newcastle disease Avian influenza caused by paramyxovirus which cause high mortality in man when occurs as an epidemic.

Newton's law This law states ' all bodies attract each other with a force that is directly proportional to their masses and inversely proportional to the square if their distance apart'

NF Abbreviation for **N**ational **F**ormulary

niacin Water soluble Vitamin B complex called Nicotinic acid is a pellagra preventing factor.

nicardipine hydrochloride Structurally related to Nifedipine is a calcium channel blocker used in Angina pectoris and Hypertension.

niche A depression seen in a radiograph such as Barclay's niche which is a deformity of the duodenal cap in duodenal ulcer.

niclosamide An anthelmintic drug used in the treatment of tapeworm infection.

Nicol prism Deflected ray of light through slabs of Iceland spar cemented together which give rise to ordinary ray and polarized ray.

Nicolas-Favre disease This refers to Lymphogranuloma venereum described by Nicolas and Favre.

Nicolle French physician and microbiologist who won Nobel Prize for his work on Typhus infection.

nicotine Derived from Tobacco has nicotinic action on the body.

nicotinic In smaller dose it stimulates nervous impulses at autonomic ganglia and neuromuscular junction. But in higher doses it inhibits the same mentioned effects.

nictitation The person winking.

nidation Implantation of fertilized ovum in the uterus.

NIDD Abbreviation for **N**on **I**nsulin **D**ependent **D**iabetes Mellitus.

NIDDM Abbreviation for **N**on **I**nsulin **D**ependent **D**iabetes **M**ellitus.

Nielsen method This is an Artificial method of artificial Respiration which is called Back pressure and Arm lift method for aiding inspiration and expiration.

Niemann-Pick disease Sphingomyelin accumulation in R.E. system causing lysosomal storage disease. This is also called Sphingomyelinase deficiency disease. There are 5 clinical types observed in clinical practice. They are:

1. Acute Neuronopathic disease
2. Chronic Non Neuronopathic disease
3. Chronic Neuronopathic disease
4. Variant of Type Chronic Neuronopathic disease
5. Adult Non Neuronopathic form of disease

nifedipine This is a Coronary Vasodilator and Hypotensive agent. Being a calcium channel blocker found useful in the treatment of Angina Pectoris.

nihilism Negative values on beliefs and traditional values. In case of medical treatment negative value or disbelief of cure.

nikethamide A respiratory stimulant used in respiratory failure or in circulatory failure.

nimodipine Calcium channel blocker used in subarachnoid hemorrhage from a ruptured intracranial aneurysm

nipple Refers to breast nipple or anything which is nipple like structure.

Nirenberg American biochemist along with Indian Scientist Har Gobind Khorana won Nobel Prize for the discovery of Genetic code and its function in protein synthesis.

Nissl bodies Granular basophilic bodies in the cytoplasm of neurons.

nit Egg stage of head louse or body louse.

nitazoxanide This drug is used in Opportunistic infection by Cryptosporidiosis of HIV/AIDS infection.

nitramine NNO_2 an amine from which a nitro derivative is present.

nitrate The Anion NO_3^- present in organic nitrates. Useful nitrate in medical practice is Nitroglycerin which is used in Chest pain.

nitrazepam This is a tranquilizer used as a sedative and anticonvulsant

nitric That which is related with nitrogen.

nitric acid A strong mineral acid, HNO_3

nitrite The Anion NO_2^- present in organic nitrites Common in clinical practice is Amyl Nitrite in chest pain.

nitrobenzene Benzene derivative used in the manufacture of aniline.

nitrofuran Antibacterial which include furazolidone, nitrofurazone, nitrofurantoin, and related compounds

nitrofurantoin An antibacterial effective against many gram-negative and gram-positive organisms like E.coli, S. pyogenes, A. aerogenes etc.,

nitrofurazone An antibacterial effective against a wide variety of gram-negative and gram-positive organisms.

nitrogen 80% of air is constituted by nitrogen. This is the main constituent of protein and nucleic acids and present in all living cells. Chemical symbol is N.

nitrogenous Substance which contains nitrogen.

nitroglycerin This is produced by the reaction of Nitric acid and sulphuric acid on glycerine. This has the property of Anti anginal, Anti Hypertensive and Vasodilator in clinical practice.

nitroprusside Chemically $[Fe(CN_5)NO]^{2-}$ Sodium nitroprusside is used in chemical analysis.

nitrous acid It is in solution form and a weak acid Formula is HNO_2

nm Abbreviation for **nano**m**eter**

NMR Abbreviation for **N**uclear **M**agnetic **R**esonance

Noack's syndrome Acrocephalosyndactyly -type I described by Noack.

Nobel prize Alfred Bernhard Nobel Chemist and an Engineer from Sweden instituted Nobel Prize to eminent scientists and eminent personality in Physics, chemistry, Medicine or Physiology and Economics. The First Prize was awarded in 1901.

Noble's position This position is useful in the examination of kidney in a patient. Patient while standing, leans forward and rests his upper body on his arms

Nocardia Gram positive aerobe that is soil borne some are pathogenic and some are non pathogenic in nature.

nociceptor These receptors are present in viscera and skin that is responsible for pain when injury or any mechanical thermal chemical or toxic stimuli occurs.

Noct. Latin word meaning at night.

nocturnal Related to or occurring in night.

nodal Related with node such as A.V. node.

node A small tissue protuberance in an organ such as Lymph node, A V Node, Heberden's node, Osler's nodes, etc.,

nodular That which is nodular or node like

nodule Small know or small node. Such as Accessory thymic nodule, Aortic nodules', Lymphatic nodule etc.,

nodus It denotes a small mass of tissue such as Nodus atrioventricularis.

noise Unwanted sound in normal atmosphere. noise pollution can result in Physical hazard in human beings.

noma This is seen in children with eaten away tissues in gingival and mouth which is called Cancrum Oris. The cause seems to be malnutrition

nomenclature Name given as per the scientific classification or grouping done such as Cancer grouping, Anatomical grouping etc.,

nondisjunction Chromosomal aberration leading to Down Syndrome or Trisomy 21.

noninfectious A disease which cannot spread by one person to another. Usually it refers to not spread either by contact or by inhalation. Hypertension and Diabetes are non infectious in nature.

Nonne-Milroy disease This is congenital Lymphoedema of the leg which is hereditary in origin.

nonparametric Explains statistical method wherein qualitative data are used in analysis and inference.

nonspecific An illness which does not found to have any known cause.

nonunion No repair or union of fractured bone .

norepinephrine It is a Catecholamine from post ganglionic nerve which is called neurohormone and acts as neurotransmitter acting on α- and β_1- adrenergic receptors.

norethandrolone This is a synthetic androgen

norfloxacin An antibacterial drug used against penicillin resistant organisms. Chemically it is a fluorinated 4-quinolone

norm Latin word meaning rule which gives an idle standard. Referable to an item, a structure, a reaction etc., which have an ideal standard.

normal Substance which is regular, that which is within physiological normalcy, that which is not pathological, When weight by volume is 1 gram in 1000 ml such as normal saline.

normotensive A person who is having normal blood pressure.

Norris' corpuscles Decolourised or Hypochromic red cells.

Norwalk virus Virus responsible in producing G.E. in a community.

noscapine This is an Antitussive agent derived from opium

nose Refers to the nostril, otherwise is known to be external nose.

nosebleed In medical practice it is known as Epistaxis.

nosegay a name applied to an anatomical structure resembling a small bunch of flowers.

A bunch of muscles that take origin from styloid process of temporal bone is called Riolan's nosegay.

nosepiece Lower portion of microscope which bears objectives that is helpful for adjustment in microscopic examination of an object without disturbing focus.

nosocomial Patient getting an infection 3 days after his/her admission to a hospital. This is also called as hospital infection.

nosology The science of the classification of diseases.

Nosopsyllus One of the genus of Rat flea which acts as a vector of Typhus and plague.

notch A depression on a bone such as acetabular notch especially one on the edge of a bone or other organ such as cardiac notch

notochord The embryonic center for development of axial skeleton which is from mesoblast of primitive node of embryo.

noxious Substance which is dangerous to tissue.

NPN Abbreviation for **N**on **P**rotein **N**itrogen.

NREM Abbreviation for **N**on **R**apid **E**ye **M**ovement under Physiology of sleep.

NSAID Abbreviation for **N**on **S**teroidal **A**nti **I**nflammatory **D**rug

NTP Abbreviation for **N**ational **T**uberculosis Control **P**rogramme

nubility Female at marriageable age.

nucha Nape of the neck.

nuchal pertaining to the nucha, or posterior aspect of the neck.

Nuck's canal Vaginal process of the peritoneum which is described by Nuck.

nuclear That which is related to a nucleus.

nuclease The enzyme which catalyses the reaction of conversion of nucleic acids to nucleotide. Nucleases are specific to RNA and DNA reactions.

nucleic acid DNA and RNA which are High molecular weight nucleotide polymers.

nucleocapsid Protein coat of nucleic acid of a virus.

nucleolus A refractile body in the nucleus of a cell that is a requisite for the synthesis of ribosome.

nucleus Central core of the cell. Central portion of a structure.

nudophobia Fear for becoming naked or unclothed.

Nuhn's glands Anterior Lingual gland described by Nuhn.

nullipara Para 'zero' denoting no viable child is produced by the woman.

number This is a figure which expresses the value by count. Common number in health sciences are: a) Chromosomal number b) Atomic number.

numbness Sensation of anesthesia by pressure effect or in the pathology of part.

nunnation Repeated use of N or hypernasality in a child which is described as speech pathology.

nurse Person who has undergone training and attained professional skills in Nursing care. This also denotes breast feeding the baby (Wet Nurse). Common nursing professionals are:

- ➢ Public health nurse
- ➢ Occupational health nurse
- ➢ Clinical nurse
- ➢ O T nurse

nurse-midwife They are certified Nurse Midwives who assist the Nurse in Obstetrical cases and in Nursing cases under treatment. They give the care for the new born and delivered mothers.

nursery A unit or a ward in maternity hospital where newborns are taken care. When young kids are given care during the day it is called day car nursery.

nursing Care given by nurse to ill patients, infants, sick, injured or the community. Common nursing area existing are:

- Paediatric nursing
- Community health nursing
- Occupational health nursing
- Medical nursing
- Surgical nursing
- Obstetrical nursing
- Psychiatric nursing
- School health nursing
- Public health nursing

Nussbaum's experiment Animal experiment conducted by Nussbaum by ligating renal arteries for isolating the glomeruli of kidneys. An experimental study on glomerular Ischaemia

nut One of the food stuff which is the source of fat in the form of oil. Ground nut, Coconut are common nuts considered in nutrition. This refers to seed element such as betel nut, areca nut

nutrient In clinical practice it refers to essential nutrients in terms of Protein, fat, carbohydrate, minerals, trace elements.

nutrition For growth and development of organisms nutrition is an important requirements. This takes in to account of nutrients. Serious patients are to be parental nutrition.

nyctalopia This refers to night blindness of a person. Common cause is vitamin a deficiency.

nylon Non-absorbable suture material.

nymph Small immature and wingless stage of insect in the life cycle of insects.

nymphomania Sexual desire in females which could be excessive and abnormal in nature.

Nyssen-van Bogaert syndrome Metachromatic Leukodystrophy among adult which was described by Nyssen and Bogaert.

nystagmus Involuntary, rapid, rhythmic movement of the eyeball

nystatin Antifungal produced by the growth of Streptomyces noursei that is used in the treatment of candida infection.

Nysten's law This is th law of Rigor Mortis i.e., changes after death. This states that rigor mortis affects the body in the following order:

1) Muscles of mastication
2) Muscles of Face
3) Muscles of Neck
4) Muscles of upper trunk
5) Muscles of arms
6) Muscles of leg
7) Muscles of feet

O

Ω Greek capital letter omega

OAP In Cancer treatment three drugs are given which are abbreviated as OAP and they are **O**ncovin, **A**ra C and **P**rednisolone.

oath A solemn declaration such as Hippocratic Oath.

oatmeal Food prepared from Oats that are used as bland diet.

OB Abbreviation for Obstetrics.

obducent That which serve as a cover.

obduction An autopsy which is M.L C.

obelion The point on the sagittal suture where it is crossed by a line which connects the parietal foramina.

Ober's operation This is surgical correction for clubfoot devised by Ober.

obese Excessively fat.

obesity Excessive deposit of fat in the body which give an increase in body weight

objective Lens system in the microscope. Effort is made for a good result. Perceptible to external sense.

obligate Pathogen which is capable of survival under certain conditions, A necessity.

oblique Inclined

obliquus Latin word meaning Oblique.

obliteration One which gets deteriorates

oblongata Refers to medulla oblongata.

observer one who watches.

obsession Persistent thought or image which occurs in spite of ignoring.

obsessive Related with obsession.

obsessive-compulsive Related with obsession and compulsion which is a personality disorder.

obsolescence Starting of non functioning of a physiological function.

obstetrician One who practices obstetrics.

obstetrics Scientific study of management of pregnancy, labour and puerperium.

obstipation This refers to severe constipation.

obstruction This denotes the blockage or closure.

obtund Dull or blunt referring to an instrument or an organ.

obturator The structure that closes an opening.

occipital That which is related with occiput.

occipitoposterior Similar to occipito anterior this also designates the position of foetus in relation to the maternal pelvis.

occlude Meaning obstruct.

occlusion Momentary closure of vocal tract, Any obstruction, Block of a vessel.

occlusive pertaining to or effecting occlusion.

occult That which is not seen or hidden.

occupancy time taken by a substance for it's excretion from the body. Number of days a patient is In Patient in a hospital.

OCD Abbreviation for **O**bsessive **C**ompulsive **D**isorder.

octa Greek word meaning eight.

octane Present in Petroleum which is an oily hydrocarbon

octigravida Gravida VIII. i.e., a woman pregnant for the eighth time;

octipara Para VIII i.e., a woman having eight viable children from eight pregnancy.

octose It is a monosaccharide containing eight carbon atoms

ocular That which is related with eyes.

oculentum An eye ointment.

oculist Refers to an Ophthalmologist.

oculomotor That which effect the movements of the eye.

OD Abbreviation for Optical Density.

Oddi's sphincter Muscle fibres of pancreatic passages to duodenum. This muscle sheath contains bile duct sphincter muscle and hepatopancreatic ampulla sphincter muscle.

odds Refers to Odds ratio which also mean the chance that a particular event will occur.

odonto That which is related with tooth.

odontoblast Connective tissue a the outer surface of dental pulp.

odontoblastoma Tumor of odontoblasts.

odontoid Resembling a tooth.

odontolith Calculus in teeth and gums.

odontologist Refers to a Dentist.

odontology It is Dentistry.

odontoma Mixed odontogenic origin with epithelial and mesenchymal cells from tooth structure.

odorant Substance that stimulates the sense of smell.

Oedipus complex Psychological disturbances in which a person show sexual attraction to opposite sex parent and show aggressive feelings towards same sex parent. The word Oedipus complex arise from Greek story in which Oedipus killed his father and married his mother without his knowledge.

oesophagus The G I tract from oropharynx to the entry of stomach.

OGTT Abbreviation for Oral Glucose Tolerance test.

Oguchi's disease This is a congenital night blindness and on examination of fundus it is found discolored.

Ohara's disease Ohara gave the clinical description of Tularaemia and is known as Ohara disease in Japan.

Ohm's law Ohm law states ' the strength of an electric current varies directly as the electromotive force and varies inversely as the resistance.

ohm This is the unit of electrical resistance described by Ohm .

oil The root word is from Latin word Oleum which defines the oil as the fat that is liquid at room temperature.

ointment A medicinal preparation for the use to apply externally which will be semisolid in nature.

Oldfield's syndrome Presence of many sebaceous cysts on the body and plenty of polyps isn the colon.

Olea This is the source of Olive Oil.

olecranon Bony projection of Ulna bone at Elbow.

oleic acid Unsaturated fatty acid present in animal fat.

oleoresin Resin and Volatile oil combination available in nature or by preparation.

oleotherapy Treatment with oil like Almond oil injection to haemorrhaoids.

oleum Latin word meaning Oil.

olfactory That which is related with sense of smell.

oligakisuria Urination occurring at long intervals.

oligo Little or scanty

oligodendroglia Neuroglia of CNS fanning out and coiling around the axon in the white matter.

oligodendroglioma Benign neoplasm derived from oligodendrocytes

oligohydramnios When amniotic fluid is less than 500 ml at early pregnancy.

oligohypermenorrhea Excessive menstrual flow but infrequent menses.

oligohypomenorrhea Menstrual flow but infrequent menses.

oligomenorrhea Disturbed and infrequent menstrual flow, occurring at intervals of 1 month to 6 months.

oligonecrospermia Condition where low quantity of semen which show dead sperms.

oligosaccharide Less monosaccharide yielding carbohydrate

oligospermia very low sperm count in the semen.

oliguria Low urine output which is defined at less than 400 ml. in a day excretion.

oliva An anatomical structure which has a rounded elevation

olivary That which is shaped like an olive.

Oliver's sign It is positive in aneurysm of the arch of the aorta which gives a pulling sensation in the trachea when the head is extended or when a finger is placed on the thyroid cartilage.

Ollier's disease It refers to Enchondromatosis described by Ollier.

Ollier-Thiersch graft Refers to thin skin graft consisting of epidermis and thin dermis. The graft is cut as broad strips and long strips.

Olshausen's operation Gynecological correction of retroverted uterus.

oma End part of the word which denotes cancer or neoplasm.

omega Ω, ω The last letter of Greek .

omentitis Infection and inflammation of the omentum.

omentopexy Suturing and fastening of omentus to other tissues in surgical practice.

omentoplasty Graft taken from the Omentum is used in abdominal surgery.

omentum The peritoneal fold which covers all abdominal or visceral organs in abdominal cavity.

omeprazole This drug inhibits gastric acid secretion. Used in duodenal ulcer.

omnivorous Animals which eat both plant foods and animal foods.

omohyoid That which is related to shoulder and hyoid bone.

omphalic Which is related with Umbilical

omphalitis Infection and inflammation of the umbilicus.

omphalocele This is Umbilical Hernia which is the protrusion at birth of part of the intestine through a large defect in the abdominal wall

Onchocerca Nematode parasites that are found on skin, sub cutaneous tissue and eyes.

onchocerciasis Human infection caused by *O. volvulus,*

oncology Scientific study of tumours in human being.

oncolytic Drug which is cytotoxic, drug in cancer treatment.

oncosis Illness due to tumour in man.

oncosphere Tapeworm larva which has six hooks called hexacanth.

oncotherapy Treatment of tumors.

oncotomy Surgical cut or the incision of a tumor

Oncovirinae RNA tumor viruses

oncovirus An oncovirus or oncogenic virus is a virus that can cause cancer. This term originated from studies of acutely transforming retroviruses in the 1950–60s, when the term "oncornaviruses" was used to denote their RNA virus origin.

ondansetron hydrochloride A drug used in cancer treatment as an adjuvant to prevent vomiting along with cancer drugs.

Ondine's curse A Mythological story in Germany that a Sea Nymph which cursed one unfaithfully lover to loose his bodily functions. Hence the name Ondine's curse. This is clinically Primary Alveolar Hypo-ventilation.

oneirism Human consciousness in Dream state is called Oneirism which is nor normal in nature.
onlay (on′la) This word is used in Organ graft and in Restoring measure of tooth. Common surgical procedure involves Epithelial only which allow new epithelial to grow out around the margin.
onomatomania Involuntary and reflexive uttering of some words which is a pathological status in mental health.
onomatophobia irrational fear of hearing a particular word or name.
onychia Infection and inflammation of the matrix of the nail resulting in Paronychia.
onychomalacia It refers to the softening of the nail.
o'nyong-nyong In East African dialect it means 'severe joint pain'. It is a viral infection transmitted by mosquito, clinically mimics Dengue and Chikungunya.
onyxis The term denotes the Ingrown nail.
ooblast This is a primordial cell from which an oocyte is developed Oocyte is nothing but ovum.
oocephalus Abnormal shape of head which resembles egg.
oocyesis This is Ovarian Pregnancy which is abnormal and ectopic in nature.
oocyst This stage is the encapsulated zygote stage in the life cycle of sporozoan protozoa, which by the process of sporogony develops into a sporozoite
oocyte This is a developing egg cell that is observed of two types. They are a) Primary oocyte wherein development is started but not complete and will be completed near the birth. b) Secondary oocyte wherein the stage develops before ovulation, developed to ootid or even seen perished.
oogamy Large non-motile oocyte is fertilized by a small motile male gamete.
oogenesis The formation of female gametes
ookinete Motile worm-shaped zygote of plasmodium parasite found in mosquito.
oophorectomy the removal of an ovary
oophoritis Infect ion and inflammation of an ovary.
oophoron Refers to egg or ovary
ootid A mature ovum
opacification By injecting contrast medium an organ is made opaque. Cornea getting opaque.
opacity Refers to opacity of lens that is cataract.
opaque Any part of item which is impervious to light rays
operable When a surgical condition is safe and appropriate for surgical removal or surgery.
operation This refers to the act of performing surgery with the help of surgical instruments.
ophthalmia Severe inflammation of the eye and the deeper structures of the eye.
ophthalmic Related with the eye.
ophthalmitis Infection and inflammation of the eye.
ophthalmo Show the relationship to the eye.
ophthalmologist The qualified person who treats the medical and surgical diseases of the eye.
ophthalmology The scientific study of Structure, Function, Pathology, Treatment and Management of The Eyes. It is an Allied subject in Surgery.
ophthalmomalacia Pathological softening of the eye.
ophthalmoplegia Clinically we observe the paralysis of the eye muscles.
ophthalmoscope The Ophthalmic instrument for the examination of interior of the eye. This is called Fundoscope.
ophthalmoscopy The Fundoscope used for the examination of the interior of the eye.
ophthalmoxerosis Dryness of the component of the eye.
opia Eye condition with defects of the eye.
opiate Opium derivative which produce sleep .
opisthion A landmark at midpoint of the posterior border of Foramen Magnum.
opistho Meaning Backward or to the back.
opisthotonos Body spasm in Tetanus which show the clinical manifestation of Hyperextension of body and head, Backward bend of heels and Forward bowing of the body.
opisthotonus Bowing of the body with spasm as described in Opisthotonos.
Opitz's disease This is clinically is called Thrombophlebitis Splenomegaly wherein spleen is enlarged due to thrombosis of splenic vein.
Opitz's syndrome An autosomal Dominant Disease which show the following clinical features:
- o Hypertelorism
- o Hernias, Heart malformations
- o Larynx and Tracheal malformations
- o Imperforated Anus
- o Kidney defects
- o Hypoplasia of Lungs
- o Downslanted palpebral fissures
- o In males hypospadias, cryptorchidism and bifid scrotum.

opium Extract from Papaver somniferum plant which yield alkaloids like Morphine, Codeine, Papaverine, Thebaine etc., which are narcotic and analgesics.
opocephalus Abnormal foetus where ears are fused and absence of mouth, nose and eyes.
opodidymus Abnormal foetus where heads are fused.
Oppenheim's, reflex This is positive in Pyramidal tract lesion. When stroking downward along the medial side of tibia, dorsiflexion of big toe occurs.
opponens Refers to muscle which help in an action of opposing
opportunistic Referred to pathogens which become pathogenic under circumstances like reduced body immunity, undergoing treatment with cortisone etc.,

opsia Denoting a condition of defective vision.

opsin They are Scotopsin and Photopsin which are proteins of the retinal rods responsible for visual pigments.

opsoclonus This is the clinical manifestation of brain stem disorder wherein oscillations of the eye is observed.

opsonin This is responsible for inducing phagocytosis by Neutrophils and Macrophages Antibodies of Opsonin like IgM, IgG1, and IgG3, Compliments like C3b, C3d, and C4b which trigger Phagocytosis.

opsonization With the help of Opsonin Rendering bacteria to phagocytosis action.

optic That which relalted to the vision or eye.

optical Pertaining to vision.

optician Opticianry Expert

optics Scientific study of vision and Light in Optics and vision corrections.

optimal Most favorable.

optimum Conditions which are conducive to the most favorable function.

optometer This is the other name for Refractometer.

optometrist Skilled person who has undergone training to diagnose, manage and treat visual system.

OPV Abbreviation for **O**ral **P**olio **V**accine

ora Latin word meaning a margin.

Oragrafin Commercial preparation which contain Calcium salt of Ipodate.

oral That which is related to mouth.

orange It is a citrus fruit which yield vitamin C to the body. Otherwise it depicts the colour between red and yellow.

Orbeli phenomenon see under In case of Fatigue, the response of Nerve Muscle Preparation comes down and at that time if we stimulates sympathetic nerve the height of contraction increases.

orbicular That which is circular

orbiculus Structure shaped like a small circle

orbit The bony cavity that contains eyeball;

orbital That which is related with orbit. It also can denote the wave function of an atom.

orcein It is a specific stain for elastic tissue.

orchidectomy Surgical removal of testes.

orchiectomy Meaning Castration i.e., excision of one or both testes

orchiepididymitis Infection and inflammation of testis and epididymis.

orchiocele Hernia protrusion of a testis.

orchiotomy Incision and drainage of testis.

Orchis Infection and inflammation of testicle.

orchitis Infection and inflammation of testis. Commonly it is associated with Mumps, gonorrhoea, Filariasis, Syphilis, Tuberculosis that is marked by pain, swelling, and a feeling of weight.

orderly Attendant in a hospital who works under of a nurse.

ordinal Item from a ranked list such as first, second, third etc.,

ordinate Distance of a point from the horizontal *(x)* axis, measured along a line parallel to the *y*-axis.

orellanine This is present in Mushroom causing Mushroom poisoning. Gastritis, Myalgia and Renal failure are common manifestations.

orelline Isolated chemical toxin from Orellanine.

organ A separate anatomical organ with it's own structure and function.

organelle They are cytoplasmic structures which are organized such as Nucleus, Mitochondria, Golgi Apparatus etc.,

organic That which is related with an organ. It also refers to substances which arise from living organisms. It also refers to chemicals which contain covalent bound carbon atoms.

organism Refers to individual plant, animal or man.

organization Organised body, organized group or organized Institution in question. That which is streamlined.

organize Formation of organic structure or an organ in nature.

organizer Term used in genetics, and chemistry which means inductor or an activator. This could be part of embryo which help in differentiation of cells and tissues.

organochlorine They are Chlorinated Hydrocarbon which have the effect of killing insects and hence are powerful insecticides. Common Organochlorine insecticides are:

1. DDT
2. Lindane
3. Aldrin
4. Endosulfan
5. Endrin
6. Methoxychlor

organogenesis Origin and development of organs.

organophosphorus Chemical with phosphorus bound to organic molecule that are commonly used as insecticides. They are called organophosphorus compound such as:

1. Chlorfenvinphos
2. Chlorothion
3. Malathion
4. Parathion
5. Diazinon
6. Temephos
7. Tetra Ethyl Pyrophosphate

orgasm The climax in sexual act.

Oribasius Medical writer and Physician from Rome who has written MAGNUM that was Medical Encyclopedia with 70 volumes.

orientation Indicate awareness of our surroundings such as Orientation of place, orientation of time and orientation of people.

orifice This could be entrance or outlet of a cavity, any foramen, any meatus in the body.

origin Proximal end of a muscle. Source of emergence of a nerve or a vessel. Beginning of any item in anatomical positions.

Ormond's disease Fibrotic lesion particularly Retroperitoneal Fibrosis. described by Ormond.

ornithine This is an amino acid produced in the urea cycle that when gets decomposed yield putrescine.

Ornithodoros Genus of Ticks which transmit Borrelia infection in man. Ornithodoros moubata is common vector in the transmission of spirochetal infections.

ornithosis Diseases of Birds often attack man .

oromaxillary Related to mouth and the maxillary region.

oropharyngeal Related to mouth and Pharynx.

oropharynx Passage from mouth to pharynx.

orotidine This is a product in Pyrimidine Synthesis.

Oroya fever It is called Bartonella fever that cause anaemia was first detected in Peru.

orphenadrine This is an antihistamine and antispasmodic drug which is called methanamine.

Orr treatment This Orthopaedic treatment is for compound fractures and osteomyelitis which include the following surgical management:

a. Wound debridement
b. Fracture alignment
c. Drained by putting petrolatum gauze
d. Limb Immobilisation by plaster of Paris

ORS Abbreviation for **O**ral **R**ehydration **S**olution.

Orsi-Grocco method This is clinical examination with palpation through percussion of the heart.

ORT Abbreviation for **O**ral **R**ehydration **T**herapy.

ortho Means normal, straight or that which is correct. This can be Ortho position in Benzene ring.

orthocresol Isomeric form of cresol.

orthodontia This is Orthodontics in Dentistry.

orthodontics This field of Dentistry deals with correction of growing dentofacial structures. It is also called Dentofacial Orthopaedics. This field can put interception, can do correction, can prevent malocclusion and can do surgical corrections.

orthodontist A specialist in orthodontics.

Orthomyxoviridae They are RNA viruses and are called Influenza viruses.

orthopedic Related to orthopaedics where correction of deformities of Muscles and bones are done.

orthopedics Science that deals with skeletal system, the Joints and other associated structures. It is a specialty.

orthopercussion This is a type of percussion wherein distal phalanx of pleximeter finger is held perpendicularly to chest wall.

orthopnea Difficulty in breathing in upright position.

Orthopoxvirus Fever and Rash producing viruses such as cow pox, monkey pox smallpox etc.,

orthopraxy Orthopaedic correction of deformities.

orthoptics Correction by exercise for visual axes for binocular vision.

orthoptist Expert in orthoptics.

orthostatic pertaining to or caused by standing erect.

orthostatism an erect standing position of the body.

orthostereoscope an apparatus for stereo radiography.

orthotherapy treatment of disorders by correction of posture.

orthotonos In case of Tetanus infection opisthotonic posture where head, body and limbs are in right position.

Ortner's syndrome Secondary to heart disease laryngeal paralysis which is due to compression of recurrent laryngeal nerve. The nerve gets compressed between dilated pulmonary artery and the aorta.

Ortolani's sign This sign is positive in developmental dysplasia of the hip. When the hip is reduced by abduction and dislocated by adduction we hear a click in and out as the hip is reduced.

os This refers to orifices of the body such as mouth, anus, vagina etc., This also refers to the naming of bones such as Os basalare, Os acromiale, os acetabuli etc., (Basal bone, Acromial bone and Acetabular bone etc.,)

OSAS Abbreviation for **O**nstructive **S**leep **A**pnea **S**yndrome.

osazone This refers to Glucosazone which are crystals of specific sugars. In the presence of Phenylhydrazine and acid when a sugar is heated, these crystals are formed which are identification point for a given sugar.

osche That which is related with Scrotum.

oscillation This is the description of a backward and forward motion, like a pendulum

oscitation It is Yawning.

ose When this word 'ose' is suffixed it indicates that the given chemical is a carbohydrate.

OSHA Abbreviation for **O**ccupational **S**afety and **H**ealth **A**dministration.

osis The word when is combined with another word it denotes a morbid process or abnormal increase of pathology.

Osler's disease This is Hereditary Haemorrhagic Telangiectasia and Polycythemia Vera described by Osler.

osmatic Related with the smell.

osmo Related with odour. Otherwise related with Osmosis.

osmolality Chemical particles in a solution (solute) (Osmole per Kg. solvent). The Osmolality depends on Osmotic pressure, Boiling point, Freezing point and Vapour pressure.

osmosis Movement of solvent from lower solute concentration to higher solute concentration through a membrane.

osmotherapy I.V.Fluid administration in dehydration.

osmotic Related to osmosis.

osseous That which is bony.

ossicle Small bone e.g., Auditory ossicles, Episternal ossicles etc.,

ossification The process of conversion of fibrous tissue or of a cartilage into bone.

ossifying Developing into bone.

ostealgia pain in a bone or in the bones.

ostectomy Excision of a bone

osteitis Infection and inflammation of a bone which involve the haversian spaces, haversian canals, and their branches.

osteoaneurysm This refers to the aneurysm in a bone.

osteoarthritic Related to osteoarthritis.

osteoarthritis Degenerative and Non inflammatory disease of joint of elderly. There will be changes in articular cartilage and synovial membrane. Pain, stiffness and inactivity are characterstic features.

osteoarthropathy Disease of the joints and bones.

osteoblast Immature bone cell which is called fibroblast that becomes a bone cell at maturity.

osteoblastoma Benign, painful vascular tumour of the bone.

osteochondritis Infection and inflammation of both bone and cartilage.

osteochondroma Bone capped with cartilage to form a benign tumour.

osteochondrosarcoma Chondrosarcoma of bone

osteochondrosis Bone pathology which is seen in ossification centers that is common in children. Necrosis followed by recalcification is seen in this process.

osteochondrous That which is composed of bone and cartilage.

osteoclasia Destruction and absorption of bone tissue.

osteoclasis Breaking the bone again or it is refracture.

osteoclast Instrument used to refracture the bone in orthopaedic surgery. Other meaning is the multinuclear cell that brings the changes of absorption of bone.

osteoclastoma Other name for Gaint Cell Tumour of the bone.

osteocranium The cranium of foetus which is yet to get ossified.

osteocystoma This is a bone cyst.

osteocyte They are responsible for bone compactness. The osteoblast in bone matrix with their slender cytoplasmic processes gives the strength to the bone.

osteodiastasis This refers to the separation of two adjacent bones.

osteodynia A clinical manifestation of bony pain.

osteodysplasty Abnormal development of bone.

osteodystrophy Defective bone formation.

osteoectasia Bow like bent of a bone.

osteofibroma Benign tumor containing Osseous and Fibrous elements.

osteofibromatosis Fibrous dysplasia of bone.

osteofluorosis Refers to osteomalacia and osteosclerosis that is caused by the consumption of excessive quantities of fluorides.

osteogenesis Process of Bone formation.

osteoid That which resembles bone.

osteology Scientific study of the bones

osteolysis Bone dissolution which is highlighted with calcium loss in the bone.

osteoma A benign tumour of membranous bones such as osteoma of skull, osteoma of facial bones.

osteomalacia Rickets of adults wherein delayed mineralization of osteoid tissue is seen.

osteomyelitis Infection and inflammation of bone by pyogenic organisms.

osteon This is the basic unit in the structure of a bone. This consists of a Haversian canal, lamellae along the long axis of the bone.

osteonecrosis This is the clinical manifestation of Ischaemic Necrosis of a bone.

osteopathology Disease of bone.

osteopathy This refers to the diseases of a bone. It also can mean a type of treatment enunciated by Andrew Taylor Still (1828–1917) to effect normal body structure that can cure illness.

osteopetrosis Bone that are abnormally dense. There are two types:

- Autosomal recessive disorder which is severe in nature
- Autosomal dominant disorder which is not severe in nature.

osteoporosis Reduced bone density which is associated with fractures.

osteosarcoma Cancer of the bone composed of malignant bone and malignant connective tissues.

osteosclerosis Hardening of bone

osteosis Connective tissue is in filtered with the bone with the formation of bone by connective tissue.

osteotome Bone cutting instrument.

osteotomy Surgical cutting of a bone.

osteotribe Surgical instrument used for rasping carious bone.

ostiomeatal Related with the opening of the urinary, nasal, or acoustic meatus.

ostitis Infection and inflammation of bone.

Ostrum-Furst syndrome Congenital abnormality syndrome associated with the following:

- o Synostosis of the neck

- o Platybasia
- o Congenital elevation of scapula

OT Abbreviation for **O**peration **T**heature. Also for **O**ld **T**uberculin.

otic Aural or that which is related with ear.

otitis Infection and inflammation of the ear, often associated with pain, fever, hearing loss, tinnitus, and vertigo

otogenic Produced by ear.

otolaryngology This is a specialty under Surgery and allied subjects. This covers Medical and Surgical treatment of the head and neck, including the ears, nose, and throat.

otologist A specialist who handles ear pathology .

otology Field that deals with the medical treatment and surgery of the ear, and its anatomy, physiology, and pathology.

otomycosis Aspergillus fungal infection of the external auditory meatus

otomyiasis Plenty of larvae infested in the ear.

otoneuralgia Neuralgic pain in the ear.

otopyorrhea Otorrhoea that is purulent in nature.

otorhinolaryngology E N T specialty which is an allied subject of surgery.

otorrhea Ear discharge which is purulent in nature.

otosclerosis Hardening of stapes bone resulting in conductive deafness.

otoscope Instrument used for examination of ear which is also called as Auriscope.

ototoxic Agent or substance which is toxic to organs of hearing and organ of balance.

Otrivin Drug Xylometazoline Hydrochloride which is nasal decongestant.

Otto's disease Arthrodesis is described by Otto.

ounce It a measure of weight (which is equivalent to 28.33495 grams.

outbreeding Cross breeding equivalent to the mating of totally unrelated individuals, which allow good survival.

outpatient Patient gets treatment after diagnosis without getting admitted to hospital.

output Final yield in a functional unit. E.g., Cardiac output, Energy output, Urinary output etc.,

ova Pleural form of Ovum.

oval Structure which is an egg shaped.

ovalbumin Albumin from whites of eggs.

ovarian Related with the ovary.

ovariectomy Surgical removal of ovary for a treatment.

ovariocyesis Ectopic pregnancy in ovary called ovarian pregnancy.

ovariopexy Elevating and Fixing the ovary to the abdominal wall.

ovariosalpingectomy Removal of ovarian tube along with ovary.

ovarium Female reproductive organ which produces ovum or egg.

ovary Similar to Ovarium, the female reproductive which produces ovum or egg.

overflow Escape of a fluid such as urine or tears.

overgrafting It is the second skin graft for reinforcing split thickness graft in plastic surgery

overgrowth It can be Hyperplasia or Hypertrophy i.e., size increase or number of cells increase.

overhydration A condition of excess fluids in the body.

overinflation Refers to Hyperventilation.

overjet It is horizontal overlapping. It is called overjet horizontal overlap.

overlay An additional or superimposed one.

overmatching In research methodology and for statistical analysis many similar variables produce problem or bias which need correction.

overstain Stain a tissue excessively

overstrain Fatigue by overwork .

overtransfusion Giving more than required blood or fluid which puts the circulation strain. Otherwise is called Hypervolemia.

overventilation Other name for Hyperventilation.

overweight More fat tissues in the body leading obesity or fay body.

oviduct They are Uterine tube which help in the transport of ovum to the uterus for conception.

oviferous Organism which produce ova for their reproduction.

oviparous Organism produce egg from which the offspring comes out.

oviposition The act of depositing eggs.

ovipositor Organ of an insect from which eggs are laid on soil or on plant.

ovoviviparous Animal which bear egg containing the young ones that later hatch to lead independent life.

ovulation Discharge of a secondary oocyte from a vesicular follicle of the ovary.

ovulatory Related with ovulation.

Owren's disease Parahemophilia described by Owren.

oxalic acid It is a common renal calculi that contain oxalic acid. Spinach and Rhubarb contain natural source of oxalic acid. It is a strong dicarboxylic acid with the formula HOOC-COOH

oxaloacetic acid This an intermediate Product in the tricarboxylic acid

oxalosis Calcium oxalate gets deposited in renal and extra renal tissues.

oxazepam Benzodiazepine used in the treatment of anxiety disorders and depression

oxidant The electron **acceptor** in an **oxidation-reduction** reaction.

oxidase They are Oxidoreductase in which molecular oxygen is the hydrogen acceptor.

oxidation State of being oxidized. Chemically it is the increase of positive charges on an atom (the loss of negative charges).

oxidation-reduction It is the chemical reaction where electrons are removed (oxidation) from atoms of the substance being oxidized and transferred to atoms being reduced (reduction).

oxide Compound of oxygen which has a radical. E.g., Nitric oxide, Ferric oxide.

oxidize Chemical reaction cause to combine with oxygen, or to lose electrons.

oxime Compounds containing the **CH([dbond]NOH)** group, formed by the action of hydroxylamine on an aldehyde or a ketone.

oximeter The instrument is used to determine the oxygen saturation of the blood. Kinds of oxymeter available are:

- Co oximeter
- Ear oxymeter
- Finger oxymeter
- Pulse oxymeter
- Whole blood oximeter

oxycephaly Colloquially it is called tower head wherein the head is conical in shape due to premature closure of coronal and lambdoid sutures.

oxychromatin Chromatin that stains with acid aniline dyes

oxygen An essential agent for respiration of plants and animals, is present in the air to the tune of 20 percent. Oxygen is required for combustion in atmosphere. Oxygen therapy is done in cardiac and respiratory emergencies.

oxygenation The reaction ending with oxygenating a substance.

oxygenator This is commonly used medical equipment called Artificial Lung. It helps in oxygenation of blood outside the body. Oxygenator are used in open heart surgery. Common types of Oxygenerator used are:

- Film oxygenator
- Disc oxygenator
- Bubble oxygenator
- I V oxygenator
- Membrane oxygenator
- Screen oxygenator
- Rotating disc oxygenator
- Pump oxygenator

oxyhemoglobin Haemoglobin when combines with bound oxygen of alveolar gas Oxyhaemoglobin is formed.

oxyhydrocephalus Hydrocephalus in which the top of the head is pointed shape.

oxymetholone This is an anabolic steroid for oral administration.

oxymyoglobin Myoglobin on exposure to atmospheric conditions forms oxymyoglobin

oxyopia Acuteness of vision

oxyopter This is the unit of measurement of visual acuity One oxyopter = 60 Snellen units = counting fingers at one meter.

oxyphenbutazone Derivative of phenylbutazone having anti-inflammatory action used in the treatment of arthritis, gout.

oxyphencyclimine hydrochloride Anticholinergic drug used in the treatment of Peptic Ulcer.

oxyphenisatin The drug used as enema before surgery on colon.

oxyphenonium bromide It is a quaternary ammonium compound used in the treatment of peptic ulcer.

oxyphonia Abnormal voice.

oxyquinoline It is a disinfectant, a fungicide and a chelating agent. Chemically it is a dicyclic aromatic compound.

oxytalan Connective tissue fiber present in tendon, ligament and adventitia that has the property of resistant to acid hydrolysis

oxytetracycline A broad-spectrum antibiotic of the tetracycline group produced by Streptomyces rimosus.

oxytocia Precipitate labour or rapid labour.

oxytocin Hormone of Neurohypophysis which promote uterine contractions and milk ejection.

Oxyuris Intestinal nematode called pinworm with generic name Enterobius vermicularis common intestinal parasite.

oz Abbreviation for Ounce.

ozena In case of atrophic rhinitis mucosal crusting leads to bad smell and a mucosal polyp, often associated with Klebsiella pneumoniae infection.

ozone A bluish explosive gas with the formula O_3 that is formed when oxygen is exposed to the silent discharge of electricity. Ozone is an antiseptic and disinfectant and is a major air pollutant and is irritating and toxic to the respiratory system.

P

PABA abbreviation for **P**ara **A**mino **B**enzoid **A**cid.

pacemaker Substance that influences the rate at which a certain phenomenon occurs. This also refers to the natural and artificial cardiac pacemaker. Substance whose rate of reaction sets the pace for a series of interrelated reactions.

Pachy This means anything that is thick.

pachymeningitis Infection and inflammation of the dura mater.

Pacini's corpuscles Lamellar corpuscle which is an encapsulated nerve ending sensitive to pressure and vibration.

pack Treatment by wrapping a patient in a blanket or a sheet or a towels. In nursing practice Ice pack, wet pack and cold pack are in use.

pad Mass of soft material. Examples are heating pad, abdominal pad etc.,

Paget's cell Large irregular anaplastic tumour cell with hyperchromatic nucleus. It is present in Paget's disease of the breast.

PAHA Abbreviation for **P**ara **A**mino **H**ippuric **A**cid.

pain It is a protective phenomenon. Pain is the result of stimulation of specialised nerve endings. Common clinical entities are:

- Chest pain
- Labour pain
- Hunger pain
- Referred pain
- Wandering pain

paint Antiseptic liquid applied for protection.

pair Identical entities

Pajot's law An inside solid body takes an adjustment of shape of outer smooth walled body. Common example is foetus in uterus.

palatorrhaphy Surgical correction of a cleft palate,

palliative Treatment which produce relief but not cure.

pallor Lowered skin colour called paleness

palm Refers to Palm tree.

palpation To feel with the hand; To feel with fingers the consistency of the parts beneath in physical examinations. Light touch palpation and Bimanual palpation are known entities.

palpebra The are protector of anterior surface of eye and they are movable folds. Upper and lower palpebrae are common terminologies. Nictitating membrane of the eye is called palpebra tertia.

palpitation Rapid heart beat which can be experienced by man. It can be physiological or pathological.

palsy This is the other name for paralysis. Common clinical entities are:

- Erb's palsy
- Facial palsy
- Saturday night palsy
- Bell's palsy
- Brachial palsy
- Pseudo bulbar palsy

PAN Abbreviation for **P**oly **A**rteritis **N**odosa.

Panacea In Greek mythology she is the daughter of Aesculapius. This is the name given to a juice which can cure any illness. Incidentally other daughter of Aesculapius is Hygeia.

pancarditis Infection and inflammation of all the three layers of the heart namely Pericardium, Myocardium and Endocardium.

Pancoast's suture It is called Tongue and groove suture where a tongue is cut in one lip of the wound and a groove in the other.

Pancoast's syndrome In case of lesion of brachial plexus and cervical sympathetic nerves, which is secondary to a pulmonary sulcus tumour, we come across of following clinical manifestations:

- o Neuritic pain in arm
- o Atrophy of muscles of hand and arm
- o Horner's syndrome features.(ptosis and sinking of eyeball, lower lid elevation, papillary constriction, palpebral fissure are narrowed , flushing of affected side of face and anhidrosis in brain stem lesion)

pancreas Organ situated behind stomach consists of Islets of Langerhans with Beta cells that produce Insulin. Pancreas in it's acini secretes pancreatic juice that help in digestion.

pancreatin A preparation from Pancreas which contains digestive enzymes like amylase, trypsin and lipase.

pancuronium bromide A muscle relaxant which has curare like action and is used in General Anaesthesia.

pancystitis Infection and inflammation involving the entire thickness of the wall of the urinary bladder

pancytopenia This is a clinical condition where there is deficiency of all cellular elements of the blood.

pandemic It is a widespread epidemic of a disease occurring through the world.

Pander's islands This is an embryonic site in splanchnopleure of embryo that is going to develop into blood and blood vessels.

panel Many individuals participating in a specific discussion or activity.

panencephalitis Viral encephalitis which produces infection and inflammatory changes in both gray and white matter. One of the devastating form of encephalitis called Sub Acute Sclerosing Panencephalitis (SSPE) due to high titers of measles virus in the serum.

panic Anxiety with disorganisation of human personality.

Panner's disease (Pan·ner's disease) This is referred to Osteochondrosis of the capitellum of the humerus described by Panner.

panniculitis Infection and inflammation of subcutaneous fat.

pannus Vascularization of the cornea with infiltration of granulation tissue. This can also refer to Inflammatory exudate overlying the lining layer of synovial cells on the inside of a joint,

panophthalmitis Inflammation of all the structures of the eye.

panus Non suppurative inflammation of lymphatic gland.

papain Enzyme that catalyzes the hydrolysis of proteins and peptides with preferential cleavage at bonds containing arginine, lysine, and glycine residues.

Papanicolaou's stain Test used to detect exfoliated cels which can say a word on malignant process. Pap smear or cervical smear is common screening test done worldwide. Respiratory and digestive secretions can also be tested with this.

papilla Nipple shaped projection of an organ.
papilledema Oedema of the optic disk (papilla), common causes are increased intracranial pressure, malignant hypertension, or thrombosis of the central retinal vein;
papilloma Benign epithelial neoplasm
papular Pertaining to a papule.
papule Circumscribed superficial solid elevation of the skin
papulopustular Characterized by the presence of papules and pustules on the skin.
para Para indicates how many pregnancies a woman has undergone. It is Latin word to denote number of viable offspring.

Para 0 = nullipara
Para I = Primipara
Para II = Secundipara
Para III = Tripara
Para IV = Quadripara

para- Greek word para is a prefix which convey the meaning beside or near such as

para Xylene
para Nitrophenol
para Amino benzoic acid
para Acetyl amino phenol
para Amino Hippuric acid
para Amino Salycylic acid

paracardiac beside the heart.
Paracelsus Paracelsus was called as "Luther of Medicine," His treatment included lead, sulphur, iron, and arsenic that are even today present in pharmaceutical chemistry.
paracentesis Diagnostic or Therapeutic aspiration of fluid by a needle introduced into a cavity.
paracetamol This is Acetaminophen which is antipyretic and analgesic.
paracholera Asiatic cholera caused by organism other than Vibrio.
paraclinical very near to clinical such as investigation by microbiologist, Biochemist or Pathologist.
paradox A Self Contradictory statement such as:

Weber paradox stretched	Elongation of a muscle which has been fully That it cannot contract further.
Simpson's paradox	An extreme confounding such that this association Between 2 variable is reversed by the adjustment For the third variable.
Opie paradox	Specific protective mechanism produced by necrotising Local anaphylaxis.

paradoxical That which occur against any normal rule.
paradysentery Mild dysentery caused by Shigella.
paraffin Solid hydrocarbons obtained from petroleum used as a stiffening agent in pharmaceutical preparations. Types of paraffin in clinical use are:

- Soft paraffin (white or yellow)
- Hard paraffin
- Liquid paraffin (usual or light)
- Synthetic paraffin

paraganglion They are chromaffin cells from neural ectoderm, situated near sympathetic ganglia. They secrete epinephrine. Other name for paraganglion is Chromaffin body.
paragnosis Diagnosis done after death on the basis of historical clinical characters available before death.
Paragonimus Trematodes of the family Troglotrematidae which have two invertebrate hosts, One is snail and the other is crayfish. Lung fluke called Paragonimus westermani is common and widely distributed.
parahippocampal That which is situated near the hippocampus.
paraldehyde A sedative and hypnotic which is used in convulsions and agitation through rectally.
parallel Straight lines that do not intersect.
paralysis Lesion of muscle and nerve produces loss of motor function in a part.
paralytic Person affected with paralysis..
paramedical Physical therapist, occupational therapist, speech therapists, medical social workers (M.S.W.), pharmacists and technicians who work with doctors and are adjunctive to their practice of medicine are called Paramedicals.
parameter Constant mathematical expression that distinguishes specific cases. There will be fixed value in one and different values in another.

E.g., 1:	**a = mx + b** suppose m and b are parameters that specify a particular straight line. Changing m changes the slope of the line. Changing b changes the point at which the line crosses the a axis.
E.g., 2:	Blood glucose and urine sugar are parameters of sugar metabolism
E.g., 3:	Pulse and B.P. are parameters of Heart disease.

paramethadione Anticonvulsant used in the treatment of Petit mal.
paramethasone acetate It is a glucocorticoid used as anti-inflammatory and antiallergic
parametritis Infection and inflammation of the parametrium.
paranoia Systematized delusions of persecution and delusions of grandeur or both.

paranoid That which resembles paranoia.

paraparesis Partial paralysis of the lower extremities.

parapertussis Whooping cough like syndrome which is clinically similar to whooping cough.

paraphasia Wrong words are used in wrong sense called paragrammatism.

paraphilia Psychosexual disorder characterized by recurrent intense sexual urges such as in conditions like exhibitionism, fetishism, frotteurism, pedophilia, sexual masochism, sexual sadism, transvestic fetishism, and voyeurism.

paraphimosis Retraction of foreskin with painful swelling of the glans

paraplegia Paralysis of the legs with paralysis of lower part of the body. Common clinical entities are

- Cerebral paraplegia
- Flaccid paraplegia
- Alcoholic paraplegia
- Spastic paraplegia
- Pott's paraplegia
- Toxic paraplegia

parasacral Near the sacrum.

parasite That lives upon another living organism and at whose expense it obtains some advantage.

parasitemia When parasites are found in blood.

parasitism Infestation with parasites.

parasitology Science of parasites and parasitism.

paraspadias Urethra opens upon one side of the penis. This is a developmental anomaly.

parasympathetic Related with ocular, bulbar and sacral divisions of autonomic nervous system.

parasympatholytic That which interrupts the parasympathetic nerve supply to a part.

parasympathomimetic Effect similar to stimulation of parasympathetic nerve supply to part.

parasystole Cardiac irregularity by two foci that independently initiate cardiac impulses at different rates

parathion Insecticide which belongs to Organophosphorus compound.

parathormone Parathyroid hormone secreted by parathyroid gland.

parathyroid Glands by the side of Thyroid gland.

paratyphoid Salmonellosis caused by serotypes other than Salmonella typhosa.

Paré French Surgeon during 1510 to 1590 popularly called Ambroise Pare has contributed in developing surgery in gunshot wound, amputation and ligation of arteries. He reintroduced podalic version into Obstetrics. His famous statement "I dressed him and God healed him" considers his devotion to mankind.

parenchyma Parenchyma denotes to the functional elements of an organ.

parental Anything derived from parents.

parenteral Drug or medicamentation through other than alimentary canal such as injection

paresis Greek word meaning incomplete paralysis.

paresthesia Abnormal touch sensation

parietal Related to the wall of a cavity, or it can be related to parietal bone or parietal lobe.

pari passu The same proportion or the same degree.

parity Denotes woman's status with respect to giving rise to a viable offspring. It can also connote that there is similarity.

Parker's fluid Fluid used to harden tissues which is composed of formaldehyde solution and alcohol.

Parkinson's disease Paralysis agitans described by Parkinson. Person showing the symptom is said to be suffering from Parkinsonism.

Parona's space In the forearm 5 cm above the wrist, this space lies between the pronator quadratus muscle and the deep flexor tendons in the forearm.

paronychia Infection and inflammation of tissue surrounding the nail.

parotid Gland situated near the ear.

parotitis Infection and inflammation of the parotid gland.

paroxysm Sudden intensification of symptoms.

Parry's disease This refers to toxic nodular goiter described by Parry.

parthenogenesis Development of a gamete without fertilization seen in invertebrates and plants.

particle One tiny mass of material. Entities of clinical importance are

- Viral particle
- Colloid particle
- Alpha particle
- Beta particle
- Dane particle
- Nuclear particle

partition Anatomical structure that divides an organ or a part into further parts.

parturition the action of giving birth to young; childbirth

parumbilical Alongside the umbilicus.

PAS Abbreviation for **P**ara **A**mino **S**alicylic Acid.

Pascal's law This physical law states "the pressure applied to a liquid at any point is transmitted equally in all directions". One pascal is equal to one Newton per square meter force in S I unit.

Paschen's bodies Inclusion body seen in Variola infection.

passage This means a passage. But commonly denoted as the act of moving from one place to another.

Pasteur French Chemist who pronounced the Germ Theory of disease, who found out the use of inoculation with attenuated microbes. His work helped Lister to develop antiseptic surgery.

Pasteur's effect Microorganisms and tissues suppress lactate accumulation and glycolysis in the presence of oxygen.

Pasteurella Gram-negative, facultative anaerobic, rod-shaped bacteria that cause plague in human beings by causing abscesses and septicaemias.

Pasteurization Process of milk purification devised by Pasteur. There are two methods. They are

1. High Temperature Short Time method called Flash method where milk is heated rapidly to 80°C and held for 30 seconds
2. Low temperature holding method called holding method where milk is heated to 62°C for 30 minutes.

PAT Abbreviation for **P**aroxysmal **A**trial **T**achycardia

patch A change in colour and texture of skin such as Ash Leaf patch, Mucous patch, Payer's patch, etc,

patella About 5 cm diameter triangular sesamoid bone in front of knee joint.

patellar That which is related with Patella.

patency That which is widely open.

patent That which is not obstructed or which is open one.

Paterson's syndrome This is referred to Plummer-Vinson syndrome described by Paterson.

Patey's operation This refers to modified radical mastectomy described by Patey.

path Route or pathway for movement.

pathogen Disease-producing microorganism.

pathogenesis During the development of a disease we observe the development of morbid condition of illness.

pathogenic That which produces disease.

pathogenicity Ability to produce pathologic changes

pathognomonic Symptoms and signs on which a diagnosis can be made.

pathological Related to pathology;

pathologist A person who is an expert in pathology.

pathology The discipline which explains the structural and functional changes in cell, tissue or organ

patient Person who is ill or who is undergoing treatment for disease.

Patrick's test This is positive in arthritis of the hip. Pain is produced with the patient supine, the thigh and knee are flexed and the external malleolus is placed over the patella of the opposite leg and the knee is depressed.

pattern Design or arrangement in cel, tissue or organ. It can also tell the behavioural pattern.

patulous Latin word meaning distended.

Pauci Denotes a few items. Such paucibacillary.

Paul-Bunnell test The diagnostic test in infectious mononucleosis. Sheep red cells are agglutinated by a given dilution of patient's serum is inferred as positive.

Pavlov Russian physiologist and experimental psychologist during the period 1849–1936; is the winner of the Nobel prize for medicine in 1904 for his work on the physiology of digestion

Pavlov's pouch A pocket of stomach which is surgically separated by a septum but retaining bagal connection is used in experimental study of gastric physiology.

pavlovian conditioning Learning by a stimulus which can evoke response by repeated pairing with another stimulus to elicit the response.

Pawlik's triangle Exactly with vesical triangle, it is within the vagina and is counted laterally by Pawlik's fold.

PBI Abbreviation for protein-bound iodine.

PCEC Abbreviation for purified Chick Embryo Cell vaccine.

pCi Abbreviation for picocurie.

PCO_2 symbol for *carbon dioxide partial pressure* denoted as P_{CO_2}, .

PCR Abbreviation for polymerase chain reaction.

PCT Abbreviation for *Patent Cooperation Treaty*.

PCV Abbreviation for Pneumococcal Conjugate Vaccine.

PDA Abbreviation for patent ductus arteriosus.

Péan's forceps He devised curved haemostatic forceps and a straight haemostatics forceps which have serrations along the entire length of the jaw.

Pearson's correlation coefficient It is product moment correlation which is the covariance of two random variables divided by the product of their S.D.

pectin Used in jam and jellies. It is obtained from inner portion of orange, apple pomace and is useful as the protective component of various formulations employed in the treatment of diarrhea

pectus Front of the chest.

pediatric Related with to pediatrics.

pediatrician A specialist in pediatrics.

pediatrics Branch of medicine which treats of the child and its development and care and of the diseases of children and their treatment.

pedicle Basal part of a tumour which is attached to normal tissue. This can also be a flap tissue through which it receives its blood supply

Pediculus Genus of sucking lice of the family Pediculidae. Head louse, Body louse nd pubic louse are medically important.

pedicure Professional care and treatment of the feet.

pedigree In the analysis of inheritance in genetics, list of a person's ancestors is used.

pediodontia Speciality called pediatric dentistry.

peduncle A swelling or a tumour is attached through a connection called peduncle.

pedunculated That which has a pedicle.

PEF Abbreviation for peak expiratory flow.

PEFR Abbreviation for peak expiratory flow rate.

peg This is a projecting structure.

pellagra Deficiency of niacin characterized by dermatitis, inflammation of mucous membranes, diarrhea, and psychic disturbances.

pellet Pill containing drugs for slow absorption.

Pellizzi's syndrome This refers to epiphyseal syndrome described by Pellizzi.

pelvic That which is related with pelvis.

pelvimeter This is an instrument for measuring the diameters and capacity of the pelvis to forecast normal delivery or cesarean. It is also called pelvimetry that can be done manually, using instrument or X-ray.

pelvirectal That which is pertaining to the pelvis and the rectum.

pelvis Lower trunk which is bounded anteriorly and laterally by the two hip bones and posteriorly by the sacrum and coccyx. Pelvis of medical importance are

- Gynecoid pelvis
- Android pelvis
- Flat pelvis
- Anthropoid pelvis
- Rachitic pelvis
- Round pelvis
- Split pelvis
- True pelvis

PEM Abbreviation for protein-energy malnutrition.

pemphigus Chronic, relapsing, sometimes fatal skin diseases characterized clinically by the development of successive crops of vesicles and bullae.

penetrability Character of penetration of X-ray.

penetration Entering deeply by an object or radiation or a chemical

-penia Abnormal reduction in number such as Leukopenia.

penicillamine A chelating agent used in hepatolenticular degeneration and rheumatoid arthritis.

penicillin Antibiotics derived from strains of fungi of the genus *Penicillium*. Common penicillin used in medical or clinical practice is Benzathine penicillin and Procaine penicillin.

penis Male sex organ of copulation homologous with clitoris in females.

pentose a monosaccharide containing five carbon atoms in a molecule.

penumbra A shadow at partial illumination and it surrounds the umbra. In radiography it suggests blurring around the edges of a structure.

pepsin Enzymes of the gastric juice that catalyze the hydrolysis of proteins to form polypeptides. Pepsin A, B and C are known entities.

pepsinogen This is a proenzyme secreted by mucous cells and pyloric gland cells. Pepsinogen is converted into pepsin in the presence of gastric acid .

peptic Related to pepsin or digestion or action of gastric juices.

peptidase Enzymes of the hydrolase class that catalyze the hydrolysis of peptide bonds

peptone Products produced by the partial hydrolysis of protein by an acid or by an enzyme.

per Latin word meaning throughout the given time or given space.

percentile Position of a value in 100 values when the values are in ascending order. For example 80th value of American children for weight (when arranged in ascending order of 100 values) is equal to 100th value of Indian child (when 100 values of Indian children weight are arranged in an ascending order) This probability value is 80th percentile for Indian children.

perception Latin word meaning that the conscious mental registration of a sensory stimulus. Perceptions of medical importance are

- Depth perception for recognition of depth
- Stereognostic perception for stereognosis
- Extrasensory perception for other than the senses.

percolation The chemical process wherein the extraction of the soluble parts of a drug causes a liquid solvent to flow slowly through it.

percuss Doing percussion.

percussion Striking a part with short blows for diagnosing a condition. The types of percussion are

- Bimanual percussion
- Deep percussion
- Direct percussion
- Finger percussion
- Hammer percussion

percutaneous injection or introduction done through skin.

perennial Referred to illness that last through several years.

Pérez's sign This sign is positive in case of aneurysm of aorta or a mediastinal tumour. When patient raises and drops the upper limbs a friction sound is heard over the sternum.

perflation Air movement from broader space to narrow space. It can be blowing air to force out secretions

perforated That which is pierced with holes.

perforation Act of piercing through a part.

performance The execution of an action.

perfuse To pour over

perfusion Passage of a fluid through the vessels of a specific organ.

periadenitis Infection and inflammation of the tissues around a gland.

perianal Around the anus

pericarditis Inflammation of the pericardium.

pericardium Fibroserous sac that surrounds the heart and the roots of the great vessels

perichondritis Inflammation of the perichondrium.

perichondrium Fibrous connective tissue which invests all cartilage except the articular cartilage of synovial joints.

pericolpitis Infection and inflammation of the tissues around the vagina.

peridural Around the dura mater.

perimetritis Infection and inflammation of the perimetrium.

perimetry Determination of peripheral visual field by using perimeter.

perinatal Period shortly before and after birth

perineum The space between the anus and scrotum

period This refer to the time for the regular recurrence of a phenomenon.

periodicity To recur at regular intervals of time.

periodontics This is the branch of dentistry that deals with the study and treatment of diseases of the periodontium.

periosteum Connective tissue covering all bones of the body

periostitis Inflammation of the periosteum.

peritoneal Pertaining to the peritoneum.

peritoneum Serous membrane lining the abdominopelvic walls which is called parietal peritoneum and that serous membrane which lines viscera is called visceral peritoneum.

peritonitis Infection and inflammation of the peritoneum. Clinical entities are:

- Bacterial peritonitis
- Bile peritonitis
- Fungal peritonitis
- Adhesive peritonitis
- Meconium peritonitis
- Perforation peritonitis
- Traumatic peritonitis
- Tubercular peritonitis

Perls' test A test to detect haemosiderin. Substance to be tested is treated with HCL and Potassium ferrocyanide. Appearance of Prussian blue is positive for haemosiderin.

permethrin Used as external application in Scabies infestation. This is a pyrethroid insecticide

pernicious Fatal

peroxidase Enzymes of the oxidoreductase class that catalyze the oxidation of organic substrates by hydrogen peroxide

peroxide Commonly refers to Hydrogen peroxide. Peroxide have the linkage as —O—O—;

per rectum By way of the rectum.

perseveration Repetition of a thought after the causative stimulus has ceased or it can be in response to different stimuli, e.g., answering a question correctly and then inappropriately. Commonly seen in schizophrenia.

personality Characteristic how a person thinks, feels, and behaves. Types are

- Dependent personality
- Antisocial personality
- Double personality
- Hysterical personality
- Paranoid personality
- Sadistic personality
- Split personality

perspiration process of excessive sweating.

Perthes' disease This refers to osteochondrosis described by Perthes.

pertussis Acute infectious whooping cough caused by Bordetella pertussis among children.

per vaginam popularly called P.V. examination which means 'through the vagina'.

perversion Abnormal course of anything. Mental perversion and sexual perversion are common entities.

pervious That which is permeable.

pessary This refers to medicated vaginal suppository. Cup pessary, diaphragm pessary and ring pessary are common types.

pest Lower animal, birds and insects that are harmful to man.

pesticide Poison used to destroy pests of any kind.

PET Abbreiation for **P**re **E**clamptic **T**oxaemia.

petechia Purple red spot caused by intradermal hemorrhage.

pethidine hydrochloride This is meperidine hydrochloride.

petit mal Minor epilepsy.

Petri dish Used for tissue culture and bacteriological culture. This will be a round shallow flat bottomed transparent glass dish with vertical sides and a similar but slightly larger dish that forms a cover.

petroleum Naturally available mixture of solid liquid and gas from below the earth. This contains a mixture of various alkanes, cycloalkanes, and aromatic hydrocarbons as well as small amounts of sulfur, nitrogen, and oxygen compounds.

petromastoid 1. pertaining to the petrous portion of the temporal bone and its mastoid process. 2. otocranium.

Peyer's patches are groupings of lymphoid follicles in the mucus membrane that lines your small intestine.

PG Abbreviation for prostaglandin; **pg (pg)** picogram.

PGD_2, PGE_2, $PGF_{2\alpha}$, PGI_2, etc. Symbols for various prostaglandins

pH It tells about hydrogen ion (H^+) concentration of a solution to that of a given standard solution. pH is approximately equal to the negative logarithm of H^+ concentration and is expressed in molarity.

pH 7 is neutral
pH 7 and above alkaline
pH below 7 acidic.

phac(o) Word denotes to a lens

phacoanaphylaxis Hypersensitivity to the protein of the crystalline lens of the eye

phacoemulsification Method of cataract extraction by ultrasonic vibrations and by irrigation and aspiration.

phagocyte Cells that ingest microorganisms such as monocytes, macrophage or microphage.

phagocytosis The cellular process of taking the material into the cell in membrane-bound vesicles (phagosomes) that originate as pinched off invaginations of the plasma membrane.

phalanx Bones of the fingers or toes

phallus This is the representation of the penis.

phantom Greek word meaning an appearance Physically a model of the body or radiologically a device that simulates the conditions

pharmaceutical Related to pharmacy or to drugs.

pharmacist Person who is licensed to prepare sell or dispense drugs

pharmacodynamics This is a branch of Pharmacology which deals with biochemical and physiological effects of drugs

pharmacognosy Branch of pharmacology which deals with the biological, biochemical, and economic features of natural drugs

pharmacologist Person who makes a study of the actions of drugs.

pharmacology This deals with the origin, nature, chemistry, effects, and uses of drugs. Pharmacology includes pharmacognosy, pharmacokinetics, pharmacodynamics, pharmacotherapeutics, and toxicology.

pharmacopeia An authoritative treatise on drugs

pharmacy This deals with preparation, dispensing, and proper utilization of drugs.

pharyngeal That which is related with pharynx.

pharyngitis Infection and inflammation of the pharynx.

phase Stages through which a disease pass.

PhD Abbreviation for **D**octor of **Ph**ilosophy.

Phelps' operation This is operation for talipes with an open and direct incision through the sole.

Phemister graft Graft done for enhancement of callus formation in case of poor cortical bone. It is a bone graft with cancellous bone chips

phenacetin Acetaminophen derivative used as an analgesic and antipyretic

phenantoin Active ingredient mephenytoin used as anticonvulsant.

Phenergan Preparations of promethazine hydrochloride.

phenformin hydrochloride Oral hypoglycemic agent

pheniramine maleate Antihistaminic

phenobarbital Long-acting barbiturate used as a sedative, hypnotic, and anticonvulsant. It is also called Phenobarbitone.

phenol This is obtained by the distillation of coal tar and is an antimicrobial agent. It is also called as carbolic acid, hydroxybenzene, and oxybenzone.

Phenolax Preparation of phenolphthalein.

phenolphthalein It is a cathartic and a pH indicator (range 8.5 to 9.0)

phenomenon Observable occurrence or a fact.

phenothiazine A veterinary anthelmintic. Antipsychotic agent

phenotype As against genotype, phenotype explains the entire physical, biochemical, and physiological makeup of an individual as determined both genetically and environmentally, Bombay phenotype, a rare blood phenotype produced by the interaction of genes of the ABO blood group and a rare recessive gene at a different locus, resulting in a complete lack of H antigen; cells of individuals with this phenotype lack A, B, and H antigens, and their serum contains anti-A, anti-B, and anti-H antigen. McLeod phenotype, a rare blood phenotype with X-linked inheritance in which several antigens of the Kell blood group are weakly expressed; affected individuals sometimes have an anemic condition called McLeod syndrome.

phenyl Chemical derived from Benzene which is the monovalent radical C_6H_5,

phenylalanine This is an aromatic essential amino acid,

phenylbutazone An analgesic, antipyretic, anti-inflammatory with mild uricosuric properties. Used in Gout, rheumatoid arthritis and ankylosing spondylitis,

phenylketonuria Clinical manifestation of hyperphenylalaninemia due to phenylalanine 4-monooxygenase deficiency. Maternal phenylketonuria, classic phenylketonuria, atypical phenylketonuria and transient phenylketonuria are known types.

phenytoin Anticonvulsant and cardiac depressant used in the treatment of all forms of epilepsy except petit mal. Because of its cardiac depressant action it is used in arrhythmia.

pheochromocytoma Benign, encapsulated, lobular, and vascular tumor of chromaffin tissue of the adrenal medulla

phial Small bottle called vial

philia Word means abnormal craving

phimosis Condition where prepuce cannot be retracted back over the glans.

phlebectomy Excision of a vein,

phlebitis Inflammation of a vein

Phlebotomus Bloodsucking sand flies which transmits diseases.

phlebotomy Surgical incision of a vein called venepuncture. blood.

phlegm Thick mucus secreted by the mucosa of the respiratory passages

phlycten Small vesicle containing lymph seen on the conjunctiva

phlyctenular That which is associated with the formation of phlycten

phobia Intense fear of a specific situation
phobia Irrational fear or an aversion to the given situation.
Phocas' disease Glandular chronic mastitis described by Phocas.
phocomelia Absence of the proximal portion of limb the hands or feet being attached to the trunk of the body
phonetic Articulated sounds of speech
phonetics The science of vocal sounds
phonogram Graphic record of a sound like ECG.
phosgene Toxic colorless gas (War gas) that causes fatal pulmonary edema or pneumonia on inhalation . Chemically it it carbonic dichloride (CCl_2O)
phospholipidemia the presence of phospholipid in the blood.
phosphoprotein This is a protein to which phosphate groups are attached at threonine residues.
phosphorylase Enzymes catalyzing phosphorolysis of glycosides, transferring the cleaved glycosyl group to inorganic phosphate.
phosphorylase kinase Enzyme of the transferase class that catalyzes the phosphorylation of inactive glycogen phosphorylase *b* to form active glycogen phosphorylase *a* a step in the cascade of reactions regulating glycogenolysis.
phosphorylation Phosphate group is introduced into an organic molecule. This is a metabolic process.
photochromogen By exposure to light pigmentation is developed in pathogens. Non Tubercular mycobacteria M.kansasii becomes yellow orange in the presence of light.
photocoagulation By using xenon arc light protein material can be condensed. Photocoagulation is done in retinal detachment and for intraocular tumour mass.
photosensitive Sensitive to sun light in an abnormal way.
photosynthesis Carbohydrates are formed from oxygen, water in the presence of chlorophyll in plants.
phrenic That which is related with diaphragm.
phthalic acid Isomer used in dye manufacture.
phthalylsulfathiazole Sulfonamide used in the infection of intestine by bacteria.
phthiriasis Infestation with pubic lice
phthisis Greek word meaning wasting commonly referred to Pulmonary Tuberculosis.
phylum Main division of Plant kingdom
physical Related to material things,
physician One who practices Medicine or internal medicine after graduation from Medical College
physics Basic science which deals with forces and general properties of matter and energy.
physiology Science that deals with the functions of human body or organisms. Types of physiology that are to be noted in medicine are:

- Human physiology
- Animal physiology
- Comparative physiology
- General physiology

physostigmine Cholinergic alkaloid obtained from seed of a plant and is used in ophthalmology as miotic . It reduces intra ocular tension. Hence used in Glaucoma.
pia Latin word meaning soft and is referable to pia mater.
pia mater Innermost covering the brain and spinal cord
picocurie Unit of radioactivity which explains the quantity of radioactive material in which the number of nuclear disintegrations is 3.7×10^{-2}
PID Abbreviation for pelvic inflammatory disease.
pigmentation Physiological or pathological deposition of coloring matter on the body.
pile Ball like structure always referable to haemorrhoid.
piles Haemorrhoids..
pill Tablet which is medicated mass for swallowing.
pilocarpine Cholinomimetic drug which produces muscarinic effects. Used in Glaucoma.
pimple Papule on the face due to acne vulgaris.
Pinard's maneuver Obstetrical method of bringing down the foot in Breech presentation.
pinch Pressing tightly between the thumb and one finger.
pineal Shaped line pine cone such as pineal body.
pinguecula Yellowish spot of proliferation on the bulbar conjunctiva near the sclerocorneal junction seen in old age.
piperazine Anthelmintic used in round worm and Thread worm infection.
pipette Glass tube used in transferring small quantities of liquid
piriform A structure which is pear-shaped.
pisiform Structure which is pea shaped.
pit A depression or indentation . Common entities are:

- Arm pit
- Ear pit
- Gastric pits
- Nasal pit
- Preauricular pit
- Pit of arytenoids cartilage

pith Piercing spinal cord called pithing done in Frog experiments in physiology or pharmacology.
pitting small depressions on pressure is seen and is called pitting oedema.
pituitary Endocrine gland consisting of anterior pituitary and posterior pituitary otherwise called adenohypophysis and neurohypophysis.
pityriasis Fine branny scales on the skin as manifestation of skin disease.
pizzle Colloquial term to denote penis of lower animals.
PKU Abbreviation for phenylketonuria.
placebo Latin word meaning 'I will please you'. Pharmacy preparation for satisfying psychophysiological aspect

of patient in an illness. This is also called dummy treatment. In clinical trial placebo are used as control study.

placenta Latin word meaning flat cake. It is a connection between mother and foetus in mammals which provide nutrients, endocrine secretions and immunological particles.

Placido's disk It is a keratoscope used in ophthalmology.

plague Bacterial infection caused by Yersinia pestis which cause bubo an epidemic plague. Plague is transmitted by rat flea. In man bubonic plague, pulmonic plague and septicaemic plague are known varieties.

plane It denotes a surface which has the straight line connecting 2 points which are wholly in the surface.

plankton Minute free-floating organisms vegetable and animal that live in natural waters.

planoconcave Flat on one side and concave on the other

planoconvex Flat on one side and convex on the other

plantar Related to the sole of the foot.

plasma Fluid portion of the blood in which the particulate components are suspended. It is cell free portion of blood from which the fibrinogen I separated.

plasmalemma Peripheral layer of the ectoplasm in a fertilized oocyte.

plasmid A structure in bacterial cell that carry genes that are double stranded DNA.

plasmin An enzyme present in plasma which is activated by plasminogen.

plasmodium Protozoa of the genus Plasmodium that cause malaria.

plasmogen An essential part of protoplasm

plasmoid an abnormal protein cellular element

plaster Gypsum material which hardens when mixed with water is used for immobilizing or making impressions of body parts.

plaster of Paris Historically plaster of paris was first made in 19th century in Paris by Gypsum deposits.

plastic High-molecular-weight polymeric organic material, that can be moulded.

plasticizer Substance that make other substance soft and flexible.

plate Bone plate or dental plate which are flat structure.

platelet Disk-shaped structure which are 2 to 4 µm in diameter, found in the blood of all mammals and chiefly known for its role in blood coagulation

Platyhelminthes Referred to trematode and cestoidean which are flatworms.

platysma Plate-like muscle of the neck which function to wrinkle skin of neck and help to depress the jaw.

pledge Any solemn statement of intention such as Nightingale pledge.

pleomorphism Different forms of an organism.

Plesch's percussion To percuss within intercostal space and avoiding ribs to have vibration. At percussion the pleximeter finger with the first interphalangeal joint flexed at a right angle.

plethora Fullness of a part with the blood which make the part red florid complexion .

pleura Serous membrane covering the potential space called pleural cavity which is moistened with serous secretion which helps the movements of lungs in the chest.

pleural That which is related with pleura.

pleurisy Infection and inflammation of pleura which are of two types. One is dry and the other is wet pleurisy. It is also called Pleurisy.

plexiform That which resembles a network.

plexor The finger which is used as a hammer in performing percussion.

plexus This can be lymphatic vessels plexus, nerve plexus or venous plexus.

plumbism This refers to lead poisoning.

Plummer's disease This refers to Toxic Multinodular Goitre described by Plummer.

PMR Abbreviation for proportionate mortality ratio.

pneumococcus Bacteria belonging to organism of the species Streptococcus pneumoniae.

pneumoconiosis It is an occupational disorders by the accumulation of dust particle in the lung which can be organic dust or an inorganic dust.

pneumonia Infection and inflammation of the lungs with consolidation.

pneumopericardium Presence of air or gas in the cavity of the pericardium.

pneumoperitoneum Presence of gas or air in the peritoneal cavity

pneumothorax Accumulation of air or gas in the pleural space

PNH Abbreviation for paroxysmal nocturnal hemoglobinuria.

pock Depressed scar left by Pustule especially of the lesions caused by dermotropic viruses. The mark produced by such viral infections in the form of depressed scar are called pockmark.

podiatry Speciality that deals with the study and care of the foot

poiesis Word termination meaning formation.

poietin Termination word used in names of hormones to indicate involvement in regulation of cells in the peripheral blood.

poikilocyte Abnormal RBC such as:

- Sickle cell
- Target cell
- Schistocytes
- Stomatocytes

- Elliptocytes
- Acanthocytes
- Burr cell

poikilocytosis Presence ofpoikilocytosis in the blood .

point A spot or an area on the body, or on the surface.

poise Unit for expressing viscosity of liquid (Number of grams per Cm. per Sec)

poison That which causes harm to the body and damage to structure.

poisonous That which is toxic.

Poisson distribution It is a discrete distribution wherein the probability of occurrence is towards impossible from theoretical point of view.

$$P = (X = x) \frac{e^{-\ddot{e}}\,\ddot{e}^{x}}{x\,!}$$

where x = a count 0,1,2,3,4,5, etc.,
e = Base of natural log = 2.7181
ë = Mean = Variance
ì = S.D.^{2}

Simplified version formula for Poisson distribution is used in fitting the distribution which denote;-

$$P_x = e^{m} \frac{m^{x}}{x\,!}$$

where e = constant
m = ì
x = Distribution
x ! = Factorial

Under the following conditions, we observe that distribution becoming poison:

- Value of P or q becomes indefinitely small
- Number of observations becomes (n) very large
- The product of (n) and (p) which is np = mean number of events is always finite.

polar Related with a pole

Polaramine Preparations that contains dexchlorphenira-mine maleate.

polarization Establishment of polarity. This also mean the separation of electric charge so that there is directionality of flow as between two poles anode and cathode of an electrolysis cell

poliomyelitis Acute infectious disease caused by a virus called poliovirus. Colloquially it is called infantile paralysis. This is caused by virus of the genus Enterovirus which has 3 serotypes . Type 1 is responsible for 85% of polio paralysis. Type 2 is responsible for 5 percent and Type 3 is responsible for 10 percent of cases.

pollen They are microspores or male fertilizing elements of flowering plants. They are known to produce allergy.

pollination When pollen are transferred from anther to stigma of a flowering plant.

pollution Refers to impurity such as air pollution, water pollution etc.,

Polya's operation Anastomosis of stomach and jejunum following subtotal gastrectomy.

polyandry Woman is concurrently married to more than one man.

polyarthritis Inflammation of several joints

polyclinic Clinic run by doctors which treats many kinds of illness. Different specialists join together in one place and treat cases.

polycystic That which is made of many cysts.

polycythemia Increase in total red cell of the blood

polydactyly Supernumerary fingers or toes on the hands or feet.

polydipsia Excessive thirst which could be pathological due to diabetes mellitus, diabetes insipidus, reaction to medication or psychological origin.

polygamy Man or woman to have more than one spouse as opposed to monogamy.

polygon Figure bounded by more than three sides

polygyny Man is married concurrently to more than one woman.

polymer Compound formed by the joining of smaller molecules called monomers. Common polymers are polypeptides, nucleic acids, polysaccharides, and plastics

polymerase Enzyme that catalyzes nucleotides to polynucleotides.

polymerization Process of formation of polymers y monomers.

polymorphic That which occurs in several forms

polymorphism Capacity to exist in several different forms.

polymyositis This is a chronic progressive inflammatory disease of skeletal muscle

polymyxin Polypeptide antibiotics derived from strains of the soil bacterium *Bacillus polymyxa*

polyneuritis Inflammation of many peripheral nerves at the given time simultaneously.

polynuclear Related to several nuclei

polyp A protruding growth from mucous membrane

polypeptide Peptide that on hydrolysis yields more than two amino acids

polysaccharide Carbohydrate that on hydrolysis yields a large number of monosaccharides.

polyvinylpyrrolidone This refers to povidone.

POMP Cancer treatment regimen which include **P**rednisone, **O**ncovin (vincristine), **M**ethotrexate, and 6-mercapto **P**urine

Pompe's disease This refers to glycogen storage disease type II described by Pompe.

pons Tissue connecting two parts of an organ. This is usually referable to the part of the C.N.S. lying between the medulla oblongata and the mesencephalon just above the cerebellum

Pool's phenomenon This is seen in Tetany. When upper limb is raised above the head with forearm extended, upper limb contracts. This is due to stretching of the brachial plexus.

pool Common reservoir for a group.

popliteal Related to posterior surface of the knee

population Category of individuals which form inhabitant of a geographic area.

porcelain When a mixture of kaolin, feldspar, quartz, whiting are mixed in high temperature we get dense ceramic material called porcelain.

porosis Callus formation during the repair of bone. In Greek it means cavity formation.

porphyria Disturbances due to porphyrin metabolism that cause neurological and cutaneous manifestations.

porphyrin Chemical that contains four pyrrole rings connected by methylidyne

Porro's cesarean section This has historical importance where caesarean section done with extirpation of the uterine corpus and ovaries.

porta designates an opening especially the site of entrance to an organ of the blood vessels

portion A part of a larger structure.

porus Any of various small openings in the body.

Posadas' mycosis This refers to coccidioidomycosis described by Posadas.

Position Bodily posture by a person to achieve comfort in certain conditions, Foetal situation in uterus of a pregnant woman.

Bodily positions are:

- Valentine - supine, hips flexed
- Trendelenburg – supine, head tilted 40 degree downwards, table angulated below the knee.
- Semi prone, on left side, , right knee thigh flexed for P V exam called Sim's position
- For kidney examination Noble's position
- Knee elbow position
- Fowler's position – head raised and knee elevated
- Lateral recumbent called English position
- Lithotomy position which dorsolateral position
- Supine or dorsal position
- Anatomical – erect face anterior, upper limb sideward, palm supinated
- Semirecumbent for radiograph called albert's position
- Left occipito anterior and Left occipito posterior in vertex presentation

Positive A value greater than zero

positron A positive electron with positive electric charge. It is represented as e^+.

posology System or science of dose in medicamentation.

posterior Back surface of the body called dorsal.

posterolateral Posteriorly and to one side.

postganglionic Autonomic nerve fibers situated distal to a ganglion.

post mortem Latin word meaning after death. This is related to time after the death.

postnatal That which occurs after birth.

postoperative That is occurring after a surgical operation.

post partum That which occurs after child birth.

postprandial That which occurs after a meal

posture This refers to the attitude of the body.

potency Ability of the male to perform sexual intercourse.

potential Not active but ready for action.

poultice Cooked cereal in layers of gauze is put on skin surface as moist heat application

pound Unit of a mass. Abbreviated as Lb meaning as under:
16 oz or 7000 grains or 453.6 grams in avoirdupois
12 oz or 5760 grains or 373.2 grams in apothecaries.

Poupart's ligament Fibrous band running from anterior superior spine of the ilium to the spine of the pubis.

povidone Synthetic polymer called Poly Vinyl Pyrrolidone used as a tablet binder in pharmacy.

powder Grinding of solid to make fine particles.

power One who is able to act, It can be a measure of magnification in microscopic examination, In statistics it is the probability of correctly rejecting N.H.

PPD Abbreviation for purified protein derivative (tuberculin)

ppm Abbreviation for parts per million.

practice Diagnosis and treatment by one's knowledge by the medical practitioner.

precancerous Pre malignant condition.

precipitation The process of precipitating.

precision Quality of being sharply defined

preclinical Period before which a disease becomes clinically recognizable.

precocious Overgrowth than expected in an individual.

precordium Anterior surface of the body covering the heart and stomach

precursor Biological process which precedes another biological process.

predator Living creature which lives on another creature.

prednisolone Synthetic glucocorticoid from cortisol,.

prednisone Synthetic glucocorticoid from cortisone,

preeclampsia Complication of pregnancy manifested in the form of hypertension, edema, proteinuria.

pregnancy By the union of male and female gametes, foetus develops in the uterus and the average period of development is about 266 days.

pregnanediol Derivatives of progesterone found especially in urine of women during pregnancy or the luteal phase of the menstrual cycle.

pregnant Female with growing foetus in her uterus.
prehension Act of grasping.
prelacteal Any thing that precedes the establishment of breast milk flow
premalignant Tumour which is precancerous.
premature Infant which is not matured to the gestational age.
prematurity Meaning underdevelopment
premedical Period of study before entry to medical course.
premedication Pre anaesthetic preliminary medication particularly to produce narcosis
premenstrual That which occurs before menses.
premolar Refers to tooth which is situated in front of the molar teeth.
premonitory Which serves as a warning
prenatal Which occurs before birth of child.
preoperative Any measure preceding an operation.
preparation That which is ready, To prepare for surgery, Material is set for the study etc.,
preponderance That which has greater influence.
prepuce Foreskin of male organ.
prepyloric Proximal to the pylorus
presbycusis Old age hearing loss.
presbyopia Hyperopia and impairment of vision due to advancing age;
prescribe Prescription for treatment by physician.
prescription Written direction for administration of a remedy. This is written as R_x (Recipe meaning take.)
presenile Early old age changes occurring.
presentation Portion of the foetus that is touched by the examining finger through the cervix .
preservative Substance added to a product for the purpose of inhibiting the multiplication of microorganisms.
pressoreceptive Sensitive to stimuli due to vasomotor activity
presumptive To presume and act such as presumptive treatment in Malaria.
presystole The interval immediately preceding systole.
prevalence Cases of a disease that are present in a population at a specified time (Point prevalence or period prevalence)
preventive To avoid the occurrence of.
PRF Abbreviation for prolactin-releasing factor.
Priapism) Persistent abnormal erection of the penis usually without sexual desire seen in spinal cord injuries.
primaquine phosphate 8-aminoquinoline compound used as an antimalarial agent.
primary First in the order such as Primary Health Care, Primary Prevention Primary Health Centre etc.,
primigravid Pregnant for the first time. Gravida I.
primipara Woman who has had one pregnancy that resulted in a fetus that attained a weight of 500 g para I.
primitive Early form which shows little evolution.
primordial Undeveloped, original and simplest.
primordium Rudimentary structure in development.
principle Regulation of the law to conduct oneself. It can be main chemical component.
prism Polygonal solid or a triangular solid glass which splits up ray of light to its constituent colours.
probability In a random independent trial chance of occurrence of an event which can be never or always. When we say P=0.05 it means chance of occurrence of an event is one in 100 or 5%.
probe Flexible instrument designed for introduction into a wound, cavity, or sinus tract for purposes of exploration.
proboscis Snout of an animal used in feeding.
procaine This is a benzoic acid derivative with local anesthetic activity.
procedure Steps by which a desired result is accomplished. Also called method, manoeuvre or technique.
process Projection of a bone; This can be steps to lead to achievement.
processus Mass projecting from a larger structure.
procidentia Prolapse of the uterus to such a degree that the cervix protrudes from the vaginal outlet.
procreation Process of bringing a new individual into the world.
proctodynia Pain in the anus.
proctology Branch of medicine concerned with disorders of the rectum and anus.
proctoscope Tubular instrument with appropriate illumination for inspecting the rectum.
prodrome Premonitory symptom of a disease
productive Refers to productive cough which brings copious sputum.
proenzyme Inactive precursor that can be converted to the active enzyme.
professional Refers to a specialist and his profession.
profile Face viewed from the side. This can be summary representing a set.
progesterone Progestational hormone of the body from corpus luteum, placenta, and adrenal cortex
proglottid A segment making up the body of a tapeworm.
prognosis Forecasting the probable outcome of an attack of disease
progression Walk forward or disease becoming more severe.
proguanil hydrochloride Drug used in the treatment and prophylaxis of malaria.
projection Act of putting forth thoughts and feelings. It can be projecting an audio visual aid in teaching.
prolactin Hormone secreted by adenohypophysis which stimulates formation of milk. It is called lactogen or lactogenic.

prolapse Displacement or falling down loosely such as prolapse of uterus.

proliferate Growth occurring by the multiplication of cells.

proliferation Multiplication of similar forms cells. This is otherwise is called hyperplasia.

proline One of the nonessential amino acid that constitute main core of collagen.

promazine hydrochloride Antipsychotic agent which is a phenothiazine derivative.

promethazine hydrochloride Antihistaminic and antiemetic which is phenothiazine derivative

prominence Projection of an anatomical structure.

pronate In a prone position

pronation Medial rotation of the hand which allow palm turn to posteriorly.

pronator Muscle that helps to pronate.

prone Lying face downward

propane Hydrocarbon present in natural gas and is an inflammable gas Chemically it is $CH_3CH_2CH_3$,

prophase First stage in cell reduplication. In mitosis,

prophylactic Steps to prevent disease occurrence. This can be concurrent, terminal or preventive in nature.

prophylaxis Intervention aimed at the prevention of disease;

propiolactone Disinfectant effective against gram-positive, gram-negative, and acid-fast bacteria, fungi, and viruses.

propionic acid Saturated fatty acid that can be fermented by several species of bacteria

proportion Relation of one part to the whole.

propranolol Beta-adrenergic blocking agent which reduces blood pressure and helps in the prophylaxis of migraine.

proprietary Drug used in treatment is protected against free competition as to name and product.

proprioceptor Terminals found in muscles, tendons, and joint capsules, which give information concerning movements

prostaglandin Derived from unsaturated fatty acids that are potent mediators of numerous different physiologic processes.

prostate Gland in the male which surrounds the neck of the bladder and the urethra. It contributes to seminal fluid.

prostatectomy Surgical removal of the prostate

prostatitis Inflammation of the prostate.

prosthesis Artificial substitute for a missing body part like tooth, limb etc.,

prosthodontics Dentistry pertaining to the restoration and maintenance of oral function

prostration Extreme exhaustion.

protamine They are basic proteins of low molecular weight, occurring in combination with nucleic acids in the sperm and has the property of neutralizing heparin.

protease This refers to endopeptidase.

protective To affort immunity. Any protective device physical, for skin, for eyes, for ears, for head etc.,

protein Organic compounds which contain carbon, hydrogen, oxygen, nitrogen, and sulphur, with main element nitrogen. 20 known amino acids with defined sequence are present. Main functions of protein are growth, differentiation, immunity, nerve impulse, coordination of movement and enzymatic catalysis.

protein kinase Enzyme that catalyzes the phosphorylation of serine, threonine, or tyrosine

proteinuria Also called albuminuria with the presence of an excess of serum proteins in the urine

proteolysis By proteolytic enzymes, splitting of protein occurs.

Proteus Gram-negative, facultative anaerobic, rod-shaped bacteria which cause urinary tract infections, wound infections.

prothrombin It is one of the coagulation factor.

proton Elementary particle of positive charge which forms the nucleus of the ordinary hydrogen atom

protoplasm Essential material of cell which is translucent colloid with water. This is composed of nucleic acids, proteins, lipids, carbohydrates and inorganic salts.

protoporphyrin An intermediate in heme biosynthesis. It is produced by oxidation of the methylene bridge of protoporphyrinogen.

protoporphyrinogen An intermediate in heme biosynthesis. Type IX isomer is produced by oxidative decarboxylation of coproporphyrinogen

Protozoa They are simplest organisms of animal kingdom which are one celled organisms.

protuberance This is a projecting part

provitamin This denotes a precursor of a vitamin.

provocation challenge

provocative Stimulating an organ or an individual for a sign, reflex, reaction, or therapeutic effect.

Prowazek's bodies Inclusion bodies seen in case of cowpox and smallpox

proximal That which is nearest. Equivalent to Proximate.

prurigo Crust or lichen form of skin lesion that cause severe itching.

pruritus Cutaneous sensation that provokes the desire to scratch the skin to obtain relief.

pseudoappendicitis Signs of appendix without actual appendicitis.

pseudocyesis Pseudo pregnancy.

pseudocyst Cavity resembles a cuts but not lined with epithelium.

pseudohermaphroditism Clinical condition where an individual has genetically and gonadally of one sex but has significant secondary sex characters of the opposite sex

pseudomenstruation Seen in newborn babies where uterine discharge unattended with endometrial changes

Pseudomonas Gram-negative bacteria which are saprophytic present in soil, water and decomposing matter.

pseudopolyp Hypertrophied mucous membrane resembling a polyp

pseudopregnancy This is false pregnancy.

pseudopuberty Because of steroid hormones by adrenocortical tumour there is development of secondary sex characters

psittacosis Respiratory and systemic disease of wild and domestic birds, transmitted to humans. Causative organism is *Chlamydia psittaci*

psoralen Photosensitizing constituents of plants that include methoxsalen and trioxsalen. They are common ingredients of perfumes and drugs.

psoriasis Chronic, squamous dermatosis which are pustular, circumscribed and erythematous. Dry scaling patches are common.

psoriatic Person affected with psoriasis.

PSVT Abbreviation for paroxysmal supraventricular tachycardia.

psyche Human faculty for thought, judgment, and emotion

psychiatry Medicine which deals with the study, treatment, and prevention of mental disorders.

psychic Related to mind.

psychoanalysis Method of investigation into the contents of the mind. To study unconscious forces such as repressed impulses, conflicts, childhood trauma etc.,

psychology Science which deals with the mind and mental processes,

Common branches of psychology are Behavioural psychology, Child psychology, Comparative psychology, Criminal psychology, Developmental psychology, Social psychology,

psychopathy antisocial personality disorder.

psychosexual That which is related with emotional aspects sexuality.

psychosis Gross mental impairment with delusion, hallucination, incoherent speech, agitated behaviour.

psychosocial That which is related with psychic as well as social aspects.

psychosomatic It denotes to clinical condition which is related both mind and body.

psychotherapy Method of treatment of mental disorders and behavioral disturbances Common methods of psychotherapy are

- Dynamic psychotherapy
- Stress response syndromes psychotherapy
- Behaviour therapy which can be cognitive or Dialectical
- Anxiety provoking psychotherapy
- Supportive expressive psychotherapy
- Time limited psychotherapy.

psychotic Person exhibiting psychosis.

psychrometer Apparatus for measuring atmospheric humidity by the reading of dry bulb and wet bulb thermometer.

PT Abbreviation for prothrombin time.

pterygium Abnormal triangular fold of membrane, in the interpalpebral fissure, extending from the conjunctiva to the cornea

ptosis Drooping of the upper eyelid from paralysis of the third nerve

ptyalin α-amylase occurring in saliva.

puberty This refers to the period during which the secondary sex characteristics begin to develop and the capability of sexual reproduction is attained.

pubic Related to the pubes,

pudendum Latin word expressing ashamed of and the word mean the external genetalia of woman.

puerperal Related to puerperium.

Pulex Refer to human flea.

pulmonary Related to the lungs.

pulmonology Science that deals with anatomy, physiology, and pathology of the lungs.

pulp Soft animal or vegetable tissue, such as dental pulp or splenic pulp.

pulsation Throb of the heart.

pulse Rhythmic expansion of an artery that is palpable with the finger. Common types of pulse that are clinically important are

- Anacrotic pulse
- Abdominal pulse
- Alternative pulse
- Bounding pulse
- Bigeminal pulse
- Carotid pulse
- Collapsing pulse
- Dicrotic pulse
- Femoral pulse
- Irregular pulse
- Jugular pulse
- Kussmaul's pulse
- Paradoxical pulse
- Radial pulse
- Water hammer pulse

pulverization Reduction to powder.

pump-oxygenator Apparatus, used outside the body that consists of an arterial pump and blood oxygenator plus filters and traps, for saturating blood with oxygen and perfusing the body tissue. This is used for cardiopulmonary bypass surgery.

punctiform That which is located in a point.

punctuation Small points or dots.

punctum Extremely small area or a point of projection.

puncture Act of piercing

pungent Acrid and disagreeable smell.

PUO Abbreviation for **P**yrexia of **U**nknown **O**rigin.

pupa Second stage in the development of an insect

pupillary That which is related with pupil.

pure That which is free from mixture

purgative Other name for cathartic.

purge To clean, To purify, To relieve of faecal matter.

purification the separating of foreign or contaminating elements from a substance of interest.

purine It is a heterocyclic compound chemically represented as $C_5H_4N_4$, Uric acid is a metabolic end product. Purine bases are:

- ✓ Adenine
- ✓ Guanine
- ✓ hypoxanthine
- ✓ xanthine

Purkinje's cells Large neurones in the cerebellar cortex that have piriform cell bodies in the Purkinje layer.

purple It is a color between blue and red.

purpura Ecchymoses or other small hemorrhages in the skin

purulent Containing pus

pus Inflammatory product of leukocytes and a thin protein-rich fluid called liquor puris.

pustular Related with pustule.

pustule Collection of pus beneath the epidermis often in a hair follicle or sweat pore.

putamen Larger, darker and more lateral part of the lentiform nucleus,

putrefaction Decomposition of proteins with the production of foul-smelling compounds like hydrogen sulfide, ammonia, and mercaptans.

PVC Abbreviation for polyvinyl chloride ,Premature ventricular contraction and pulmonary venous congestion.

PVP Abbreviation for polyvinylpyrrolidone.

PVS Abbreviation for persistent vegetative state.

PWA Abbreviation for person with AIDS.

pyelitis Infection and inflammation of the pelvis of the kidney.

pyelocystitis Infection and inflammation of the renal pelvis and of the bladder.

pyelogram Radiograph of the kidney and ureters

pyelography Radiography of the renal pelvis and ureter after the structures have been filled with a contrast solution.

pyelolithotomy Operation of excising a renal calculus from the pelvis of the kidney.

pyelonephritis Infection and inflammation of the kidney and its pelvis because of bacterial infection

pyelonephrosis Disease of the kidney and its pelvis.

pyemia General septicaemia with multiple abscesses.

pyknocyte Distorted and contracted RBC present in haemolytic disorders.

pyknocytosis Increased number of pyknocytes in the blood.

Pyle's disease metaphyseal dysplasia described by Pyle.

pylorus Distal aperture of the stomach surrounded by a strong band of circular muscle,

pyocolpos Collection of pus within the vagina.

pyoderma Purulent skin disease.

pyogenic Producing pus

pyometra Accumulation of pus within the uterus.

pyometritis Infection and purulent inflammation of the uterus.

pyonephritis Purulent inflammation of the kidney.

pyorrhea This is referred to as marginal periodontitis.

pyosalpinx Collection of pus in an oviduct.

pyothorax Other name for empyema

pyramidal That which is shaped like a pyramid.

pyrantel Broad-spectrum anthelmintic effective against pinworms and roundworms

pyrazinamide Anti tubercular drug from nicotinic acid.

pyrethrin Esters, *pyrethrin I* and *pyrethrin II*, found in the flowers of Chrysanthemum (pyrethrum), is an insecticide and topical pediculicide.

pyrexia fever.

pyrogen Fever-producing substance.

pyrogenic That which causes fever.

Q

q This represents Long Arm of Chromosome in Cytology.

q.d. Abbreviation for the prescription writing meaning To Give Every Day

Q fever First identified in Australia in 1935, this is rickettsial infection by Coxiella burnetti which is transmitted as air borne infection and no known vector of transmission is established. This is referred to as Nine Mile fever as a colloquial usage. Usually mild and self limited but can cause complications like pneumonia, hepatitis and endocarditis.

q.h. Abbreviation for the prescription writing meaning To Give Every Hour.

q.i.d. Abbreviation for Quarter In Die meaning To Give Four Times a day.

q.s. Pharmacy prescription abbreviation meaning To Give in Sufficient Quantity.

quack Native Medicine Practitioner who is not qualified but practicing by family tradition. One who practices medicine without proper license.

quadrant In anatomical description it signifies one quarter of a part such as:

- Quadrant in the Field ov Vision
- Quadrant in Abdominal area
- Quadrant on the Tympanic membrane (Ear drum)

quadratus An organ which has four sides or which looks like a square.

quadriceps Thigh muscle which has four heads and is called Quadriceps Muscle.

quadrigeminal That which is related with Corpora Quadrigemina.

quadrilateral Anatomical structure which has four side.

quadriplegia Paralysis of both lower limbs and upper limbs due to trauma, infection Nerve lesions.

quadruplet Four offspring birth at one time which are conceived in one conception. Quadruplet refers to one of these four offspring.

qualitative That which is related with quality of an item such as Qualitative analysis in chemistry.

quantitative That which is related with quantity such as Quantitative Analysisi in chemistry.

quarantine As per International Public Health Measures person who is having some specified infections are not allowed to move freely and are kept isolated under observation for the period of Incubation Period of that infection. This is to avoid spread of infection from one country to another country.

quartan Which repeats once in 3 days such as Quartan Malaria where fever and rigor recurs once in 3 days.

quartile When values are arranged in ascending order or descending order, the values which lies in 25th place, 50th place, 75th place are called Quartile. That which related to every 1/4th value.

quasi Prefix meaning that which resembles such as Quasi-government.

quaternary Chemical that contains four elements such as Quaternary ammonium compound.

Quatrefages' angle Parietal angle described by Quatrefages.

quenching In occupation health quenching refers to rapid chilling of a hot metal by plunging into cold liquid. In coal mine burning coal is brought into cold by quick plunging cold. In Biochemistry it is bringing down fluorescence of a molecule In Radiology quenching the ionizing detector to make it sensitive for operation.

Quick's test Liver Function Test. By administration of Sodium Benzoate excretion of hippuric acid is checked for the estimation of liver function.

quickening During 16th to 18th weeks of pregnancy mother starts feeling the first foetal movement which is called Quickening.

quicklime This refers to Calcium Oxide which antiseptic property.

quinacrine hydrochloride A chemotherapeutic agent used in the treatment of malaria, in Amoebiasis and against intestinal worms.

Quincke's edema This pertains to Angioedema described by Quincke.

quinidine This is derived from Cinchona bark which has the effect in the treatment of malaria and in heart problems.

quinine An Antimalarial drug derived from the alkaloid which is derived from Cinchona bark.

quinoline Alkaloid from Quinine which has the property of antiseptic and anti-fever property.

quinsy Refers to Peritonsillar abscess.

quintuplet Five offspring in a single conception in a pregnancy lady. One of five offspring produced in one gestation period.

quotient The mathematical expression to demarcate ho many times one number is contained in another number. In Medical sciences, various Quotients are known. They are:

- Calorie Quotient
- Intelligence Quotient
- Protein Quotient

R

R_x This is the prescription symbol in Pharmacy or drug prescription.

ρ The symbol for Spearman's correlation coefficient by using this Greek letter.

rabid Animal which is infected with rabies.

rabies Rabies is **a preventable viral disease most often transmitted through the bite of a rabid animal**. The rabies virus infects the central nervous system of mammals, ultimately causing disease in the brain and death.

race This means the genealogic line of descent of people who have a common lineage. This is spoken of as an ethnic group of people in a country or in a geographical area.

racemose That which resembles a bunch of grapes.

rachial This refers to spinal

rachicentesis This is L.P. or Lumbar Puncture.

Rachiopagus Back to back united conjoined twins where union will be at trunk and cervical region.

rachitic That which is related with rickets.

racial Related to one type of race.

rad This is a notation for the words Radiation Absorbed Dose in ionizing radiation. This measures about 100 ergs per gram of any absorbing material in tissues.

radial It is referable to Radius bone which also mean any thing spreading outward from center in upper limb.

radiant Emitted away from centre which is called radiation transmission.

radiate When a thing is arranged in a radiating manner.

radiathermy This refers to Short Wave Diathermy.

radiation Electromagnetic radiation where stream of particles like electrons, neutrons, protons and alpha particles spread in a radiate fashion. Common types are alpha radiation, beta radiation, gamma radiation, X-ray radiation and Ultra violet radiation.

radical Referable to a) Radical treatment b) Acid radical c) Alcohol radical d) Colour radical e) Free radical in its descriptions.

radioactivity When nuclear disintegration occurs electromagnetic radiations are emitted which is one of the natural property of elements.

radiobiology This deals with the effect of light and radiation on living organisms.

radiocarbon Radioactive isotope of carbon like ^{11}C or ^{14}C.

radiodermatitis Skin manifestations due to the exposure to radiations.

radiodiagnosis Radiological diagnosis by X-rays, imaging and radiographs.

radioencephalography This is called REG. By injecting tracers through brain blood vessels, they can studied for pathology.

radiograph This refers to a film produced by radiography.

radiography By passing X-rays and Gamma rays, internal structures of the body can be studied. This is also called roentgenography.

radioimmunoassay A radioimmunoassay (RIA) is an immunoassay that uses radiolabeled molecules in a stepwise formation of immune complexes. A RIA is a very sensitive in vitro assay technique used to measure concentrations of substances, usually measuring antigen concentrations (for example, hormone levels in blood) by use of antibodies.

radioimmunosorbent It is a radio immuno assay to measure Immunoglobulin E in blood sample.

radioiodine Radioactive isotopes of iodine such as ^{131}I, ^{125}I, and ^{123}I

radioisotope Isotopes which emit radiation are used in diagnosis and therapy .

radiologist Specialist and consultant who has specialized in S ray, Ultra sound, CT scan and MRI for the radiological diagnosis of lesions.

radiology Field of speciality that deals with diagnosis and treatment with X-ray, Ultra sound, CT scan, MRI scan.

radiopaque Where X-rays cannot penetrate.

radiophysics Physics that is related to radiology.

radiopraxis Light and electricity are used in disease treatment.

radiotherapy Treatment with radiation called irradiation.

radium Element which has radiant quality in uranium series. It releases radon and emits á particles. From Radium B and C â and ã particles which are used in clinical therapy.

radius Latin word meaning wheel. It is the length of the segment from centre to circumference of a circle.

radix Part by which a structure is anchored. E.g., radix of accessory cranial nerve.

radon Radioactive element which is heavy, colourless and gaseous. Isotopes of this therapy ^{219}Rn and ^{220}Rn.

Radovici's sign Scratching the palm produces twitching of the chin which is also called as Marinescu Radovici reflex.

RAE Abbreviation for **R**ight **A**trial **E**nlargement

Raeder's syndrome Para Trigeminal Syndrome described by Raeder.

raffinose This was called maltose which is a non-reducing trisaccharide present in sugar beets.

rage This is the state of violent anger.

rale Short notice which not continuous heard during inspiration. Common types of rales recorded are:

- Bubbling rale
- Mucous rale
- Tracheal rale
- Vesicular rale
- Crackling rale
- Cavernous rale
- Gurgling rale
- Atelectatic rale
- Amphoric rale

Raman effect Raman's effect is described as under; "When a substance is irradiated with monochromatic light, the spectrum which the substance scatters contains, in addition to a line of the same wavelength as the incident radiation, lines which are satellites of the primary line moving with it when the wavelength of the primary radiation is altered."

RAMC Abbreviation for **R**oyal **A**rmy **M**edical **C**orps.

ramification Set of branches of nerve, a vessel or any other anatomical structure.

Ramon's flocculation test In a series of test tubes containing toxin, antitoxin is added in increasing concentration and the tube in which neutralised mixture of toxin and antitoxin is noticed which is taken as end point.

Ramond's sign This is positive in pleurisy with effusion. The positive sign is rigidity of the erector spinae muscle.

Ramóny Cajal Spanish physician and histologist who won Nobel prize for his work on the discovery of structure, staining and neuronal branches in nervous system in the year 1906.

Ramsay Hunt paralysis This refers to Progressive cerebellar paralysis described by Ramsay Hunt.

Ramsden's eyepiece This is lens containing two plano convex lenses which are put together with their convexities facing each other. This is a positive eye piece.

Ramstedt operation This refers to Pyloromyotomy operation devised by Ramstedt.

rancid This refers to decomposed fatty substances.

Randall's plaques Calcium oxalate crystals deposited in renal papillae which are common urinary salts.

random A thing that can happen according to natural probability distribution such as simple random or stratified random selection process which is called randomisation.

range This is one of the measures of dispersion where the difference between lowest and highest numbers are taken.

ranitidine hydrochloride Drug used in gastric ulcer, duodenal ulcer, gastroesophageal reflux. Mechanism of action is that it antagonises histamine H_2 receptors

rank When sequence of samples are arranged in an ascending order, the position of a value considered becomes it's ranking.

ranula Retention cyst in the floor of the mouth. It is a burrowing mucocele due to obstruction of the ducts of submaxillary glands.

rape Latin word meaning to seize. Sexual intercourse by force or by threat on a woman who has not given consent.

raphe When two symmetrical parts urine, the area of union is called raphe. E.G., Palpebral raphe, Abdominal raphe etc.,

rapport Good relation between doctor and patient, or between 2 persons.

rarefaction Reduction in density and weight but not by volume.

rash Skin eruption due to urticarial, drug or viral infections.

rat Black and white small rats belonging to Rattus rattus and Rattus norvegicus which are responsible for the diseases like Weil's disease and Plague in a community.

rate This describes the change in physical number of occurrence of an event per unit time such as IMR, MME, Death rate or Birth rate.

Rathke's columns This refers to two cartilages at the anterior end of the notochord.

ratio Ratio is the relationship of one quantity to another expressed as the quotient. E.g., Staff population ratio, Albumin Globulin ratio, Body weight ratio etc.,

ration Limited quantity of food in the form of raw material, or bread or drink allowed per person in national emergencies such as World War etc.,

rational Action taken based on a reasonable conclusion.

rationale Latin word meaning logical basis of a procedure.

rationalization If a person justifies without reasoning that normally is not acceptable in society or community

Rauwolfia enus of tropical shrubs which provide alkaloids of medical importance like reserpine, called Rauwolfia serpentine

Ray General term to denote radiant energy such as á rays, â rays, ã rays, Cosmic rays, X-rays, Ultra violet rays etc.,

Raymond's apoplexy a type of stroke where paraesthesia of hand occurs and is followed by paralysis of that part.

Raynaud's disease It is gangrene occurring which is a idiopathic vascular disorder manifested by bilateral attacks of ischaemia.

RBC Abbreviation for **R**ed **B**lood **C**orpuscle.

RCA Abbreviation for **R**esearch **C**um **A**ction type of Latrine.

RDA Abbreviation for **R**ecommended **D**ietary **A**llowance.

Re Latin prefix meaning once again.

reabsorption Selective absorption of glucose, protein or sodium by kidney

react Refers to chemical reaction. Other meaning is response to a stimulus.

reaction It is a chemical process showing counter action in chemicals.

reagent A chemical which detect a reaction, which measure a chemical reaction or which produce a chemical reaction.

reagin It is an antibody that mediates type I hypersensitivity reaction. It denotes the outcome of Wassermann test.

Réaumur's scale It is the temperature scale from 0 to 80 degree Reaumurs, where 0 is ice temperature and 80 is boiling temperature expressed in Reaumur scale. as degree Reaumur.

rebound This is a reversed response on the withdrawal of a stimulus

recalcification Correction and returning to normalcy of calcium content of bone and other tissues.

recall It is the process of recollection. Getting back events to consciousness.

recanalization In case of vessels which are obstructed, new path is formed for the blood flow.

receptor That which binds with a specific substance such as nuclear receptors, membrane receptors, chemoreceptors, photoreceptors etc.,

recess A hollow space in the body where specific anatomical structure is not found. E.g., Anterior recess of tympanic membrance, Infundibular recess.

recession Organ or tissue drawn back from it's normal place.

recessive A genetic term denoting the non possibility of expression of characteristics.

recipe Written at the top of a physician's prescription and indicated by the symbol [rx].

recipient Person who receives blood in transfusion or a tissue or an organ graft.

recirculation Venous blood is allowed to circulate in arterial to reduce gradient concentrations across the dialyser membrane in Haemodialysis.

Recklinghausen's disease This refers to Neuro-fibromatosis described by Recklinghausen.

recombinant A cell with a new combination of genes not found together in either of its parent

reconstruction Re doing the job of construction in surgery to restore physiological function as in the case of By pass heart surgery.

record Device either mechanical or electronic to keep the data or material permanently to view whenever needed.

recrudescence Recurrence of symptoms in a disease.

recrudescent To occur as a fresh event which is referred to a disease.

rectoscope The other name for Proctoscope.

rectovaginal That which is related to rectum and vagina such as Rectovaginal fistula.

rectum This is the continuation of Sigmoid colon upto the anal canal. Rectum starts from just anterior to third sacral vertebra as the distal portion of large intestine.

recumbent This is the posture of lying down.

recuperation This refers to Recovery of health and physical strength.

recurrence It is called relapse or re appearance of an attack of illness. E.g., recurrence of typhoid.

recurrent It is repeated occurrence of an episode of illness called frequent relapse of disease.

red One of the primary colours Common chemical available are:

1. Basic red
2. Aniline red
3. Bromophenol red
4. Cresol red
5. Congo red
6. Neutral red
7. Methyl red
8. Sudan red

reduce Refers to reduction of the fracture, to reduction in chemical reaction, to restore to its normal place, to get reduced to original weight.

reducible Capable of being reduced referable to hernia.

reductase They are enzymes of the oxidoreductase group which is responsible for reduction of metabolite in the body.

reduction Referred to the reduction of weight, to the reduction of fracture, to the addition of H ion in chemistry.

Reed's cells Their presence indicate the presence of Hodgkin's disease. On microscope examination it is giant histiocytic cells, multinucleate.

reef Infolding of tissue

Rees' test The test for the detection for albumin. To the test sample, solution of tannic acid in alcoholic solution produces precipitates.

reflection Latin word meaning bending back. Ray reflection, Heat reflection, etc.,

reflex This is a reflected movement when a jerk is given on the muscle or tendon. E.g., are Accommodation reflex, Abdominal reflex, Plantar reflex etc.,

reflux This refers to return flow such as Hepatojugular reflux, Venous reflux etc.,

refraction Determination of refractive error of the eyes. Done for the giving of glass correction.

refractionist A trained person to give correction for refractive errors.

refrigeration Other name for cooling by using refrigerator.

regeneration Renewal of tissue after a tissue loss.

regimen To obtain good healing or cure of disease, regulated scheme of diet, of exercise, etc., are given to patient.

region An anatomical area which has boundaries, used for anatomical descriptions. E.G., are Anal region, Abdominal region, Axillary region etc.,

registrar A resident specialist who acts as assistant to the specialist.

regression Any thing that returns to its original or normal position or state.

Common terms in use are:

- Logistic regression
- Linear regression
- Multiple regression

regurgitant To flow back in the opposite direction such as Aortic regurgitation, Pulmonary regurgitation etc.,

rehabilitation This is tertiary level of prevention where restoration of normal form and function is tried for restoration

rehydration To give I V or Oral replacement of fluid in case dehydration.

reimplantation Re fixing of a structure in the site from where it is lost.

reinfection Getting the same type of infection second time in an organ or in an area.

Reissner's fiber These fibres are present in smallest bronchi.

Reiter's syndrome This seems to be an abnormal immune response of the body which is manifested by a) urethritis b) conjunctivitis and c) arthritis.

rejection Body when rejects the graft due to an immune response

rejuvenescence Renewed strength in a person.

relapse Return of a disease after its apparent cessation.

relation Anatomical relationship. It also means the state of one in comparison with another.

relaxant Drug that cause relaxation by reducing tension.

relief This refers to relief from pain, relief from pressure,

REM Abbreviation for **R**apid **E**ye **M**ovements

rem (rem) The device of potential danger to health that is equivalent to Rad + Factor of potential danger. It is also calculated by the following formula;

1 rem = 1 rad x RBE (Relative Biological Effectiveness)

Remak's ganglion It is S.A. ganglion in the heart wall which is a sympathetic ganglion near superior vena cava.

remedy Drug or the substance that help in curing preventing disease.
remission Reduction in the intensity of illness called abatement of disease.
remnant A vestigial organ or tissue which is a residue of the development process.
Rendu-Osler-Weber syndrome This refers to Hereditary Haemorrhagic Telangiectasia.
renin Enzyme that is responsible in the conversion of Angiotensinogen to Angiotensin I. This enzyme is synthesised in kidney (as protein) which is released to blood by various body stimuli. This is different from Rennin which chymosin.
renography Radiography of the kidney.
Reoviridae RNA virus which is transmitted through night soil, through fomites and through arthropods. Common viruses are Rotavirus, Orthoreovirus, Orbivirus, Coltivirus and Aquareovirus.
repair Restoration of damaged tissues by the growth of healthy new cells
repellent Chemical agent or organic agent which makes insects fly away from its source such as mosquito repellent.
repercussion When inflammatory swelling gets distorted, when skin eruption gets driven in. This also denotes ballottement.
replication This is the production of an exact copy of an item e.g., replication of DNA OR RNA.
repolarization This refers to Polarity establishment.
reproduction Production of offspring by organism
RES Abbreviation for **R**eticulo **E**ndothelial **S**ystem
resect to remove part or all of an organ or tissue.
reserpine Alkaloid isolated from the root of Rauwolfia serpentine.
reserve To keep some without using for future use. Cardiac reserve and alkali reserve are common examples in physiological process.
reservoir A place for keeping alive of organisms. This is referable to reservoir of infection.
reshaping Restoration of shape
resident a Medical graduate receiving training in a hospital.
residual Remaining after its use such as residual chlorine in water.
resin Exudation of trees or a synthetic resin which contains carboxylic acids, terpenes..
resolution When an inflammation or an infection resolute or subsides.
resonant On percussion we hear a vibrant sound.
respiration This physiological process involves inspiration and expiration where exchange of oxygen takes place in the lung which is called ventilation . This is a necessity for life. Types of respirations are:

- Thoracic respiration
- Abdominal respiration
- Thoracoabdominal respiration
- Artificial respiration
- Cheyne Stokes respiration
- Cogwheel respiration
- Kussmaul's respiration
- Paradoxical respiration
- Tissue respiration or internal respiration.

response Reaction to a stimulus.
rest Taking to the position of ease after an exertion.
restoration Anatomical and physiological reconstruction of tissue or organ. The process can be surgical restoration or prosthetic restoration.
resuscitation This is the process of restoration to life or restoration to consciousness. This can mean cardiac resuscitation, respiratory resuscitation or other conditions like anoxia, hypothermia, electrocution.
retardation This can mean physical growth delay or mental growth delay. Intra uterine growth retardation is common term used in day to day practice.
retching This is physiological or pathological process of an effort for vomiting.
retention To keep or to possess or to hold in position such as urinary retention, denture retention etc.,
reticular That which relates to a network .
reticulocytosis Increase in the number of reticulocytes in the peripheral blood.
reticuloendothelial Tissues which have both reticular and endothelial attributes. The System is called R.E. system. .
reticulum This refers to protoplasmic network in a cell.
retina The innermost layer of the eyeball which surrounds the vitreous body and continuous with optic nerve. The main parts have been Pars optica, Pars ciliaris and Pars iridica. The Pars optica has two main parts called pigmentary part and nervous part. The nervous part has following nine parts:

1. Internal limiting membrane
2. Nerve fibre layer
3. Ganglion cell layer
4. Inner plexiform layer
5. Inner nuclear layer
6. Outer plexiform layer
7. Outer nuclear layer
8. External limiting membrane
9. Rods and cones layer which responds to photochemical reaction.

retinaculum This anatomical structure retains a tissue or an organ in its place.
retinal That which is related with retina. This also refers to retinol derived from carotenoids in food which has vitamin A activity.

retinitis Infection and inflammation of the retina which can be any one of the following types:
- o Diabetic retinitis
- o Actinic retinitis
- o Cytomegalovirus retinitis
- o Syphilitic retinitis
- o Retinitis pigmentosa
- o Solar retinitis
- o Suppurative retinitis

retinoblastoma Cancerous growth from retinoblast which is called retinal glioma.

retinol It is the form of vitamin A from dietary sources .

retraction Any tissue or organ which is brought back .

retrobulbar Position indicating posterior to the eyeball.

retroflexion Refers to posterior bending of uterus called retroflexion of uterus.

retrograde Moving in opposite direction than its normal direction.

retroinfection Infection of the mother by the foetus.

retroperitoneal Posterior to the Peritoneum.

retropharyngeal Posterior to pharynx.

retroversion Backward bend of uterus in relation to pelvis.

retrovesical Posterior to the urinary bladder.

Retrovir Commercial preparation of Zidovudine drug which is used in the treatment of HIV/AIDS.

Retroviridae It is RNA viruses called retroviruses. They contain major polypeptide reverse transcriptase. Main public health problem from this virus is HIV/AIDS.

Rett syndrome A developmental disorder in females which is called cerebral atrophic Hyperammonemia. Grey matter of the brain is involved producing pathology. Common manifestations are:
- Ataxia
- Dementia
- Seizures
- Loss of purposeful use hands
- Hyperammonemia
- Autistic behaviour

Retzius' fibers Hard fibres made of Deiter's cells in the organ of Corti.

Reuss' colour charts This is used in testing colour vision where colour charts are used which are printed in colour letters that will have a colour background.

revaccination Vaccination on second time to a person.

revascularization After By pass blood supply restored. In wound healing re blood supply to the area.

Reverdin's graft This refers to Epidermal graft described by Reverdin.

Reye's syndrome As sequel of viral infections distinctive changes in liver and viscera produces fatal outcome in children

RF Abbreviation for **R**heumatoid **F**actor.

Rh antibody *Rhesus* monkeys, whose blood was found to contain the factor discovered in 1940. They are antibodies against human RBCs. Normally they are not ato be seen but are produced when Rh negative persons receive Rh positive blood. Pregnant woman who is Rh negative who has foetus which is Rh positive

rhabdomyoma Striated muscle which is benign tumour.

rhabdomyosarcoma Striated muscle which is malignant tumour

Rhabdoviridae RNA viruses having a bullet shape in which Lyssavirus and Vesiculovirus are prominent.

Rhazes Persian physician known for his medical treatment. His writing on medicine and surgery are complied by his pupils.

rheostat Instrument used to control the current entering a circuit.

rhesus Referred to Rhesus monkey and Rh factor.

rheumatism Inflammation, degeneration and metabolic derangement of connective tissues, joints and related structures.

rheumatologist Specialist who treats rheumatic conditions.

rheumatology This is the branch of medicine dealing with rheumatic disorders, their causes, pathology, diagnosis, treatment, etc.

rhinitis Infection and inflammation of the mucous membrane of the nose. Common clinical entities are:
- Allergic rhinitis
- Atrophic rhinitis
- Dry rhinitis
- Tubercular rhinitis

rhinophyma Thick lobulated overgrowth of sebaceous glands and epithelial connective in lower half of nose.

rhinoplasty Plastic surgery of nose for therapy and cosmetic purpose. Known types are Indian rhinoplasty, English rhinoplasty and Italian rhinolplasty.

rhinosporidiosis Fungal infection of the nose by Rhinosporidium seeberi.

Rhinovirus Virus belonging to Picornaviridae that cause U R I and common cold.

Rhizopoda They are protozoa comprising of amoebae.

rho [ρ] Greek alphabet that represent the Spearman's Rank Correlation coefficient.

rhodopsin It is Chromoprotein in rods of retina which act on the stimulation of retinal sensory endings.

rhomboid having a shape similar to a rectangle that has been skewed to one side so that the angles are oblique.

rhonchus Low pitched snore like sound which is continuous heart on auscultation on throat, bronchial tube.

rhythm To occur in regular interval such as circadian rhythm, ventricular rhythm, Atrioventricular rhythm, Sinus rhythm etc.,

RIA Abbreviation for **R**adio **I**mmuno **A**ssay

rib Bone of thoracic cage which are called costa. Common terms that are in use are:
- ❖ Cervical rib
- ❖ Thoracic rib
- ❖ Abdominal rib
- ❖ Floating rib
- ❖ False rib
- ❖ True rib

ribavirin Anti viral preparation used in the treatment of respiratory syncytial viral infection (severe pneumonia).

Ribbert's theory This theory of Ribbert postulates that because of reduced tension in the surrounding tissues a tumour can develop in the area of that tissue.

riboflavin Water soluble vitamin B_2 which is present in milk, meat, egg, green leafy vegetables.

ribonuclease This enzyme is catalyser in ester linkages in ribonucleic acids.

ribonucleic acid RNA commonly called is responsible for the flow of genetic information in the living body.

ribose Pentose sugar found in riboflavin and ribonucleic acid

ribosome It is found at the site of protein synthesis . Usually it is ribosomal RNA product.

rice One of the seed grain which contains main starch.

Richards American physician who won Nobel prize for medicine for his discovery of cardiac catheterisation.

Richet French physiologist winner of the Nobel Prize for medicine in 1913 for his research on anaphylaxis.

Richet's aneurysm This refers to a fusiform aneurysm described by Richet.

rickets Vitamin D deficiency in children causing interruption in development and mineralisation of bone.

Rickettsia Small rod shaped or coccoid pleomorphic microorganisms that produce typhus fevers. Common pathogens are a) R.burnette, b) R. akamushi c) R. mooseri d) R. prowazekii e) R. tsutsugamushi

Rickettsiaceae Family of bacteria of the order Rickettsiales. The tribe of this family is called Rickettsieae.

Rideal-Walker coefficient It is called Phenol coefficient. It is the measure of bactericidal activity of a chemical. This is found out by:

$$\text{R.W. coefficient} = \frac{\text{Concentration of test chemical at which is kills the test bacteria in 10 min.}}{\text{Concentration of phenol that kills the organism under the same conditions}}$$

ridge This refers to a projecting structure called crista. Usual terms in clinical practice are:
- ➢ Bony ridge of maxilla
- ➢ Bicipital ridge
- ➢ Deltoid ridge
- ➢ Dental ridge
- ➢ Dermal ridge
- ➢ Epicondylar ridge
- ➢ Mammary ridge

Riegel's pulse The pulse that diminishes in size during exhalation.

Rieux's hernia This is referred to Retrocecal hernia described by Rieux.

rifampicin Rifamycin group of antibiotics .

rifamycin Antibiotics biosynthesized by a strain of Streptomyces mediterranei used in the treatment of tuberculosis.

rigidity Stiffness of muscle in disease and after death. Common terms in use in clinical practice are;
- ✓ Cog wheel rigidity
- ✓ Cadaveric or post mortem rigidity
- ✓ Catatonic rigidity
- ✓ Decorticate rigidity
- ✓ Hemiplegic rigidity
- ✓ Lead pipe rigidity
- ✓ Clasp knife rigidity

rigor Latin word meaning chills in certain infections or as body reactions. Other varieties are due to acid, calcium excess, heat, depletion of ATP in dead muscle and water.

rim Edge of an anatomical structure.

rimantadine hydrochloride Antiviral agent used in the prophylaxis of influenza type A.

rimose Cracks and fissures.

ringworm The fungal infection which is manifested in the form of ring lesion. Tinea in man and dermatophytosis in animals are common.

Rinne's test Hearing test done with the help of tuning fork. Three frequency of tuning form used are 256 Hz, 512 Hz and 1024 Kz. The stem of vibrating tuning form is placed on mastoid process and later 1 cm from external ear till the noise or vibration is no longer heard. It is inferred as under:
- Rinne positive: When air conduction is greater than bone conduction it is positive and infers that it is normal hearing.
- Rinne negative: When bone conduction is greater than air conduction it is negative and infer that it is conductive deafness.

Risk French word denoting the danger or hazard existing such as Diabetic risk, Cardiovascular risk etc., In Epidemiological approach we used Relative risk and Attributable risk

risus Latin word meaning laughter seen in Tetanus infection called risus sardonicus.

Ritgen maneuver In this maneuver the foetal head is delivered by extending the head upward and forward through vulva in between contractions, by pressing the perineum behind anus.

ritonavir Drug used in HIV/AIDS. It is a protease inhibitor active against the Human Immunodeficiency Virus.

Ritter's disease This is referred to Staphylococcal scalded skin syndrome described by Ritter.

Rivinus' ducts The ducts of Rivinus, **a group of excretory ducts**, drain the sublingual gland. The largest sublingual gland excretory duct called the sublingual duct of Bartholin joins Wharton's duct near the sublingual caruncle.

riziform That which resembles the grain of rice.

RLF Abreviation for **R**etro **L**ental **F**ibroplasia

RMA Abbreviation for **R**ight **M**ento **A**nterior the position of the foetus.

RNA Abbreviation for **R**ibo **N**ucleic **A**cid.

RNA polymerase Enzyme that catalyses RNA chain.

ROA Abbreviation for **R**ight **O**cciput **A**nterior the position of foetus.

Robbins American paediatrician, won Nobel prize in medicine for 1954 for the discovery that poliomyelitis viruses can be grown in tissue culture and thereby be isolated and studied, making possible the production of vaccines.

Robert's ligament Posterior femoral ligament described by Robert.

Roberts American biochemist won Nobel prize for medicine in 1993 for his discoveries about the structure of genes and the transmission of genetic information.

Robison ester This refers to Glucose 6 Phosphate discovered by Robison.

rodenticide Poisons used to kill rats and other rodents. Common ones are Zinc oxide, Warfarin.

roentgen dissemination of ion emission per 0.001293 gram of dry air

roentgen rays X-rays discovered by Roentgen.

Roger's reflex This refers to Esophagus salivary Reflex described by Roger.

Role Behaviour pattern of an individual which is presented to others.

Roller's nucleus This refers to Sublingual nucleus described by Roller.

roller Refers to Cotton roll (rolled cotton) a small cylinder of rolled cotton,

Romanovsky's Stain used for blood smear staining and for Malaria smear staining.

rongeur Instrument for cutting tough tissue, particularly bone.

Röntgen German physicist won Nobel Prize for his discovery of X-rays in 1895, while experimenting with a cathode ray tube, he received the first Nobel prize for physics in 1901.

rooming-in Keeping a newly born infant in a crib near the mother's bed,

rootlet Small root or root like structure

ROP Abbreviation for **R**ight **O**cciput **P**osterior position of the foetus.

Rose's position This position is used on patients in whom blood swallowing is to be prevented and who has sustained injury. Supine and head hanging over the end of the table in full extension.

Rosenbach's sign It is positive in inflammatory diseases of the intestine where abdominal skin reflex is absent.

Rosenthal's test Test for the blood in urine. It demonstrates hemin crystals.

Rosenthal's vein This refers to Basal vein described by Rosenthal.

Roseolovirus Herpes group of viruses.

rosette Rose like anatomical structure. This is seen in symmetrical segmenter stage of Plasmodium malariae.

Ross British physician and protozoologist who won Nobel prize for medicine in 1902 for his demonstration of the life history of the malarial parasite Plasmodium in the stomach of the Anopheles mosquito and its transmission by the bite of the female anopheline mosquito.

Rossbach's disease This refers to Hyperchlorhydria described by Rossbach.

rostellum Fleshy protuberance of scolex of tapeworm.

ROT Abbreviation for **R**ight **O**ccipito **T**ransverse position of the foetus.

rotation This is turning round an axis. It can be foetal rotation.

Rotavirus They are wheel like shaped viruses which produce infantile G E and diarrhoea.

roughage High fibre diet containing fibers, cellulose etc.,

Rougnon-Heberden disease This refers to Angina Pectoris or chest pain a symptom of ischaemic heart disease, by Rougnon and Heberden.

rouleaux are stacks or aggregations of red blood cells (RBCs) that form because of the unique discoid shape of the cells in vertebrates.

RPF Abbreviation for **R**enal **P**lasma **F**low.

rpm Abbreviation for **R**evolutions **P**er **M**inute.

RQ Abbreviation for **R**espiratory **Q**uotient.

rRNA Abbreviation for **R**ibosomal **RNA**.

rub Movement on a smooth surface with friction such as pericardial rub or pleural rub.

rubefacient Passive Hyperaemia by subbing a substance on the skin.

rubella Acute infectious disease by toga virus in children characterised by red skin rash called German measles.

rubeola Acute viral infection called Measles.

Rud's syndrome Congenital syndrome which is manifested with

- Ichthyosis

- Mental retardation or deficiency
- Epilepsy
- Infantilism

rudiment If a structure remains undeveloped it becomes rudiment.

rugosity Many folds or wrinkles present.

rump Colloquial word for the buttock.

rupture Forcible tearing of tissue or organ.

Russell's bodies They are seen in cancer cells and chronic inflammation cells. They are globular plasma cell inclusions.

RV Abbreviation for **R**esidual **V**olume.

Rye classification The classification of Hodgkin disease and is based on histopathological classification. They are:

- o Lymphocyte predominance type
- o Mixed cellularity type
- o Lymphocyte depletion type
- o Nodular sclerosis type

Ryle's tube This is used in Test meal which is made of a thin rubber tube with an olive shaped end.

S

S_1 S_2 S_3 S_4 Symbol refer to heart sounds I, II , III and IV respectively.

σ Greek word symbol for S.D.

SA Abbreviation for Sino Atrial.

Sabin's vaccine This refers to Live Oral Polio vaccine, popularly called OPV.

saccharic acid This is dicarboxylic sugar acid.

saccharide They are sugars and depending upon number of saccharide group ($C_nH_{2n}O_{n-1}$) we have Mono, Di and Poly saccharides.

saccharin A sweetening agent which is hundreds of time sweeter than sucrose. They are available as salt of saccharin either by calcium or sodium.

saccular That which is shaped like a sac.

sacculated Organ with the presence of saccules.

Sachs' disease It is a ganglioside storage disease among infants or children. This is characterized by

- Doll face
- Early blindness,
- Macrocephaly,
- Seizures,
- Hypotonia

sacral That which is related with sacrum

sacralgia Pain in the sacrum.

sacralization Fusion of the fifth lumbar vertebra to the first segment of the sacrum and thus sacrum consists of six segments.

sacrococcygeal Located in the region of the sacrum and coccyx.

sacrum Triangular bone just below the lumbar vertebrae

sadism Gaining pleasure from inflicting physical or psychological pain on another

sadistic Characterized by sadism.

safranin O Basic red aniline dye for nuclear stain and as a counterstain in Gram's stain.

sagittal That which resembles an arrow. This refers to anteroposterior plane of the body.

Sahli's method Common method of estimating Hb% called Acid Haematin Method. By adding HCl, haemoglobin is converted into acid haematin and colour developed is compared to a standard colour scale.

Saint's triad Three conditions seen simultaneously in a patient. They are:

- o Hiatus hernia
- o Colonic diverticula
- o Cholelithiasis

sal Latin word meaning salt.

salicylic acid It is ortho hydroxybenzoic acid obtained from wintergreen leaves. It has the property of anti bacterial, antifungal and keratolytic.

saline That which is the nature of a salt.

saliva Clear, alkaline, viscid secretion from the parotid, submaxillary, sublingual, and smaller mucous glands of the mouth.

salivary Pertaining to the saliva.

Salk vaccine Injectable vaccine for the prevention of poliomyelitis.

Salmonella Gram-negative, facultatively anaerobic bacteria of the family Enterobacteriaceae usually motile with peritrichous flagella. They ferment glucose but not sucrose or lactose. S. typhi, S. paratyphi and S. enteritidis cause enteric fevers namely typhoid and paratyphoid. Salmonella can cause food poisoning.

salmonellosis Disease caused by infection with a species of Salmonella which cause G.E., typhoid and paratyphoid.

salpingitis Infection and inflammation of the uterine tube.

salpingo-oophorectomy Uterine tube and ovary are removed by operation.

salt This refers to sodium chloride or common salt.

salubrious Conducive to health

salvage Treatment undertaken late in the treatment process after other measures have failed.

sample Representative part taken to typify the whole population or a universe in studies and research. Simple random sample, stratified sample, multistage sample are common types of samples.

sampling Selection of a sample.

sanatorium Older term for open air treatment of TB patients. Sanare from Latin means to cure the sick in an establishment.

Sanders' disease This refers to Epidemic Kerato Conjunctivitis described by Sanders.

sandfly Fly of genus Phlebotomus which transmits sand fly fever.

sane Latin word meaning healthy mind. Opposite of insane.

Sanger English biochemist, born 1918; winner of the Nobel prize for chemistry in 1958 for his discovery of amino acids order identification in insulin.

sanitary Clean environment that is required for good health.

sanitation Establishment of environmental conditions favorable to health.

Sansom's sign This is positive in pericardial effusion. It is marked by increase of the are of dullness in the second and third intercostals spaces.

saponification Chemical process of converting fats into soaps and glycerol by heating with alkalis.

sarcoidosis Occurrence of hard tubercle in skin, lungs, lymph nodes, liver, spleen, eyes and bones which is a chronic, progressive, systemic granulomatous reticulosis of unknown etiology

sarcolemma Delicate plasma membrane which covers all striated muscle fiber.

sarcoma Malignant tumours from connective tissue. Depending upon involvement of tissues they can be;

- ❖ Lymphosarcoma
- ❖ Chondrosarcoma
- ❖ Fibrosarcoma
- ❖ Osteosarcoma
- ❖ Myxosarcoma
- ❖ Rhabdomyosarcoma

sarcomere Contractile unit of myofibrils

sarcoplasm Interfibrillary matter of the striated muscles

Sarcoptes Itch mite that causes scabies.

sarcosis Abnormal increase of flesh.

sardonic Involuntary smile produced in spasmodic contraction of facial muscles. It is common in Tetanus. Root of the word is from Greek which mean facial distortion by eating poisonous Sardinian herb.

sarsaparilla It contains sarsasapogenin which is used as flavouring agent in beverages.

satellite Latin word meaning companion which refers to smaller body that is under influence of a larger body.

satiety Full gratification of appetite

saturated If a solution contains very much solute it is called saturated. If a chemical compound is satisfied with all chemical affinities it is called saturated.

saturation Condition of being saturated.

saucer A round plate with shallow depression.

saucerization Shallow shelving is produced to facilitate drainage from infected area.

Saunders' disease Digestive disturbances in infants with the following manifestations:

- ▪ Vomiting
- ▪ Cerebral symptoms
- ▪ Circulatory failure.

saw Cutting instrument with serrated edge. Common surgical saw in use are:

- ❖ For trephining crown saw is used
- ❖ For amputation, amputation saw is used
- ❖ For enlarging orifices in bone, Hey's saw is used

SBE Abbreviation for **S**ub acute **B**acterial **E**ndocarditis.

scab Crust formed on the surface of a wound.

scabicide Drugs used in killing scabies mite.

scabies A contagious skin infection by Sarcoptes scabiei associated with eczema and associated bacterial infection.

scalar Latin word pertaining to a ladder which is denoted in different cadre system in administration.

scald Burns caused by hot liquid

scale A device by which some property may be measured For example linear surface in inches or centimeters.

scale This refers to any of the following

- ✓ A plate of bone
- ✓ Piece of enamel
- ✓ Scale of epidermis
- ✓ A fragment of tartar of tooth
- ✓ Calcareous deposts of teeth gingival margin

scalene Refers to muscle which is uneven in shape.

scaling It is dental scaling where plaque are removed from surface of tooth.

scalp Skin of head excluding face and ears which is covered with hair.

scalpel (skal'p[schwa]l) Surgical knife with a straight handle and blade.

scan Refer to organ scan such as brain scan, kidney scan, thyroid scan etc., With the help of sensing device information on an organ is obtained.

- – On cathode display the scan is called A scan.
- – On cathode display two dimensional display is called B scan.
- – Computerized Axial Tomography is called CT scan
- – Gastric mucosa demonstration is called Meckel scan.
- – For mono dimentional section of heart it is called M mode scan
- – Inhalation of radionuclide and imaging of perfusion of lung is called V.Q. Scan

scanner Equipment used for scanning. The act of examining with a sensing device is called scanning.

Scanzoni's maneuver An obstetrical maneuver with forceps by rotating foetal head when it is in the posterior position of the occiput.

scaphoid Boat shaped bone in proximal row of carpal bones.

scapula Flat, triangular bone in the back of the shoulder

scar Wound caused by burning

scarification In early decades superficial scratches for introducing smallpox vaccine was called scarification. Now that smallpox is eradicated, the term is not in use.

scarlatina Other name for Scarlet Fever.

Scarpa's fascia Subcutaneous membranous abdominal stratum described by Scarpa.

SCAT Abbreviation for **S**heep **C**ell **A**gglutination **T**est.

scatter Change in momentum of radiation particles

Schafer's method Artificial Respiration method described by Schafer.

Schäffer's reflex It is positive in organic Hemiplegia. On pinching the Achilles tendon at its middle third produces dorsiflexion of the great toe.

schedule Other name for time table or a formal list or a plan of procedure

schematic Diagram or model.

Schick's sign Diphtheria toxin intra dermal test with control. Positive, negative and pseudo reactions are observed. Area of redness appearing in 24 hours at test site and persists for 5 days which leave an area of brownish pigmentation. .

Schilling test Diagnostic test for pernicious anaemia and disorders of vitamin B_{12} metabolism. Oral administration of radioactive cyanocobalamin, parenteral non radioactive vitamin and later determination of radioactivity in the urine are the procedure in Schilling test.

Schistosoma Blood flukes from the genus of trematodes of the family Schistosomatidae. Common species are:

- Schistosoma haematobium
- Schistosoma japonicum
- Schistosoma mansoni.

schizogony Asexual reproduction characteristic of sporozoa in which daughter cells are produced by multiple fission of the nucleus of the parasite

schizont Multinucleate stage in the development of sporozoa during schizogony.

schizophrenia Mental disorder comprising psychotic disorders and characterized by disturbances in form and content of thought, particularly delusions and hallucinations

schizophrenic Person affected with schizophrenia.

Schönlein's purpura This refers to Rheumatic purpura descried by Schonlein.

Schuchardt's incision This refers to Para Vaginal incision described by Schuchardt.

Schüffner's dots They are characteristics of plasmodium vivax infection with the presence of minute granules in RBC which are infected and are demonstrable with romanowsky stain.

Schwann's cell Large nucleated cell which enwraps the axons of myelinated peripheral neurons. They are the source of myelin.

schwannoma Neoplasm originating from Schwann cells of the myelin sheath of neurons. Acoustic schwannoma is common clinical entity.

sciatica Protrusion of lumbar intervertebral disc produces pain radiating from the back into the buttock and into the lower extremity along its posterior or lateral aspect

science Knowledge accumulated by the systematic observation of natural phenomena. Basic science, applied science, behavioral science, pure science are notable terminologies

scientist Learned scholar in science.

scintillation Emission of sparks or emission of particle in the disintegration of a radioactive element.

scirrhous Means Scirrhous carcinoma or hard cancer.

scissors Surgical cutting instrument with two opposed shearing blades such as canalicular scissors, cannula scissors, craniotomy scissors, Fox scissors, Liston's scissors, Smellie scissors etc.,

sclera Tough white outer coat of the eyeball continues anteriorly with cornea and continues posteriorly with external sheath of optic nerve.

scleredema Face, head and neck pathology manifested as diffuse, symmetrical, wooden-like, nonpitting induration of the skin. Cause is not known.

scleritis Infection and inflammation of sclera.

scleroderma Chronic hardening and thickening of the skin,

sclerokeratitis Infection and inflammation of the sclera and of the cornea.

sclerosis an induration or hardening, such as hardening of a part from inflammation, increased formation of connective tissue, or disease of the interstitial substance. Common types of sclerosis are:

- Arterial sclerosis
- Amyotrophic lateral sclerosis
- Disseminated sclerosis
- Multiple sclerosis
- Progressive systemic sclerosis
- Systemic sclerosis

sclerotome Instrument used in the incision of the sclera.

sclerotomy Incision of the sclera.

scolex Anterior end of tapeworm.

scoliokyphosis Combined lateral curvature and posterior curvature of the spine.

scoliosis Lateral deviation in the vertical line of the spine.

scoop Instrument for evacuating cavities.

scopolamine Anticholinergic alkaloid from Atropa belladonna. It's action is called atropine action.

score Numerical rating according to degree of quality or condition.

- Condition of newborn assessed by Apgar score
- Prospects of induction of labour in primi assessed by Bishop score
- Severity of illness assessed by APACHE score

- Clinical state of stroke patient assessed by stroke score

scotoma An area of no vision surrounded by area of normal vision. Common types are:
- ✓ Annular scotoma
- ✓ Absolute scotoma
- ✓ Central scotoma
- ✓ Hemianopic scotoma
- ✓ Peripheral scotoma
- ✓ Physiological scotoma
- ✓ Positive scotoma
- ✓ Ring scotoma

scratch To scrape a surface lightly with the nails or with a sharp instrument to relieve itching.

screen Curtain or partition for patient examination. A barrier for protection against radiation exposure.

screening Examination or testing of a group of individuals to identify apparently health and sick for the required measure.

screw Cylinder with a helical thread to hold two objects together.

scrofuloderma Skin tuberculosis.

scrotum Pouch which contains the testes in males.

scurvy Clinical condition with deficiency of ascorbic acid or vitamin C

scutellum Chitinous plates making up the dorsum of the thorax of an insect.

scutum Hard chitinous plate on the anterior portion of the dorsal surface of Hard Ticks.

SD Abbreviation for **S**tandard **D**eviation.

SE Abbreviation for **S**tandard **E**rror.

sealant Protects against access from the outside or leakage from the inside

sebaceous Pertaining to sebum.

seborrhea Excessive secretion of sebum

sebum Secretion of the sebaceous glands composed of fat and epithelial debris from the cells of the malpighian layer.

secondary Second in line such as secondary prevention.

secretin It stimulates the secretion of pancreatic juice. Secretin is secreted by by the mucosa of the duodenum and upper jejunum

secretion Product produced as a result of activity of a gland.

secretomotor Nerves that is responsible for exciting or stimulating secretion .

section Latin word meaning to cut such as cesarean section, abdominal section, coronal section, frozen section, paraffin section, sagittal section etc.,

sectorial That which is related with sector.

sedation Medical method of producing calmness.

sedative Agent that takes away excitement. Depending on the site of action they are gastric sedative, intestinal sedative, cardiac sedative, nerve trunk sedative, cerebral sedative, spinal sedative, vascular sedative or respiratory sedative.

sedentary Simply becoming inactive and not involving in any activity.

sediment Deposit of solid matter in the liquid. E.g., urinary sediment.

sedimentation With the help of centrifuge, deposits of sediment is made to settle down the liquid.

segment Portion of a structure which may have a natural or artificial boundary. In anatomical descriptions, we have superior segment, inferior segment, anterior segment, posterior segment, apical segment, basal segment, bronchopulmonary segment, cranial segment, frontl segment, renal segment, sacral segment, spinal segment, uterine segment, venous segment are commonly used.

segregation Separation of different elements of a population, or separation of allelic genres in meiosis.

Sehrt's clamp This clamp is used to arrest haemorrhage of a limb or of an aorta by compression.

Seidel's scotoma It is an arcuate scotoma which extends at both ends.

seizure One episode of epilepsy. An acute attack of disease.

selection Forces that determines the performance of the various genotypes in a population.

selene Moon-shaped structure.

self Ones own with reference to tissue constituents.

self-analysis Psychoanalysis of oneself

self-antigen Other name for auto antigen.

Selivanoff's test Test done for the presence of fructose in urine. Urine with resorcinol in presence of HCl, boiled for 10 seconds give dark red colour for positive test.

sella Saddle-shaped depression referable to sella turcica.

semantics This field is the study of the meanings of words and the rules of their use

semen Thick whitish secretion of the testes composed of spermatozoa

semicanal Channel which is open on one side.

semilunar That which resembles half moon.

seminiferous That which coveys semen.

seminoma Malignant neoplasm of the testis

semipermeable Refered to a membrane which allow certain molecules and hinders others.

Semliki Forest Disease Named after Semliki Forest in western Uganda, where mosquitoes transmit this viral infection. It is an arboviral infection transmitted by Aedes mosquitoes. The virus belongs to alphavirus that is known to cause encephalitis.

Semmelweis was a Hungarian physician. He proved that puerperal fever is a form of septicemia, thus becoming the pioneer of antisepsis in obstetrics in the year 1846.

senescence Old changes occurring in man.

senile Old enough with changes.

senility Physical and mental deterioration associated with old age.

senna India senna and Tinnevelly senna are used as cathartic which contain sennosides.

sense Refers to special sense and somatic sense. It is a brain process by which stimuli are received, transduced, and conducted as impulses to be interpreted in the brain

sensitive One who is able to receive or respond to stimuli quickly and acutely often used to mean abnormally responsive to stimulation

sensitivity Of a test which identifies persons having disease correctly by the screening test.

$$\text{Sensitivity} = \frac{\text{True +ve}}{\text{True +ve + False –ve}}$$

sensitization Exposed to antigen to induce immunity or show the development of hypersensitivity.

sensor A device to respond to light, heat, pressure.

sensorium Human consciousness or mental clarity.

sensory That which is related to sensation.

separation To make items apart such as shoulder separation, separation of adhesion etc.,

sepsis Greek work meaning decay indicating the presence of pathogens and their toxins in the area.

septal Related to a septum.

septic Infected with pathogens and decomposed.

septicemia Presence of pathogens and toxins in the blood of a patient.

septum Dividing wall

sequela Further lesion following an attack of disease.

sequence Connected series of events

sequestration Formation of a sequestrum.

sequestrectomy Removal of a sequestrum.

sequestrum Dead bone that has become separated during the process of necrosis from the sound bone.

series Objects or substances arranged in succession.

seroconversion Change in serologic test from negative to positive which indicates the development of antibodies in response to infection or immunization.

serodiagnosis Diagnosis by serologic tests.

seroflocculation Flocculation produced in serum by an antigen.

serogroup Presence of common antigen which demonstrates more than one serotype that help in classification of bacteria.

serologist An expert in serology.

serology This field is the study of agglutination, precipitation, complement fixation, antibody titres determination in infections, and clinical correlation of antibody titre in diseases.

seropositive High antibody titre in infections called serologically positive

serosanguineous That which is related with blood and serum.

serotonin It is produced in intestine, neurons, and CNS. Serotonin is a vasoconstrictor. It has the following properties:

- Gastric secretion inhibition
- Smooth muscle stimulation
- Neurotransmitter

serotype Based on antigens microorganisms are classified.

serous Resembling serum.

serum Clear portion of any body fluid

sesamoid Referred to bone embedded in a tendon.

setup Arrangement.

Sever's disease This refers to epiphysis infection of the calcaneus.

sewage Waste water from human settlement containing liquid waste and human excreta.

sex Male and female characterized by the presence of gonads and secondary sexual characters. Types of sex in use are:

- o Genetic sex determined by chromoses
- o Morphological sex by external genitalia
- o Gonadial sex by whether ovarian or testicular tissue present.
- o Nuclear sex by XX or XY genotype
- o Phenotype sex by secondary sex characters

sexology Study of sex from evolutionary, physiological, developmental and sociological aspects.

sexual That which is related to sex such as erotic desires.

sexuality Constitution of an individual in relation to sexual attitudes

SGOT Abbreviation for **S**erum **G**lutamic **O**xaloacetic **T**ransaminase .

SGPT Abbreviation for **S**erum **G**lutamic **P**uruvic **T**ransaminase.

SH Abbreviation for **S**erum **H**epatitis.

shakes Chills and rigors in fever.

Sharp British biochemist, Co-winner, the Nobel prize for medicine in 1993 for his discoveries about the structure of genes and the transmission of genetic information.

Shaver's disease This refers to Bauxite Pneumoconiosis described by Shaver.

sheath Tubular structure surrounding an organ such as carotid sheath, dural sheath, femoral sheath, Sheath of Henle, medullary sheath, mitochondrial sheath, Myelin sheath, nerve sheath, rectal sheath, sheath of Schwann, synovial sheath,

Sheehan's syndrome This refers to Post Partum Pituitary necrosis described by Sheehan.

sheet Linen or bed covering.

Shenton's line Top of obturator foramen form a curved line seen in X-ray of normal hip.

Sherrington English physiologist co-winner of the Nobel prize for medicine in 1932 for their work on the function of the neuron

Sherrington's law A nerve impulse to contract a muscle is received, at the same time an antagonist receives an impulse to relax.

shield Protecting structure. E.g., Eye shield, Lead shield, nipple shield, etc.,

shift Change of position

Shigella Gram-negative, facultative anaerobic, rod-shaped bacteria of the family Enterobacteriaceae that causes dysentery. Common strains are Shigella flexneri, Shigella boydii, Shigella sonnei, and Shigella dysenteries.

shigellosis Bacillary dysentery caused by shigella organisms.

shin Anterior aspect of the leg below the knee.

shingles Other name for herpes zoster.

shiver Tremble from a chill.

shock Disturbance of mental or physical equilibrium that occur all of a sudden in a person. Types of Shocks are

- Septic shock due to loss of vasomotor tone
- Neurogenic shock due to loss of vasomotor tone
- Cardiogenic shock due to loss of heart function
- Hypovolemic shock due to loss of blood volume.

shortsightedness This is Myopia.

shoulder Junction of the arm and trunk

shoulder-blade Common term for Scapula.

shoulder slip Colloquial term for suprascapular paralysis.

show Appearance of blood as a forerunner of menses or labour.

shudder Involuntary shake.

shunt Bypass meaning anastomosis between two natural channels between blood vessels. Common shunts that are being done are:

- Cardiovascular shunt
- Arteriovenous shunt

sialadenitis Infection and inflammation of a salivary gland.

sialagogue That promotes the flow of saliva.

sibling Offspring of the same parents called a brother or a sister.

siccus That which is dry.

sick Person afflicted by disease or illness.

sickness Other name for disease. Some of the associated terminologies are:

- Morning sickness
- African sleeping sickness
- Aviation sickness
- Motion sickness
- Mountain sickness
- Radiation sickness
- Serum sickness
- Sea sickness

side Lateral portion of the body or of a structure.

side effect Adverse effects produced by a drug

siderosis Lung changes produced by the inhalation of iron particles.

SIDS Abbreviation for **S**udden **I**nfant **D**eath **S**yndrome.

sieve Device with perforations of uniform size used for separating particles of different sizes.

Sigh Latin word meaning audible and prolonged inspiration which is followed by an audible expiration.

sight Vision

sigmoid Refers to sigmoid colon which is S shaped or C shaped.

sigmoidoscope Flexible endoscope with appropriate illumination for examining the sigmoid colon.

sign An objective evidence of a disease,

Positive findings	Sign
Miotic, responds o accommodation effort. Do not respond to light	Argyll Robertson pupil sign
Lowered Achilles tendon reflex in sciatica	Babinski's sign
Outward and upward rolling of eye when eye is closed on facial palsy side	Bell's sign
Uterine contraction painless and irregular in the beginning, becomes more rhythmic and painful in third trimester of pregnancy	Braxton Hick's sign
Pulse respiration ratio is reduced from4:1 to 2:1 in scurvy	Cardiorespiratory sign
Purple red and congested vaginal and cervical mucosa in pregnancy	Chadwick's sign
Sinking in of epigastrium on inhalation found in paralysis of diaphragm	Duchenne's sign
Free up and down movement of head of femur in congenital dislocation	Dupuytren's sign
Tender upper inner angle of orbit in obstruction of outlet of frontal sinus	Ewing sign
Dyspigmentation of hair as band of light hair in children in kwashiorkar	Flag sign

Softening of lower segment of uterus in pregnancy	Hegar's sign
In supine position when lower limbs are hanging and patient coughs, it produces flexion of the thigh and extension of paralysed lower limb; seen in upper motor neuron lesion	Huntington's sign
Interstitial keratitis and discoloured cornes in congenital syphilis	Hutchinson's sign
Distension of jugular veins during inhalation in constrictive pericarditis	Kussmaul's sign
Tenderness on McBurney point in appendicitis	McBurney sign
Red triangle at tip of tongue in typhoid	Marfan's sign
Inability to keep eyeballs converged in Graves' disease	Mobius's sign
Pressure on right costal margin interrupts deep inhalation in gallbladder disease	Murphy's sign
Presence of palpable click in abduction of hip joint in dysplasia of hip	Ortolani sign
Rapid rise of CSF pressure is not seen when veins in the neck are compressed in patients with block in vertebral canal	Queckenstedt's sign
Acrocyanosis	Raynaud's sign
No abdominal reflex in intestinal inflammation	Rosenbach's sign
Cherry red spot	Tay's sign
Pulse, respiration and temperature	Vital sign
Spastic Hemiplegia on opposite side of lesion and paralysis of oculomotor nerve on the same side	Weber's sign

significant When event occur not by chance but as though occurring in nature. The term is used in statistics.

silhouette The contour of a thing or an organ such as cardiac silhouette,.

silicosis Pneumoconiosis due to the inhalation of the dust of stone, sand, or flint containing silica

Silverman's needle Needle used for tissue specimen taking. Inner split needle holds the tissue when the needle and cannula are withdrawn.

Simmonds' disease This refers to Panhypopituitarism described by Simmonds.

Simons' disease This refers to Partial Lipo Dystrophy described by Simons.

Simpson's forceps It is an obstetrical forcepts.

Sims' position Semiprone position used for vaginal examination.

simulation Mimicking of disease .

Simuliidae Small flies of the suborder Nematocera, medical impotence are black flies

Sindbis fever A viral infection transmitted by culex mosquitoes which is characterized by fever, rash and arthritis.

single blind Clinical trial in which subjects do not know which treatment they are receiving.

sinister Situated on the left side of the body.

sinoatrial That which is related with sinus venous and the atrium of the heart.

sinoventricular That which is related with sinus venous and the ventricle of the heart.

sinuous That which is found winding .

sinus Anatomical cavity such as air sinus, carotid sinus, cavernous sinus, venous sinus etc.,

sinusitis Infection and inflammation of a para nasal sinus,

siphon For the transfer of liquid from higher to lower level by using atmosphere pressure, a bent tube with two arms of unequal length is used.

Siphonaptera This include Rat flea, Dog flea, Cat flea, human flea.

Sippy diet Diet containing bland diet with milk, cream etc., for peptic ulcer.

sister The nurse in charge of a hospital ward .

site This refers to a place or position,

situation All factors with which an individual is confronted

situs Describes the position

SIV Abbreviation for **S**imian **I**mmunodeficiency **V**irus

Sjögren's syndrome A condition which is due to abnormal immune response described by Sjogren includes the following:

- Dry keratoconjunctivitis
- Xerostomia
- Systematic lupus erythematosus
- Sometimes scleroderma or polymyositis

skatole An a crystalline amine present in human excreta which has a characteristic odor. It is produced by the decomposition of proteins in the intestine

skeleton Bony framework of the body

skew Deviation or asymmetrical. Skew to the left or skew to the right is used in case of not symmetric about the mea which is called skewness.

skiagram Other name for Radiograph.

skimming It is the process of removing of floating matter from a liquid.

skin Outer covering of the body. Common terminology used are:

- Glossy skin
- Elastic skin
- Fish skin

skinfold This is the yardstick for the estimation of percentage of body fat. Usually sites of skinfold thickness taking are over biceps, over triceps, above iliac crest and subscapular region.

Skinner classification Based on edentulous space, edentulous conditions are classified.

skull Skeleton of the head which includes cranium and the mandible

slant Slope; usually refers to the sloping surface of agar in a test tube

SLE Abbreviation for **S**ystemic **L**upus **Er**ythematosis.

sleep When a person takes complete rest for his body and mind. During this period bodily functions are suspended. There are two types of sleep. They are

- ❖ Non Rapid Eye Movement Sleep (deep sleep)
- ❖ Rapid Eye Movement Sleep. (dreaming sleep)

sleepwalking This status is called Somnambulism.

slice Cross-sectional plane of the body for imaging.

slide Used for microscopic examination. Another type is used for projection.

sling Bandage for supporting part of the body.

slit A narrow incision.

slope his is an inclined plane

slough Dead tissues that is separated from living tissues. The process is sloughing.

sludge Semisolid particles in a fluid. Always refered to active sludge in night soil disposal.

SMA Abbreviation for **S**equential **M**ultiple **A**nalyser.

smear Material spread across the glass slide for examination. E.g., Cervical smear, Pop smear, skin smear etc.,

smegma Cheesy desquamated epithelial cells found beneath the prepuce.

Smith's dislocation Dislocation of metatarsals and medial cuneiform bone backward and upward direction.

Smith's sign The sign is positive if a murmur is heard over the manubrium with patient's head thrown back in case of enlarged bronchial glands.

SMR Abbreviation for **S**tandardised **M**ortality **R**atio.

snap Sharp sound of short duration.

sneeze Involuntary sudden violent audible expulsion of air through the mouth and nose.

Snellen's chart Chart used to test visual acuity. It is 6/6 if all size letters can be read by the person. The chart contains black letters of decreasing size.

snore Noisy breathing during sleep. This is due to vibration of the uvula and soft palate

SNS Abbreviation for **S**ympathetic **N**ervous **S**ystem.

SOAP Abbreviation for **S**ubjective data, **O**bjective data, **A**ssessment of patient's status and **P**lan for patient care.

soap Compound of fatty acids with an alkali and is a detergent.

socialization Person learns to behave in socially acceptable ways. There are three types namely Primary, Secondary and Re-socialisation.

sociologist Person who is trained in sociology.

sociology It deals with the science of social relations and social phenomena.

sociometry Measurement of human social behavior.

socket A depression into which a corresponding part fits such as eye socket, tooth socket etc.,

soda Commonly referred to sodium bicarbonate or baking soda. This is also applicable to sodium hydroxide or caustic soda and to sodium carbonate or washing soda.

sodomy It is referable to anal intercourse and the word is derived from the name of a city called Sodom.

SOFAS Abbreviation for **S**ocial and **O**ccupational **F**unctioning **A**ssessment **S**cale.

solar That which is related to sun.

solder Fasten together pieces of metal through the use of fusible metals

soluble Which can get dissolved.

solute Substance dissolved in a solvent

solution It is a liquid preparation containing one or several soluble chemical substances usually dissolved in water such as heparin solution, alcohol solution, Benedict's solution, aqueous solution, buffer solution, Drabkin's solution, Formaldehyde solution, Fehling solution, Hypobaric solution, hyperbaric solution etc.,

solvent A liquid capable of dissolving

somatic That which is related to body.

somnambulism Performing motor bahaviour during sleep.

sone Unit of loudness

sophistication Adulteration of medicine.

sorbic acid An antimicrobial preservative which contains 2,4-hexadienoic acid

sorbitol A sugar alcohol present in fruits which is a precursor of the fructose

sore Term for almost any lesion of the skin or mucous membranes.

sore throat Colloquial term for Pharyngitis.
S.O.S. Abbreviation for when it is necessary.
souffle Soft blowing auscultatory sound
sound Effect produced on the organ of hearing, Common sounds of clinical importce are:
- Heart sound
- Adventitious sound
- Breath sound
- Friction sound
- Ejection sound
- Metallic sound
- Korotkoff sound
- Gallop sound
- Percussion sound

soybean A legume which contain 40% of protein.
Spalding's sign Positive in case of death of foetus. X-ray film of foetus in uterus overriding of the bones of the vault of the skull.
span Distance in a fully extended hand between the tips of the thumb and little finger.
sparfloxacin Broad-spectrum antimicrobial agent
spasm Sudden violent muscle contraction producing pain and functional interference. E.g., Facial spasm, Esophageal spasm, Torsion spasm, titanic spasm.
spasmodic Having the nature of spasm.
spastic Refers to Spastic paraplegia of cerebral palsy which show stiff muscles and has awkward movements.
spatula Flat flexible instrument used for mixing ointments
Spearman's rank correlation coefficient It is a statistical Rank correlation by giving each sample a unique rank. It is represented as Rho.
specialist Doctor who is specialized his area of practice either in medical field or in surgical field.
specialization When the medical practice is limited to some special branch of medicine or surgery.
specialty Field of practice of a specialist.
specificity Person not having a disease will be correctly identified by a clinical test by number of true negative results
specimen Sample taken for the laboratory examination in terms of urine specimen, blood specimen, tissue specimen etc.,
SPECT Abbreviation for **S**ingle **P**hoton **E**mission **C**omputed **T**omography .
spectacles Pair of lenses in a frame to assist vision.
spectinomycin Antibiotic derived from Streptomyces spectabilis and used against many gram-positive and gram-negative organisms
spectrophotometer It measures the quantity of light absorbed by a liquid thereby estimating the quantity of coloring matter in that solution.
spectroscopy Spectra is analysised by means of this device.
spectrum By means of refraction and diffraction we can get the wavelengths of electromagnetic vibrations that can depict the range of action. Common clinical entities are:
- Chemical spectrum
- Colour spectrum
- Absorption spectrum
- X-ray spectrum
- Anti Bacterial spectrum

speculum This instrument is used to enlarge an opening and exposes the interior of a cavity of of a passage for direct examination.

Name	Use
Sim's speculum	Vaginal examination
Cook's speculum	Rectal examination
Fergusson speculum	Cylindrical speculum for P V
Duck billed speculum	Two valved speculum for P V
Bozeman's speculum	I valve speculum when parallel separation is needed
Eye speculum	To separate eye lids
Grave's speculum	Two valved speculum for P V
Kelly's speculum	Rectal examination
Martin's speculum	P R
Mathew speculum	Four pronged speculum used for P R

speech Utterance of vocal sounds called phonation. Known clinical entities are:
- ✓ Cerebellar speech
- ✓ Cleft palate speech
- ✓ Esophageal speech
- ✓ Slurred speech
- ✓ Staccato speech

sperm Male gonad and is the testicular secretion.
spermatic That which is related with semen.
spermatogenesis Process of formation of spermatozoa
spermatorrhea Discharge of semen without copulation.
spermatozoon Mature male germ cell,
spermicide Chemical used as an agent to destroy spermatozoa.
Sperry American psychobiologist who won Nobel prize for medicine in 1981 for his studies of functional specialization of the cerebral hemispheres.
sp gr Abbreviation for **S**pecific **Gr**avity.
sphenoid That which is wedge-shaped.
sphere A globe which is a three dimensional round body;
spherical That which is sphere-shaped.

spherocytosis Presence of spherocytes in the blood;
spheroid That which is resembling a sphere.
spherometer Instrument to measure the curvature of a surface.
sphincter Band of muscle fibers that constricts a passage such as cardiac sphincter, anal sphincter.
sphygmomanometer Instrument for measuring blood pressure
sphygmometer Instrument for measuring the force as well as frequency of the pulse.
spica Figure-of-8 bandage at the shoulder joint or or hip joint.
spike Upward deflection of a curve in ECG or EEG .
spinal That which is related with spinal cord.
spindle Microtubules radiating from centrioles occurs during the metaphase of mitosis.
spine Projections of vertebral column.
spiral Which is winding about a center like a coil
spiramycin One of the Macrolide antibiotics.
Spirillum Bacteria which is curved and spiral that are motile and found in salt water or water containing organic matter.
spirit Volatile liquid such as alcohol.
Spirochaeta Belong to family spirochaetaceae and are present in mud, sewage and polluted water. They are pathogenic to man.
spirogram This is graph of respiratory movements.
spirometer Instrument used in pulmonary function tests. Measurement of such lung function test is called Spirometry.
spironolactone This is 17-spirolactone steroid used in the treatment of C C F, Liver failure, kidney failure, in hypokalemia, and primary hyperaldosteronism.
spleen This is largest lymphoid organs in the body. It is the reservoir of blood that produces plasma cells and lymphocytes.
splenalgia Pain in the spleen.
splenectomy Excision of the spleen.
splenomegaly Enlargement of the spleen.
splenorrhaphy Surgical repair of the spleen.
splicing In genetic term it is the attachment of individual DNA molecules to each other.
Splint Hard and rigid device to hold broken bones as first aid procedure, Useful to ease pain in certain rheumatic diseases rigid appliance to put a safeguard fractures, appliance used in first aid, immobilisation of part of the body.
splinting Treatment of fractures and injuries by splints.
splitting Division into two or more parts.
spondylitis inflammatory changes of the vertebrae. Types of spondylitis are:

- Ankylosing spondylitis
- Muscular spondylitis
- Post traumatic spondylitis
- Rheumatoid spondylitis

spondylosis Degenerative spinal changes due to osteoarthritis or ankylosis of vertebral joint.
sponge Absorbent pad of gauze such as Gelatin sponge, Fibrin sponge, Bernay's sponge.
spongiform That which resembles sponge.
spool Surgical instrument around which suture material is put
sporadic Diseases occurring occasionally in an isolated manner.
spore This is the resting stage during the life history of the cell which is resistant to environment.
sporocyst Sac like stage in the life cycle of trematodes produced by metamorphosis of a miracidium which gives rise to rediae.
sporogony Multiple fission in protozoa giving rise to sporozoites or sporocysts.
Sporozoa Spores like organisms such as microspore or ascetospora under protozoa.
sporozoite Sporozoites of malaria parasite are liberated from the oocysts in the mosquito, accumulate in the vector's salivary glands, and are transferred to the definitive host by the bite of the infected anopheles female mosquito.
spot (spot) Circumscribed area distinguished by its color.

Descriptions	Spots
Foamy gray spots on conjunctiva	Bitot's spot
Cherry angiomas	De Morgan's spot
Mental scotoma	Blind spot
Sclerosed spots in bones	Carleton's spot
Bright red spots on buccal and lingual mucosa	Koplik's spot
Rose macules on skin of abdomen and thighs	Rose spots of typhoid
Oval white spots of coagulated fibrin	Roth's spot
Spots of ecchymosis under pleura in suffocation	Tardieu's spots

sprain Joint injury in which some of the fibers of a supporting ligament are ruptured
spray Nebulized as by a jet of steam.
sprue Chronic form of malabsorption syndrome
spurious Not genuine.
Spurway's syndrome This is referred to Osteogenesis imperfecta described by Spurway.

sputum This is expectoration or ejected matter from lungs, bronchi and trachea.

squama Scale or plate like structure. Commonly called squamous.

square A plane with four equal sides and four right angles.

squatting Position of defecation among Indians. It is a position of flexion of the knees and hips, the buttocks being lowered to the level of the heels.

squeeze Subject to compression.

squint Colloquial word for strabismus.

SSPE Abbreviation for **S**ubacute **S**clerosing **P**anencephalitis.

stability Showing stable status or resistance to change.

stabilization Creation of a stable state.

staccato Speech delivered in a quick, jerky manner, with an interval between each two syllables.

staff Professional personnel of a hospital.

staggers Vertigo occurring in decompression sickness.

stain Dye or reagent producing coloration. Common stains are:

- Acid stain
- Basic stain
- Contrast stain
- Counter stain
- Differential stain
- Acid fast stain
- Albert's stain
- Giemsa stain
- Gram's stain
- Leishman's stain
- Papanicolaou's stain
- Romanovsky's stain
- Z.N. Stain

staining Artificial coloration of tissues for examination under microscope.

Common types of staining are:

- Simple staining
- Differential staining
- Bipolar staining
- Supra vital staining
- Fluorescent staining
- Multiple staining
- Polar staining
- Vital staining

stalk Elongated slender anatomical structure called peduncle.

stamina Vigor

stammering Colloquially called stuttering wherein the speech is marked by involuntary pauses.

stance Posture and bodily orientation of a person when he is standing.

standard An established model to which other things should conform.

standardization Setting up the formulation of standards for a substance or for a procedure.

standardize An act of comparing with standard.

standstill Suspension of movement.

Stanley American biochemist, 1904–1971 who won Nobel prize for chemistry in 1946 for isolating virus crystals and for isolating nucleic acid

stapes The auditory ossicle which is shaped like a stirrup.

Staphylococcus Gram-positive, facultative anaerobic bacteria of the family Micrococcaceae which are like grapes bunch at observation under microscope. Common Staphylococcus are:

Staphylococcus aureus, Staphylococcus haemolyticus, Staphylococcus pyogenes,

staphyloma Defect in the eye inside the cornea leading to protrusion of the cornea

stapling Process of fastening with staples.

starch Polysaccharides represented with - $C_6H_{10}O_5)_n$, . Starch is the chief storage form of energy reserve in the form of cárbohydrates in plants.

stasis Diminution of the flow of blood in any part.

stat. 'immediately'.

state This is the condition of patient in his disease status. Clinical states that are often used are:

- Persistent vegetative state
- Acute confusional state
- Refractory state

stationary Not subject to variations

statistic Item of numerical data.

statistics Collection, analysis, and interpretation of numerical data for the purpose of inference about characteristics.

statoacoustic Related to balance and hearing.

status Used in reference to a morbid condition.

stavudine Drug used in HIV infection which is a nucleoside analogue of thymidine that inhibits human immunodeficiency virus replication.

STD Abbreviation for **S**exually **T**ransmitted **D**isease.

stearic acid Saturated fatty acid occurring in most fats and oils

steatoma Fatty mass or a Lipoma.

steatorrhea Fats in the feces in malabsorption syndromes.

stenosis Abnormal narrowing of a canal which is called stricture.

stent Acrylic mass of slender device used to provide support for a tubular structure that are anastomosed.

stercobilin Bile pigment derivative that contribute to the color of feces and urine.

stercobilinogen Precursor of stercobilin that is formed by reduction of urobilinogen.

sterility Inability to produce offspring. Male cannot induce conception or female cannot conceive.

sterilization For pathogens it is physical or chemical methods to destroy them. For humans it is vasectomy or Tubectomy.

sterilizer Apparatus used for the destruction of microorganisms.

sternum Single central bone in anterior wall of thorax which articulates with clavicle and first seven ribs.

steroid They are lipids such as progesterone, adrenocortical hormones, the gonadal hormones, cardiac aglycones, bile acids, cholesterol

stethoscope Doctor's instrument to auscultate and arrive at clinical diagnosis. Stethoscope helps in identifying sounds of respiratory, cardiac, pleural, arterial, venous, uterine, foetal and intestinal pathology.

Stevens-Johnson syndrome Fatal form of erythema multiforme showing severe mucocutaneous lesions.

stiffness Rigidity of an anatomical organ.

stigma Personal trait that is perceived as physically, socially, or psychologically disadvantageous.

stillbirth Delivery of a dead child.

stillborn Born dead.

stimulant Agent that produces stimulation.

stimulus Agent that produces functional reaction in tissue.

stippling Dark dots or a spotted appearance.

stochastic Random process used particularly to refer to a time series of random variables.

stoma Orifice or opening on a free surface.

stomach Other name for gaster. This is in continuation with oesophagus above and duodenum below.

stomatitis Inflammation of the oral mucosa due to local or systemic factors .

Stomoxys Genus of flies of the family Muscidae.

stone Colloquial word for calculus.

strabismus Deviation of the eye which the patient cannot overcome.

strain Excessive effort or undue exercise.

strangle Choke

strangulated In case of hernia, stricture blood supply is reduced .

strangulation Arrest of the circulation in a part

strap Adhesive used for attaching parts to each other.

strapping Strips of adhesive tape used as bandage.

stratum Other name for layer

Strauss' sign Fatty food usage increases fat in chylous ascites.

strength Denotes power.

Streptobacillus Anaerobic, gram-negative, rod-shaped bacteria which is known to cause rat bite fever.

Streptococcus Gram-positive, facultatively anaerobic cocci occurring in pairs or chains from the family Streptococcaceae. They are pathogenic to man.

streptokinase Protein produced by β-hemolytic streptococci;

streptolysin Exotoxin produced by streptococci, particularly those of group A, that destroys RBC.

streptomycin Effective antibiotic on gram-negative bacilli and some gram-positive bacteria, including mycobacteria.

stress An exerted pressure.

stretcher Portable bedlike structure for carrying the sick

striation Marked by stripes

stricture Other name for stenosis.

stridor High-pitched respiratory sound seen in acute laryngeal obstruction.

stroke Sudden and severe attack with paralysis.

Strongyloidea Family of hookworms which includes Ancylostomatidae, Strongylidae,

structure Manner in which components are arranged in a unit.

strychnine Poisonous alkaloid obtained from Nux vomica which is used in killing stray dogs in the prevention of Rabies.

STS Abbreviation for **S**erologic **T**est for **S**yphilis.

Student's *t*-test British mathematician Gossett under pseudonym postulated 't' test which is a statistical test of significance.

stump Distal end of the limb left after amputation.

stun Render unconscious by a blow .

stunning Unconsciousness.

stunt Retardation referred to the growth in terms of height.

stupor Lowered level of consciousness or reduced responsiveness,

stuttering This is a speech disorder

stye Colloquial word for hordeolum.

subacute Between acute and chronic.

Subarachnoid Situated between the arachnoid and the pia mater.

subclavian Situated below the clavicle,

subclinical Early stage of disease when we cannot see signs and symptoms.

subconscious Partially conscious.

subcostal Situated below the rib.

subculture Preparing a fresh culture from an existing one.

subcutaneous Beneath the skin. Referred to injection.

subdural Structure situated between the dura mater and the arachnoid mater.

subject In an experiment, either animal or man considered for observation and treatment.

sublimation Direct change of state from solid to vapor.

sublingual Medication given beneath the tongue

subluxate Partially dislocate. Commonly called subluxation.

submucosal Situated beneath the mucous membrane.

subphrenic Situated below the diaphragm

substitute Substance which may be used in place of another.

substitution Use or replace one for the another.
subtile Keen and acute.
succinate Salt of succinic acid.
succinic acid Intermediate product of Tricarboxylic acid cycle. Chemically it is 1,4-butanedioic acid,
succussion Splashing sound is indicative of the presence of fluid
suckle Breast feeding the baby for nourishment.
sucrose Disaccharide made of glucose and fructose. Natural sources are sugar cane, sugar beet and sorghum.
suction Aspiration of gas or fluid
Sudafed Preparations of pseudoephedrine hydrochloride..
Sudan Azo compounds which are used to stain fats.
sudation **sweating.**
SUDS Abbreviation for **S**udden **U**nexplained **D**eath **S**yndrome.
suffocant Agent that causes suffocation.
suffocation Latin word meaning asphyxiation.
sugar They are monosaccharides and oligosaccharides, very often used specifically for sucrose.
suggestion Idea for action
suicide Taking of one's own life.
suit Outer garment covering the entire body.
sulcus Groove on the surface of the brain separating the gyri.
sulfadiazine This is a sulfonamide used in in the treatment of meningitis caused by **Haemophilus influenzae**, chancroid, acute urinary tract infections, early manifestations of lymphogranuloma venereum, and falciparum malaria caused by chloroquine-resistant plasmodia.
Sulfadoxine Long-acting sulfonamide used in the treatment of leprosy and falciparum malaria.
sulfaguanidine Sulfonamide used in gastrointestinal infections especially bacillary dysentery
sulfamethoxazole sulfonamide used in acute urinary tract infections, pyodermata and infections of wounds and soft tissues
sulfone Referable to Dapsone which has chemical formula 4,4′-sulfonylbisbenzenamine and is a leprostatic.
sulfonylurea Used to control hyperglycemia in type 2 diabetics who cannot be treated solely by diet and exercise.
sulfuric acid This a strong mineral acid with the formula H_2SO_4,
sullage Liquid waste without mixing of human excreta.
Sullivan's test This is a qualitative test to detect Cysteine. A brilliant red indicate positive test.
summit Denotes apex of an anatomical organ.
sunstroke One of the hazard due to physical agent sun heat. This carrys considerable mortality.
super Latin word meaning more than normal.
superactivity Hyperactivity.
superalimentation Therapeutic treatment wasting diseases.
superciliary Related with the eyebrow.
superego Personality acting as a self monitor and show self-criticism,
superfecundation By two separate coital acts, fertilization of two or more ova
superfetation Fertilization of ova during different ovulatory cycles and yielding fetuses of different ages.
superficial Situated near the surface.
superinfection New infection occurring in a patient having a preexisting infection
superior Upper or that which is situated above
supernatant Overlying liquid after precipitation of a solid
supernumerary More than a normal number.
superscription A sign used before a prescription and is symbolized as R_x
supersonic Speed greater than the velocity of sound . The sciences of this is called supersonics.
supination In case of Hand, turning the palm forward by lateral rotation of the forearm.
supine Lying on the back.
suppository Medicated mass for introduction into the rectal, vaginal, or urethral orifice of the body
suppressant Agent that stops secretion
suppression Act of holding back
suppuration Formation of pus
sural Related to calf of the leg.
surface External part or an outer part of an organ.
surfactant This refers to Lecithin and Sphingomyelin from Type II cells of alveoli that has the property of reducing the surface tension of pulmonary fluids and this help in elastic properties of lung tissues.
surgeon Doctor who specialized in surgical treatment.
surgery Field that treats diseases, injuries, and deformities by manual or operative methods.
surgical Related to surgery
surrogate This means a substitute such as surrogate mother.
surveillance Watching and monitor infectious diseases. Which is an Epidemiological process.
susceptibility Diminished immunity to a disease particularly an infection.
susceptible At risk of infection.
suspensory That which holds a part such as a ligament, muscle, or a sling.
suture Catgut used to secure apposition of the edges of a wound;
SVT Abbreviation for **S**upra **V**entricular **T**achycardia.
swab An absorbent material used for applying medication
swaddler Wrapping for an infant's body.
swallowing Taking in of food through the mouth through the esophagus and into the stomach.

sweat Liquid secreted by the sweat glands
swelling Abnormal enlargement of a body part
sycosis Inflammation of the hair follicles of the beard.
Sydenham's chorea Self limited child disease which is linked with Rheumatic fever. This shows involuntary movements in gait, arm movement, speech. It can be hemichorea or paralytic chorea.
symbiosis Living together of two organisms. Types of symbiosis are:
- ✓ Mutualism (benefit to both)
- ✓ Commensalisms (beneficial to one, no effect on the other)
- ✓ Parasitism (beneficial to one and harmful to the other)
- ✓ Amensalism (Harmful to one and no effect on the other)
- ✓ If harmful to both it is called Synnecrosis.

symblepharon Adhesion occurring between the tarsal conjunctiva and the bulbar conjunctiva.
symbol A letter or combination of letters representing an atom or a group of atoms.
symbolism Act of representing something by a symbol.
symbolization It is a defense mechanism in which one object comes to represent another because of similarity
Syme's amputation Ankle is disarticulated by removing both malleoli
Symmers' disease This refers to Nodular Lymphoma described by Symmers.
symmetrical That which exhibits symmetry.
symmetry Similar arrangement from the point of view of form and relationships around a common axis
sympathectomy Surgical transection of the sympathetic nervous pathways.
sympathetic Refers to Sympathetic nervous system.
sympathomimetic Substance, item, drug or a nerve which mimic the effects of impulses conveyed by adrenergic postganglionic fibers of the sympathetic nervous system.
symphysis Named for Fibrocartilaginous joint.
symptom Subjective evidence of disease of a patient's condition,
symptomatic Pertaining to symptom.
symptomatology Scientific study of symptoms.
synapse An area of functional apposition between neurons, at which an impulse is transmitted from one neuron to another.
synchondrosis Union between two bones formed by either hyaline cartilage or fibrocartilage;
syncope Faint due to cerebral ischemia.
syndactyly Webbing between adjacent fingers which is an autosomal dominant trait.
syndrome Pathologically related multiple symptoms producing various types of clinical manifestations.
syndromic Occurring as a syndrome.
synechia Adhesion of the iris to the cornea or to the lens.
synergistic Two substances act together.
synovectomy Surgical excision of a synovial membrane
synovia White of an egg like liquid secreted by the synovial membrane.
synovitis Inflammation of a Synovia.
synthesis Integrated synthesis by the combination of simpler entities.
syphilis Chronic infection by Treponema pallidum through sexual contact that lead a man to be crippled. The word has the origin in 1530 with *Syphilis,* a shepherd infected with the disease in the poem of Fracastorius. Primary secondary and tertiary stages are known in this disease.
syphilitic Related with syphilis.
syringe Glass instrument or Polythene instrument for injection of medication.
syringobulbia Syringomyelia in which the cavity extends to involve the medulla oblongata.
syringomyelia Slowly progressive illness of cavitation in the central segments of the spinal cord . It is characterized by muscular weakness, atrophy and sensory loss .
syrup Solution of sucrose in purified water which is used as a flavored vehicle in pharmaceutical preparations.
system Inter connected objects, organs or organisms which function together. E.g., Cardio vascular system, Respiratory system etc.,
systemic Affecting the body as a whole.
systole Period of contraction of the heart. The pressure build up in such contraction of the heart is called systolic blood pressure.

T

T_4 Symbol for Thyroxine.
tabacum Latin word meaning Tobacco.
tabes Progressive atrophy of the body as in Tabes dorsalis.
table Data arrangement in rows and column for statistical inference.
tablespoon 15 ml holding spoon.
tablet Medicine containing solid and of varying weight, size, and shape formatted for oral administration of drugs.
taboo Negative traditions and behaviors that are harmful to society.
Tachy Anything that is rapid and swift
tachycardia Heart rate above 100 per minute in adult that has to be further examined as to its origin
tachyphylaxis Quick reduction of toxicity of serum reaction or toxic reaction.
tachypnea Increased rate of breathing.

Tachysterol From irradiation, an ergosterol produced which is an isomer of ergosterol. An isomer of ergosterol produced by irradiation.

tactile Latin word meaning that which is related with touch.

Taenia Latin word meaning tape, Large tapeworms of the family Taeniidae.

T. solium and T. saginata are important species of tape worm.

tag It refers to label like skin tag, Radioactive tag, etc.,

tail Tail is an appendage that extends from posterior trunk of animals. It is also an appendage of an anatomical organ.

Taka-diastase By the reaction of wheat and aspergillus fungus, Taka diastase is formed which is an amylolytic enzyme. It is named after Japanese chemist Jokichi Takamine.

Takahara's disease This refers to Acatalasia described by Takahara.

talc It is magnesium silicate powder plus small quantity of aluminium silicate. Common dusting powder is nothing but purified form of talk.

talipes Congenital deformity of the foot called club foot. When turned outward it is called talipes valgus. When turned inward it is talipes varus.

talus Tarsal bone that articulates with the tibia and fibula to form the ankle joint

tampon A cotton pad used in surgery to plug the nose or vagina for the control of bleeding or the absorption of secretions.

tamponade It refers to cardiac tamponade by compression of heart by intrapericardial pressure. This also can refer to esophagogastric tamponade which has triple lumen tube and two inflatable balloons during aspiration of blood clots.

tanapox Pox virus infection which cause fever and skin eruption. The name is derived from a river name called Tana in Kenya where disease is common.

tannic acid An astringent for the mucous membranes of the mouth and throat. Suppositories for the treatment of hemorrhoids

tantrum Display of wild temperament.

tap Draining off fluid by Paracentesis such as ascetic tap, spinal tap etc.,

tape This refers to adhesive tape having tensile strength used in dressings or in immobilization.

tapeworm Flat and band like intestinal worm called tape worms such as Taenia solium (Pork tapeworm), Taenia saginata (Beef tape worm

Tapia's syndrome Because of injury to vagus and hypoglossal nerves unilateral paralysis of the tongue and larynx is produced. Soft palate function will be normal.

tar Black viscid liquid which is carcinogenic is the by prouct of destructive distillation of bituminous coal. Tar is the source of many organic substances.

Tardieu's spots This is the sign of death due to suffocation wherein spots of ecchymosis under the pleura is seen.

target Degree of achievement of health activity .

Tarnier's forceps This is axis traction forceps devised by Tarnier.

tarsorrhaphy Suturing upper and lower eyelids to shorten the palpebral fissure. There are five surgical types of tarsorrhaphy which are a) External b) Internal c) Partial d) total and e) Median

tarsus Bony tarsus is the articulation between foot and leg. Connective tissue tarsus is the framework of eyelid.

tartaric acid This is cathartic chemically 2,3-dihydroxybutanedioic acid

Tarui disease This refers to glycogen storage disease type VII described by Tarui disease.

taste It is a special sense called taste sense that are sweet, sour, salty and bitter.

tattooing Permanent colors are introduced to skin through punctures.

taxonomy Classification of animals or plants in an orderly manner by using generic name and species name.

Tay-Sachs disease A ganglioside storage disease described by Tay and Sachs. The disease is characterized by

- o Doll face
- o Cherry red macular spots
- o Early blindness
- o Macrocephaly, convulsions

Td Adult type of double antigen containing toxoid against tetanus and diphtheria .

t.d.s. Ter die sumen dum meaning take three times a day, used as medication abbreviation.

tea Decoction of tea leaves which contain tannic acid used as a drink which is called stimulating beverage.

Teale's amputation In the limb amputation, an effort is made to preserve long rectangular flap is preserved on one side and short rectangular flap on the other side is preserved.

tear Ripping apart of tissue which is called laceration.

tears Watery secretion of the lacrimal glands which help to moisten the conjunctiva

technical That which is related to technique.

technician Skilled person who performs skilled procedures in health care system.

technique Technique is the mode of conducting a maneuver, a method, an operation, a procedure, a treatment or a lab test. Examples are Fluorescent antibody technique, computed tomography image technique, Begg's orthodontic technique, Coronary arteriography technique, Aseptic technique for surgery, Western blot technique etc.,

technologist Person skilled in the theory and practice of a technical profession

technology Scientific knowledge of a technique such as Assisted Reproductive Technology.

teething The process of the eruption of the teeth.

Teflon Preparation of polytetrafluoroethylene.

telangiectasia Capillaries, arterioles or venules get dilated that are irreversible are seen on the skin as red lesions.

telangiectasis Skin lesion produced by telangiectasia

tele- Meaning to operat from a distance.

telemedicine Off site discussion of high fi information by consultants with the help of a closed circuit television.

telepathy Extrasensory perception of the mental activity

telestethoscope With the help of electric amplification provision is made to auscultate heart and lung from a distance. A useful deice for demonstration to a medical audience.

telophase Last of the four stages of mitosis

temephos Insecticide used against larvae which belong to organophosphorus compound.

temperament This refers to the type of personality wherein a person reacts to external stimuli.

temperature Usually refers to fever. Otherwise hotness or coldness of atmosphere is specified and expressed in thermal units. Different types of temperature we come across in clinical practice are

- Basal body temperature
- Maximum temperature
- Minimum temperature
- Optimum temperature
- Room temperature
- Atmosphere temperature

template RNA or DNA strand, it designates a mold or a pattern, A curved plate in dentistry.

temple Lateral region on either side of the superior part of the head , the part above the zygomatic arch

temporal Related with time, related to lateral side of head.

temporalis The part related to lateral side of head above zygomatic arch.

tenderness Pain and abnormal sensitiveness to touch or pressure.

tendinitis Inflammation of tendons

tendon Fibrous connective tissue by which a muscle is attached; such as Achilles tendon, Hamstring tendon, Patellar tendon,

tenesmus Strain experienced in defecation and urination.

Tenon's capsule It is called bulbar sheath which cover eye ball. This is continuous with muscular fascia of the eye.

tenoplasty Repair of a defect in a tendon.

tenoreceptor Proprioceptor that are stimulated by contraction.

tenorrhaphy Suture put to a divided tendon.

tenosynovitis Inflammation of a tendon sheath.

tenotomy Surgical cutting of any tendon.

tension Stretching. Partial pressure of a gas. Mental strain. Common clinical terms are: Intra ocular tension, Arterial tension, Surface tension, Muscular tension, etc.,

tent Covering designed to enclose an open space such as Oxygen tent, Sponge tent, steam tent etc.,

tentacle A sense organ of animals which function in prehension and feeding.

TEPP Abbreviation for **T**etra **E**thyl **P**yro **P**hophate.

teratocarcinoma A testicular tumor which is a malignant neoplasm.

teratogen That which produces congenital defects.

teratology Study of abnormal development or congenital anomalies.

teratoma A germ cell tumor.

terbutaline sulfate A β-adrenergic receptor agonist used as a bronchodilator

teres Refers to a muscle which is long and rounded.

ter in die Three times a day used in prescription of drugs.

Term Limit of a boundary, At the period of 38 weeks of conception.

terminal That which is placed at the end.

terminology Art and science that deals with terms, their constructions and arrangements.

Terramycin This preparation contains oxytetracycline.

Terry's syndrome This refers to retinopathy of prematurity described by Terry.

tertian That occurs once in third day such as malaria vivax fever.

tertiary Third in order or third level.

tesla Magnetic flux density expressed in webers per square meter.

test Examination of trial done such as agglutination text, aptitude test, Association test,
Benedict's test, Casoni test, Montou test, Tuberculin test etc.,

testis Male gonad that secretes male hormone.

test meal Diagnostic examination of the stomach by giving a meal and examination of stomach content.

testosterone Major male hormone of testes or male gonad.

tetanus Acute infectious disease caused by tetanus bacilli that produce tonic contraction of body.

tetany Low serum calcium level that produces hyperexcitability of nerves and muscles

tetrachloroethane Industrial solvent formed from acetylene and chlorine

tetracycline Both natural and synthetic are available. The group consists of Chlortetracycline, Oxytetracycline, Rolitetracycline.

tetralogy Combination of four elements such Fallot tetralogy.

thalamus Large ovoid mass in the posterior part of the diencephalon forming most of each lateral wall of the third ventricle

thalassemia Hereditary anomalies of RBC which are two types. á and â Thalassaemia.

thalidomide Now a banned drug because it is teratogenic. It was a sedative and hypnotic

Thaysen's disease This refers to Non Tropical Sprue described by Thaysen.

thenar Mound on the palm at the base of the thumb

theobromine It is a diuretic and smooth muscle relaxant.

theophylline Present in tea leaves and prepared synthetically used as smooth muscle relaxant.

theory Principles underlying an art and science or a formulated hypothesis. Common theories are Darwin theory, atomic theory, Germ theory, Natural selection theory.

therapist Person skilled in some of the treatment such as speech therapist, physical therapist etc.,

therapy Treatment of disease such as Convulsive therapy, Serum therapy, Diet therapy, Electo convulsive therapy, Gene therapy, Radiation therapy etc.,

thermal That which is related with heat.

thermocautery Cauterisation by hot wire.

thermocoagulation Coagulation of tissue by the action of high-frequency currents

thermocouple Thermocouple is used to measure temperature differences. Thermocouple is constructed by joining dissimilar electrical conductors of copper. Here thermoelectric effect produces thermoelectromotice force.

thermodynamics Under basic science Physics this deals with heat, energy, work and their interconversions.

thermometer Instrument for determining temperatures. Alcohol, mercury or ether are used in different thermometers. Common thermometers of practical importance are;

- Clinical thermometer
- Maximum thermometer
- Minimum thermometer
- Maximum and minimum thermometer
- Kata thermometer

thermostasis Maintenance of body temperature in warm-blooded animals.

thermostat It is a device interposed in a heating system by which the temperature can be automatically maintained between certain levels.

Thévenard's syndrome This refers to Hereditary Sensory Radicular Neuropathy described by Thevenard.

thiabendazole Benzimidazole anthelmintic used against roundworms, pinworms, threadworms, whipworms, and hookworms

thiamine Present in legumes and whole grain called vitamin B_1 which is a water-soluble vitamin. Deficiency of this produces Beri Beri.

thiazide This acts as diuretics by inhibiting the reabsorption of sodium in the proximal renal tubule and stimulating chloride excretion, with resultant increase in excretion of water.

Thiersch's graft Very thin skin graft consisting of epidermis and thin layer of dermis which is cut in long and broad strips.

thigh Portion of the lower extremity extending from the hip above to the knee below

thinking Flow of ideas, associations and symbols for getting a concept or for reasoning. Different types of thinking are:

- Primary Process thinking
- Secondary Process thinking
- Abstract thinking
- Magical thinking
- Pre operational thinking
- Concrete thinking

thiopental sodium Ultra–short-acting barbiturate used as G A of brief duration, used in narcoanalysis

thiouracil Thiourea derivative used in hyperthyroidism, angina pectoris and congestive heart failure.

Thomas' sign This sign is positive in finger to nose test which is diagnostic in cerebellar leision. When patient is directed to raise the upper limb over the head and is then suddenly told to let it fall to the head, the limb will rebound.

Thomas' sign The flexion deformity is seen in hip in this test.

thoracic That which is related with thorax.

thoracolumbar Related with thoracic and lumbar parts of the spine.

thoracopagus Conjoined twins united in or near the sternal region.

thoracostomy Opening in the wall of the chest for the purpose of drainage is done.

thoracotomy Surgical incision through the wall of the chest.

thorax Part of the body between the neck and the thoracic diaphragm.

Thorn's syndrome This refers to Salt Losing Nephritis.

threadworm Enterobius vermicularis a slender nematode

threonine An essential amino acid which is chemically α-amino-β-hydroxybutyric acid necessary for growth and nitrogen equilibrium.

threshold Perception which comes just within the limits of perception such as auditory threshold, Neuronal threshold, Renal threshold etc.,

thrill Vibration felt by the examiner on palpation of the body such as over the heart , over the aortic area

throat Anterior part of the neck.

throb Pulsating movement felt on examination.
thrombin This is an activated form of coagulation factor II called Prothrombin.
thrombocytopenia Decrease in the number of Platelets. This can be thrombocytopenic purpura or Neonatal thrombocytopenia
thromboembolism Obstruction of a blood vessel with blood clot.
thrombolysis This refers to the lysing of thrombi
thrombophlebitis Inflammation of a vein associated with thrombosis. This can be intra cranial, iliofemoral.
thrombosis Formation, development and presence of a thrombus.
thrombus A stationary blood clot along the wall of a blood vessel
thrush Candidiasis of the oral cavity. Common among immunocompromised, among antibiotic users and among patients with poor health.
thymidine A pyrimidine nucleoside . The term is restricted to ribonucleoside.
thymine A pyrimidine base which is nucleoside deoxythymidine, a component of deoxyribonucleic acid
thymus Lymphoid organ consisting of two pyramidal lobes situated in the anterior superior mediastinum. It is the site of production of T lymphocytes.
thyroid An endocrine gland.
thyroidectomy Surgical removal of the Thyroid gland.
thyroiditis Inflammation of the Thyroid gland.
thyrotoxic Body effects of thyroid hormone excess.
thyrotoxicosis It is Hyperthyroidism which is caused by excessive quantities of thyroid hormones or Graves' disease which is overproduction originating outside the thyroid or loss of storage function and leakage from the gland.
thyroxine Major hormone called Tetra Iodothyronine is the hormone secreted by Thyroid gland.
TIA Abbreviation for **T**ransient **I**schemia **A**ttack.
tibia The inner and larger bone of leg called shin bone.
tic Involuntary, compulsive, rapid, repetitive movement experienced by a person. They are either neurogenic or psychogenic in origin.
- Simple tic such as blinking, shrugging the shoulder, grunting
- Complex such as echokinesis, facial gestures.

tick Blood-sucking parasite belonging to family Ixodoidea. Dermacentor andersoni is common hard tick.
t.i.d. abbreviation for L. *ter in di'e which means* three times a day in prescription.
tincture Alcoholic solution prepared from animal origin, vegetable origin or from chemical substances. Common tincture are belladonna, benzoin, cardamom, Iodine, Opium.
tinea Ringworm such as tinea barbae, tinea capitis, tinea corporis, tinea pedis, tinea cruris
tinnitus Ringing noise in the ears Usually it is called subjective tinnitus.
tissue Similar group of cells in their morphology which go to perform a specific function.
titer In qualitative analysis of chemicals it refers to the amount of one substance required to correspond with a given amount of another substance.
titration Determination of a given component in solution by addition of a liquid reagent of known strength until a given endpoint is reached. The end point is by the change in colour.
TMST Abbreviation for **T**read **M**ill **S**tress **T**est.
tobacco From plant Nicotiana an alkaloid nicotine is present.
tocopherol Compounds that are methyl-substituted tocols, some of which have biological vitamin E activity.
Todd's palsy Post epileptic paralysis described by Todd.
toe Any of the five digits of the foot.
toilet Cleansing of obstetrical patient, traumatic wound or surgical wound.
tolbutamide Sulfonylurea compound used as a hypoglycemic agent in the treatment of non–insulin-dependent diabetes mellitus
tolerance Diminished response after prolonged exposure or ability to endure to large doses of drug, toxin or poison.
toluidine Compound used in dyemaking and chemical manufacturing.
tomography When radiography is taken at different section of the body. Computarised axial tomography, Electron beam computed tomography, High resolution computed tomography,
Positron emission tomography, Single photon emission computed tomography, Spiral computed tomography, Ultrasonic tomography, are common in practical uses.
tone Vigor and tension in muscles
tongue Special organ in mouth which give taste sense.
tonic Nutrients and minerals that give the normal tone to tissue.
tonsil Round lymphoid tissue in oral cavity which protect the entry of infection.
tonsillar That which is related to tonsil
tonsillectomy Surgical removal of tonsil .
tonsillitis Infection and inflammation of the palatine tonsils. Common clinical entities are Acute, chronic, follicular, streptococcal and Vincent's tonsillitis.
tooth Refers to milk set and permanent set of teeth in man. Each tooth consists of Crown, neck and root and the solid part of tooth is dentin.
toothache Pain in a tooth.
topical certain area of skin such as topical application on the skin.
topography Description of an anatomical region.

TORCH Abbreviation for **T**oxoplasmosis, **O**ther agents, **R**ubella, **C**ytomegalovirus, **H**erpes simplex;

Torek operation Two stage operation for cryptorchidism.

Torre's syndrome Cancer of G I tract with cancer of sebaceous gland.

torsion Twisting or turning of an organ such as torsion testes.

torticollis Wry neck due to contracted sternocleidomastoid muscle.

Toti's operation This refers to Dacryocystorhinostomy described by Toti.

touch Sensation by mechanoreceptors of skin and mucous membrane. The tactile senses are light touch, coarse touch, tickling, pressure touch, vibration sense and pain sense.

tourniquet Used for compression of a blood vessel by application around an extremity to control the circulation and prevent the flow of blood to or from the distal area.

toxemia Caused by spread of toxin in the body such as toxaemia of pregnancy.

toxic That which is poisonous or toxic.

toxicity It is the degree of virulence of a toxic microbe or of a poison.

toxicology This is the scientific study of poisons, their actions, their detection, and the treatment of the conditions produced by them.

toxin Poison of bacteria, certain animals.

toxoid Inactivated bacterial exotoxin that has lost toxicity but retains the properties of stimulating the formation of antitoxin.

toxoid-antitoxoid a toxoid mixed with an equivalent amount of antitoxic serum, the precipitate being suspended in saline.

Toxoplasma Protozoa comprising of intracellular parasites of many organs and tissues

TPHA Abbreviation for **T**reponema **P**allidum **H**aemagglutination **A**ssay.

trabecula Supporting strand of connective tissue

tracer Agent by which certain structures can be identified

trachea This is cartilaginous and membranous tube from the larynx to bronchi. Colloquially called windpipe.

tracheostomy Opening in the anterior trachea for insertion of a tube to relieve upper airway obstruction

tracheotomy Surgical creation of an opening into the trachea through the neck

trachoma Chronic infectious disease of the conjunctiva and cornea, producing photophobia, pain, and lacrimation, caused by a strain of Chlamydia trachomatis organism.

tract Some length of an organ, A collection of nerve fibre, Common tracts of importance are:

- Bulbar tract
- Alimentary tract
- Digestive tract
- Pyramidal tract
- Urinary tract
- Uveal tract
- Vestibulospinal tract

traction Pulling force along the long axis of a structure.

training Preparation by instruction and practice.

trait Genetically determined characteristic.

trance a state of altered consciousness characterized by heightened focal awareness and reduced peripheral awareness .

tranquilizer Drug used to produce calmness in a patient.

transaminase That which catalyze the transfer of an amino group from an amino acid to a 2-keto acid.

transamination the reversible transfer of an amino group from an amino acid to what was originally an α-keto acid

transcript This is usually a strand of nucleic acid that has been synthesized using another nucleic acid strand as a template.

transcriptase This denote a DNA-directed RNA polymerase.

transcription Chemical process by which a single-stranded RNA complementary to one strand of a double-stranded DNA is synthesized.

transdermal Administration of a drug applied to the skin in ointment.

transducer Device that translates one form of energy to another

transdural Meaning through the dura mater.

transferase Enzymes that transfer a chemical group from one compound to another compound .

transformation Conversion from one form to another.

transfusion Introduction of whole blood or blood components directly into the bloodstream. This can be direct, exchange, fetomaternal, placental, replacement or autologous transfusion.

transgenic Pertaining to the experimental splicing of a segment of DNA

transillumination the passage of light through body tissues for the purpose of examination

transition This word is used in molecular genetics. This can represent a point mutation in which a purine base replaces a purine base or a pyrimidine base replaces a pyrimidine base

translation This is the process by which polypeptide chains are synthesized

translocation By the repair in abnormal arrangement in which one segment of a chromosome is transferred to a nonhomologous chromosome

transmigration change of place from one side of the body to the other side. This can be external and internal

transovarial Transmission of pathogens from infected ovary to individuals of the next generation seen among mites and ticks. This is one of the method of biological transmission.

transpiration This refers to the discharge of air, sweat, or vapor through the skin

transplacental Transmission through the placenta.

transplant Organ or tissue from one body taken for grafting into another area of the same body or into another individual

transplant The process of transfer of tissue from one part to another.

transplantation Grafting of tissues which can be from the same person or from the other person. Common transplantations are Bone marrow transplantation, Living donor transplantation, Cadaver organ transplantation

transsexual External anatomy of a person has been changed to that of the opposite sex.

transsexualism Gender identity disorder in adults. They have desire to relinquish their primary and secondary sex characteristics and show desire to acquire those of the opposite sex.

transvestism Desired to assume the appearance of opposite sex.

trapezium Irregular four-sided figure.

trapezoid A shape with four side out of which 2 sides are parallel and two sides diverging.

trauma Physical injury or psychological damage

Trautmann's triangle A triangular space with anterior angle at the prominence of labyrinth, posteriorly by transverse sinus and superiorly by inferior temporal line.

tray Hospital utensil with a flat surface which is used to carry examination equipment's or other objects.

treatment Medical or Surgical management of a patient in the effort of cure of a disease.

Trematoda They are Platyhelminthes or flukes such as Fasciola, Fasciolopsis, and schistosoma groups of flukes.

tremor Involuntary trembling . Common clinical entities are:

Fine tremor, Course tremor, Parkinsonian tremor and arsenic tremor.

Trendelenburg's operation Surgery on varicose veins by ligation of great saphenous vein..

trephine Electrically operated saw for the removal of a circular area of skull bone to relieve pressure within the skull. It also mean an ophthalmic instrument for the removal of circular area of cornea in corneal transplant operations.

Treponema They belong to the family Spirochaetaceae that are gram-negative spiral microorganisms. Syphilis, yaws and pinta are common diseases that are caused by treponema organisms. Treponema pallidum causes syphilis; Treponema pertenue causes yaws.

triad In case of element it will be trivalent. In case of disease it is group of symptoms.

Common triads are as under:

- **Charcot's triad** –1. nystagmus, 2. tremor 3. staccato speech (Multiple sclerosis)
- **Beck's triad** - (1) a high venous pressure, (2) a low arterial pressure, and (3) a small quiet heart. (Cardiac compression)
- **Hutchinson's triad** - 1. diffuse interstitial keratitis 2.labyrinthine disease 3. Hutchison teeth (syphilis)
- **Virchow's triad** – 1. change in vessel wall 2.change in pattern of blood flow 3. change in blood constituent (Thrombosis)
- **Osler's triad** – 1. telangiectasia 2. capillary fragility 3. hereditary haemorrhagic diathesis (Hereditary haemorrhagic telangiectasia).

triamcinolone Synthetic glucocorticoid used in adrenal insufficiency and as an anti-inflammatory

triangle Three-cornered area such as Ilio femoral triangle, carotid triangle, Anal triangle, Einthoven's triangle, Facial triangle, Cervical triangle, Inguinal triangle, etc.,

tribadism Simulated heterosexual intercourse in women.

triceps Three headed triceps muscle.

Trichinella A nematode parasites of the family Trichinellidae

trichobezoar Hair ball in stomach which gets concreted and gives rise to surgical problem.

trichomonad Protozoan of the order Trichomonadida.

Trichomonas Parasitic flagellated protozoa of the order Trichomonadida T.V. infection is common genitourinary infection .

Trichophyton Fungus causing infection of skin, nails,

Trichuris Whipworms belonging to nematodes of the family Trichuridae

tricuspid Having three cusps such as tricuspid valve of the heart.

trigeminal Refers to Fifth cranial nerve.

triiodothyronine Iodine-containing Thyroid hormone which is tissue active form of thyroid hormone.

trilogy Combination of three elements like Fallot's triology (pulmonary stenosis, atrial septal defect and right ventricular hypertrophy).

trimester Period of three months.

trimethoprim Used in combination with a sulfonamide in case of urinary tract infections due E.coli infection and Pneumonia by pneumocystis carinii

trinitrophenol This is a dye and a tissue fixative

trinitrotoluene Explosive obtained by nitrating toluene called TNT.

Tripier's amputation Amputation of foot where calcaneus, talus and parts of tarsus are removed.

triple-angle Referred to dental instrument which has three angles or angulations in the shank connecting to handle, shaft and the working portion

triple blind In case of a clinical trial doctor, patient and even pharmaceutical company do not know which treatment is given to whom. Nowadays TIPLE MASK is used as a better term to triple blind.

triplet Three are produced in a single birth.

tripod A device which has three feet such as tripod stand used in laboratory.

trisaccharide Carbohydrates composed of three glycosidically linked monosaccharide groups.

trismus Spasm of the masticatory muscles, with difficulty in opening the mouth a common symptom of tetanus.

Trisomy Presence of an extra chromosome of one type in an otherwise diploid cell . For example Trisomy 21 the known Dawn's syndrome.

tRNA Abbreviation for Transfer RNA

trocar A pointed instrument with a cannula to puncture the wall of a body cavity and withdraw fluid.

trochanter Processes below the neck of the femur called greater and lesser trochanter.

trochlea Pulley shaped organ such as Trochlea of humerus, Trochlea of calcaneus, Trochlea of fibula etc.,

Troisier's node First sign of abdominal tumor which is an enlarged supraclavicular lymph node.

Trombicula This is the genus of mites of the family Trombiculidae;

trophoblast Trophoblast attaches the blastocyst to the endometrium of the uterine wall and supplies nutrition to the embryo.

trophozoite Active, motile, feeding stage of a protozoan organism,

tropical Geographical regions of the earth bounded by the parallels of latitude 23° 27′ North and South of the Equator.

Trousseau's sign One of the sign in tetany where spasmodic contractions of muscles provoked by pressure upon the nerves which go to them is seen.

truncus Major trunk of a nerve or vessel or a duct.

Trunk Central portion of human body to which limbs and head are attached. This also refers to main trunk of a nerve, or of a vessel.

Trypanosoma Protozoa comprising hemoflagellates which are pathogenic. In man the stage is Trypomastigote stage is seen. Other stages like amastigote, promastigote and epimastigote are seen in blood sucking invertebrates. They produce trypanosomiasis and Chagas' disease.

trypsin This enzyme is secreted by pancreas which becomes active in small intestine that help in protein digestion.

trypsinogen Proenzyme of trypsin secreted by the pancreas that gets activated in the duodenum

tryptophan This is an essential amino acid present in proteins, from which it is set free by tryptic digestion Tryptophan is necessary for optimal growth in infants and for nitrogen equilibrium in human adults.

tsetse African fly of the genus Glossina.

TSH Abbreviation for **T**hyroid **S**timulating **H**ormone.

TU Abbreviation for **T**uberculin **U**nit.

tubal That which is related with tube such as tubal pregnancy.

tube Elongated hollow cylindrical organ such as Auditory tube, Buccal tube, Air tube, Drainage tube, Endotracheal tube, Eustachian tube, Fallopian tube, Feeding tube, Nasogastric tube, Neural tube, Ryle's tube, Tracheal tube, etc.,

tubectomy Surgical cut to produce discontinuity of Fallopian tubes which is a procedure for permanent sterilisation.

tuber Anatomical protuberance such as prominence of calcaneus, of Ischium or of maxillae.

tubercle Granulomatous lesion with central caseation, with macrophages and a rim of mononuclear cells.

tuberculin An antigen used in skin test that contain growth of Mycobacterium tuberculosis organism. Old Tuberculin (O.T.) and Purified Protein Derivative (PPD) are commonly available antigens.

tuberculosis Infection by M. Tuberculosis with the formation of tubercles and caseous necrosis in the tissues. Pulmonary and non pulmonary tuberculosis are common types in clinical practice.

tuberosity A protuberance such as Gluteal tuberosity of femur, Iliac tuberosity etc.,

tubocurarine Alkaloid isolated from the bark of chondrodendron tomentosum which is the active principle of curare.

tuboplasty plastic repair of uterine tube or the auditory tube

tubule Refers to a small tube such as renal tubule, Malpighian tubule, Seminiferous tubule etc.,

tuft This refers to a small clump such as Hair tuft, synovial tuft, etc.,

tularemia Infection by bacillus Francisella tularensis first reported in a place called Tulare in California and hence the name. This is mainly disease of rabbit, muskrats and is transmitted by the bite of fleas, ticks or deer flies.

tumefacient Drug or a substance which cause swelling.

tumescence Means swelling

tumor (too'm[schwa]r) Growth of tissues with uncontrolled multiplication. Types of tumor in clinical practice are:

✓ Malignant tumor

- ✓ Benign tumor
- ✓ Burkitt's tumor
- ✓ Cystic tumor
- ✓ Desmoid tumor
- ✓ Fibroid tumor
- ✓ Wilms' tumor

tunica This refers to a lining of a part or of an organ.

turbid Cloudiness of a liquid such as water is turbid. This is due to scattering of light by colloidal particles which are suspended particles.

turgid If an organ is swollen and congested. The word turgor is also used for this nature.

turmeric From a rhizome that contains curcumin an orange yellow coloring principles used as a condiment.

Turner's syndrome A gonadal dysfunction. The patient is phenotypically female. But gonads are undifferentiated. Other abnormalities seen are

- ❖ Short stature
- ❖ Webbing of neck
- ❖ Cubitus valgus
- ❖ Heart defects

turnover Rate at which something is replaced.

turpentine An volatile oil Turpentine oil present in plant Pinus palustris which has an oleoresin.

Tween It is polysorbate preparation. *Tween 80 which is commonly used is* a trademark for polysorbate 80.

twin Two offspring produced which may be monozygotic or dizygotic but fertilized at the same time.

tympanectomy Surgical excision of the tympanic membrane.

tympanoplasty Surgical reconstruction of the hearing mechanism of the middle ear with restoration of the drum membrane to protect the round window from sound pressure and establishment of ossicular continuity between the tympanic membrane and the oval window.

typhoid Bacterial infection called Typhoid or Para typhoid which causes delirious condition of brain.

typhus Caused by rickettsia through arthropods. Tick typhus is commonly seen.

tyrosine Nonessential amino acid found in most proteins and synthesized metabolically from phenylalanine This is a precursor of thyroid hormones, catecholamines, and melanin.

U

U Symbol for Unit

u Denotes the Atomic Mass Unit.

uberty This is the stage of fertility in humans or animals.

udder The milking organ the mammary organ of cattle which have teat.

UDP Abbreviation for **U**ridine **Di** **P**hosphate.

ulalgia Pain in the gum or Gingiva.

ulcer Ulcer is produced by sloughing of necrotic tissue which is usually followed by severe inflammatory changes.

ulceration Formation of an ulcer.

ulitis Infection and inflammation of gum

Ullrich-Feichtiger syndrome Multiple defect syndrome associated with Micrognathia, Hexadactyly, Small eyes, Depressed nose, Genital anomalies, Hypertelorism, and ear protuberance.

Ullrich-Turner syndrome This is Male Turner's syndrome which the phenotype of Turner's syndrome which do not show gonadal dysgenesis.

ulna Firearm bone which is towards inner side and is larger than the outer bone of forearm.

ulnar Related to the medial side or ulnar side of forearm

ultra- That which is excess or beyond

ultracentrifuge Centrifuge with high speed of rotation which will separate and sediment the molecules of a substance.

ultrafilter That filters through semi permeable membrane

ultrafiltration Filtration through semi permeable membrane constitute ultra filtration. Natural ultra filtration like Plasma filtration through capillary membrane; artificial Ultra filtration like Blood Dialysis are well known examples. Latest technique of artificial ultra filtration involves use of pressure gradients for bulk movement of solute and solvent across the membrane.

ultramicroscope This laboratory method is called Dark field Illumination which require special type of microscope for colloidal particles.

ultramicroscopic Minute organisms or particles which cannot be seen by ordinary microscope but need special type of microscopes.

ultrasonic They are supersonic radiant energy which has the frequency of above 20,000 Hertz which are not audible by ordinary human beings.

ultrasonics This refers to Medical Diagnostic Ultra Sonography where ultrasonic waves with above 500 Kilo Hertz .

ultrasonogram The recordings of ultrasonography.

ultrasonography In routine process it is called scanning in Medical Diagnosis. When U.S. Waves are directed to tissues, they are reflected and are called as "Echoes". Depending on the tissues exposed this can be 'Echo cardiography' 'Echo Encephalography etc., In Radiodiagnosis the term used as synonyms like Echography or Sonography. Latest additions of Ultrasonography are:

- Doppler Ultrasonography which include Pulsed wave Doppler ultrasonography, Continuous wave Doppler Ultrasonography, Colour Flow Doppler Imaging.

- Duplex Ultrasonography
- Endorectal
- Endoscopic
- Gray scale
- I.V.

ultrasound They are ultrasonic radiant energy with more than 20000 Hertz

ultraviolet They are popularly called a U.V. rays which are perceived beyond the violet end of the light spectrum with wavelength from 200 nm to 400 nm. Following natural phenomenon are seen:-

I. Act on the skin to produce Vitamin D (17 dehydrocholesterol)
II. Produce tanning of skin
III. Produce sun burn of skin
IV. Has actinic property
V. Has chemical property

umbilical That which is related to Umbilicus.

umbilication Depression similar to the umbilicus observed in anatomical organs.

umbilicus Colloquially it is called Naves which is the site of umbilical cord attachment in intra uterine life.

umbra In sharp contrast radiography it is the area of shadow where there is no illumination.

uncomplemented That which is active by itself. But becomes active when it is combined with a complement.

unconscious Person who is not responding to sensory stimuli and one who is in coma. Mind that is not accessible to present awareness. It can be Freud's Topographic model of human mind.

unction Cream or ointment that is applied on to the skin which can act by the process of inunctions.

uncus Anatomical organ which is hook-shaped

undernutrition Generally it means malnutrition. But different stages of malnutrition are Sub nutrition, Under nutrition and Frank starvation. In public health activities grades of malnutrition are expressed which give precise picture.

understain Refers to pathological slides stained which are less stained than normal.

undertoe This refers to Hallux Valgus where big toe is displaced under other toes.

undifferentiated This is Oncology terminology which explain the cellular arrangement of cancerous tissue.

undifferentiation Anaplasia of tissues where pattern of arrangement is gone.

Undritz anomaly This refers to Hereditary Hypersegmentation of Neutrophils described by Undritz.

undulant Refers to Undulant fever which has fluctuations.

undulation Refers to wave like motion of an item such as a Pulse.

ungual Pertaining to the nails.

unguent An ointment This is also called Unguentum.

unguis They refer to finger nails or toe nails which are horny cutaneous plates.

uni- Means 'One' used as a prefix

uniarticular Related with one joint.

unicellular Organism made of one single cell such as Amoeba, Bacteria.

unicornous Organ which has one horn.

unidirectional Refers to fluid which flows in one direction.

uniflagellate Organism which has one flagella

unilateral Situated or affected one side only.

unilobar Single lobed structure or organ.

unilocular That which has one compartment.

unimodal Having only one mode.

union Repair after an injury, The process of healing, Continuity in a broken bone or between the edges of a wound.

uniovular Monozygotic or with single ovum.

unipolar Person who is found to have only depression in life. Nerve cell having single pole.

unisexual Either Male or Female.

unit It refers to a standard measurement such as Bodansky unit of Alkaline Phosphatase, British Thermal Unit,

univalent Monovalent chemicals

unmyelinated Nerve fibre which do not possess a myelin sheath

Unna's paste boot In the treatment of Varicose Ulcers, a paste prepared from a) Gelatine b) Zink Oxide and c) Glycerine I pasted to leg and covered with a spiral bandage. Pasting and spiral bandaging is repeated till one gets rigid feeling of the leg. Sometimes 3 to 4 coating of pasting and 3 to 4 spiral bandaging is required in patients.

unsaturated Always referred to Unsaturated fatty acids which have Carbon to Carbon bonding In organic compound multiple pairs of shared electrons are present to form Unsaturated compound. This also refers to the solution in which a solute can be dissolved.

unstriated Muscles which are not having striations.

Unverricht's disease Myoclonic Epilepsy described by Unverricht.

UPPP Abbreviation for **U**vulo **P**alato **P**haryngo **P**lasty in Plastic Surgery.

upsilon [Υ, υ] The Greek alphabet.

uptake Absorption as well as intake of a substance by tissues. e.g., Radioactive Iodine uptake,

urachovesical Related with urachus and the urinary bladder.

urachus This anatomical structure is from Allantoic stalk in intra uterine life that connects umbilicus and urinary bladder. At later date this is seen as fibrous cord called Median Umbilical Ligament.

uracil This is a component of RNA that is required in body metabolism.

uracratia Clinical condition of Urinary incontinence.

uragogue Diuretics used for increasing urinary flow in a patient.

uraniscochasma Clinical condition of Cleft Palate

uraniscoplasty Correction in plastic surgery called Palatoplasty.

uraniscorrhaphy Repair in Plastic surgery called Palatorrhaphy.

uranium Radioactive Metallic element which is hard and heavy which contains three isotope entities which are U 234, U 235, and U238.

uranoschisis Clinical condition called Cleft Palate and the condition is called Uranoschism.

urarthritis Arthritis of Gout.

urate Salt of uric acid .

Urbach-Wiethe disease Lipid Proteinosis described by Urbach.

urceiform Pitcher-shaped.

urea Deamination of amino acids in liver via Urea Cycle produces the compound which has the formula $CO(NH_2)_2$. Increased Urea in blood is called Azotaemia that occurs in chronic renal diseases.

urease This is an enzyme that catalyses the hydrolysis of urea to CO_2 and ammonia concentrations.

uremia Collection of excess quantity of products of protein metabolism such as Urea, Uric acid and other nitrogenous waste products in the blood. Clinical features of uraemia are:

- Nausea vomiting and metallic taste in mouth
- Sweet disagreeable smell of breath
- Pruritus
- Pain and twitching of muscles
- Mental confusion
- Electrolyte imbalance

ureolysis The chemical process of decomposition of urea to carbon dioxide and ammonia.

uresis The act of urination

ureter This is the fibro muscular tube which conveys the urine from the kidney to the bladder.

ureterocele It is due to stenosis of ureteral meatus, calculation of the terminal portion of the ureter occurs

ureterocervical That which is related with ureter and cervix.

ureterocystoscope The Cystoscope used for catheterising ureter.

ureterogram Radiograph of the ureter.

ureterography Opaque medium is injected into the ureter and radiographed for diagnostic purpose.

ureterolith A calculus in ureter.

ureterolithiasis A calculus formation in ureter.

ureterophlegma Mucus in the ureter.

ureteroplasty Surgical repair of ureter.

ureteropyelography Radiography of the Pelvis and Ureter of the Kidney.

ureteropyelonephritis Infection and inflammation of the ureter and the pelvis of the kidney.

ureterorrhaphy Suturing the ureter.

ureteroscope Endoscopic examination of ureter by using endoscope.

urethra Passage from urinary bladder to outside by a canal which is made of membranous tissue.

urethral That which is related with urethra.

urethrism Spasm of the Urethra.

urethritis Infection and inflammation of the urethra.

urethrobulbar Related with the urethra and bulbus penis.

urethrocele Diverticulum of urethral wall upon vagina. Prolapse of female urethra through urinary meatus.

urethropenile Related with urethra and the penis.

urethroperineal Pertaining to the urethra and the perineum.

urethroperineoscrotal Pertaining to the urethra, perineum, and scrotum.

urethrorrhagia Blood flow from Urethra.

urethroscope The instrument used for viewing the interior of the urethra.

urethroscopy Direct visual observation of interior urethra.

urethrospasm Urethral Muscle tissue spasm.

urethrostenosis Stricture of the urethra.

urethrovaginal That which is related with urethra and vagina. Pertaining to fistula connecting the urethra and the vagina.

urethrovesical That which is related with urethra and urinary bladder. Pertaining to fistula connecting the urethra and urinary bladder.

urgency Urge to urinate or to defecate.

-uria Suffixing word to denote nature of urine such as Oliguria, Proteinuria etc.,

uric acid This is the end-product of purine Metabolism. Gout is related with the disorder of this metabolism.

uricopoiesis This refers to the formation of uric acid.

uridine This is related with the biosynthesis of polysaccharides and is the component of RNA.

urinal Any receptacle for the collection of urine. a vessel or other receptacle for urine.

urinalysis Qualitative and quantitative analysis of urine in terms of physical, chemical, Biological, Radiological or microscopic analysis or examination of urine.

urination The Act of Micturition.

urine It is the output of fluid after excretion from the kidneys that pass through ureters and stores in urinary bladder. Urine output and urine constituents are described for normal and abnormal or pathological variations

uriniferous That which convey the urine such as Uriniferous tubules.

urobenzoic acid Other name for Hippuric acid.

urobilin It is present in stool and urine which is an oxidised form of urobilinogen.

urobilinogen This is produced in the intestine by the reduction of bilirubin Some portion of urobilinogen is excreted in stool, other portion is reabsorbed to get excreted as bilirubin.

urocele Swollen scrotum which contain extravasated urine.

urochrome This is urinary pigment which is responsible for the yellow colour of the urine.

urochromogen A precursor of urochrome. Urochromogen on oxidation becomes urochrome.

urodialysis When urine output is reduced we use the word uro dialysis.

urodynia Urination is associated with pain.

uroerythrin Urates of red colour in urine called purpuria.

urogaster In Embryology it is described as a part of allantoic cavity of the embryo.

urogastrone Other name for Human Epidermal Growth Factor.

urogenital Otherwise called Genitourinary.

Urografin Used in Radio diagnosis as contrast medium which is Diatrizoate Meglumine.

urogram This is Urinary tract Radiograph.

urography This can be Ascending Urography, Cystoscopic urography, Descending Urography or Retrograde urography. By using opaque medium Urinary tract is made opaque for diagnosis.

urokinase It is chemically an activator called U Plasminogen Activator.

urolith Refers to Urinary calculus.

urolithiasis Kidney disease following urinary calculi.

urologist A specialist and consultant in Urology.

urology Science that deals with male and female urinary tract and genital tract diseases.

uronephrosis Pelvis of the kidney and Tubules of the kidney are distended with urine giving rise to pathological conditions.

uronic acid Uronic acids or alduronic acids are **a class of sugar acids with both carbonyl and carboxylic acid functional groups**. They are sugars in which the hydroxyl group furthest from the carbonyl group has been oxidized to a carboxylic acid. Usually the sugar is an aldose, but fructuronic acid also occurs.

urophilia Urine is linked with sexual arousal.

uropoietic Connected with the production of urine in a person.

uroporphyria porphyria in which there is excessive excretion of uroporphyrin.

uropsammus Presence of gravel in the urine.

urorhythmography Recording the urine flow from ureteral orifices by radiography.

uroscopic Related with Uroscopic examination .

urosepsis Pathogens of urinary tract entering into blood stream causing sepsis with clinical manifestation of fever, chills.

urotoxia Urine is found to be toxic by containing toxic substances.

urotoxin Presence of poisonous substances in the urine.

urticant Itching and wheat formation by a substance.

urticaria Local oedema of skin with increased vascular permeability along with wheals. Urticaria can be any one of the following:

1) Immune mediated
2) Complement mediated

US Abbreviation for Ultra Sound.

Usher's syndrome An autosomal recessive disorder which show the following manifestations:

i. Congenital deafness
ii. Retinitis pigmentosa
iii. Blindness
iv. Mental retardation
v. Gait disturbances

USP Abbreviation for **U**nited **S**tates **P**harmacopeia.

USPHS Abbreviation for **U**nited **S**tates **P**ublic **H**ealth **S**ervice.

uta Indian name derived from Peru for Cutaneous Leishmaniasis. This is mild self limiting skin ulcer manifested disease cause by the parasite Leishmania.

uteri The name of Uterus major female reproductive organ.

uterine That which is elated with uterus.

uterogenic That which is formed in the uterus.

uterogestation Pregnancy occurred in the uterus. Intra uterine development of foetus.

uterography Radiography of uterus for the purpose of diagnosis which is called Hysterography.

utero-ovarian That which is related with uterus and ovary.

uteroplasty Surgical repair of uterus or any reconstructive surgery on uterus.

uteroscope Device to observe the uterus directly for diagnostic purpose. which is called Hysteroscopy.

uterotomy Cutting open of the uterus called Hysterotomy.

uterotonic The Drug that increases the tonus of the uterine muscle.

uterovaginal That which is related with uterus and vagina.

uterovesical Pertaining to the uterus and the bladder.

uterus Anatomical structure called major reproductive organ in females which helps in the development of embryo/ foetus after conception. Fundus, Isthmus and body are three parts of this organ. It has direct connection with vagina below and abdominal cavity above. Indirect attachment with pelvic structure is called Metra.

utilization Any item or substance which is found useful and used.

utriculus This is a component of Vestibule which is a sac like structure in Membranous labyrinth that gives information about position and movements of man .

utriform Any organ or anatomical structure which is having the shape of a bottle.

uva If a structure is looking like grape or a fruit

uvea This refers to the covering of the eye ball .

uveitis Infection and inflammation of the uvea which also involves sclera, cornea and retina

uveomeningitis Infection and inflammation of Uvea and Meninges.

uviform That which has the form of a grape.

uvula Pendent and fleshy mass attached to the posterior aspect of palate.

uvulectomy Surgical excision of the uvula.

uvulitis Infection and inflammation of the uvula which is also called as staphylitis.

V

VA Abbreviation for **V**isual **A**cuity

VAC Cancer treatment regimen with **V**incristine, **A**ctinomycin, and **C**yclophosphamide chemotherapy.

vaccinate Inoculation with vaccine for Active Immunization

vaccination Originally it meant to inoculate cowpox vaccine to prevent smallpox infection. Now it is generalized to include other vaccines also.

vaccine Attenuated or killed microorganisms like Bacteria, Virus and Rickettsia when introduced to the body produce antibodies that can prevent the development of diseases. Common vaccines used in National Immunization Programme are:

- o DPT called Triple Antigen
- o OPV
- o BCG
- o Measles

Other vaccines used are:

- ▪ Cholera
- ▪ Typhoid
- ▪ Plague
- ▪ Anti Rabies
- ▪ Meningococcal
- ▪ Japanese Encephalitis
- ▪ Anthrax
- ▪ Hepatitis A
- ▪ Hepatitis B
- ▪ Influenza
- ▪ Measles, Mumps and Rubella
- ▪ Yellow Fever

VACTERL Abbreviation used for birth defects following birth control pills, which include the following;-

- **V**ertebral defects
- **A**nal defects
- **C**ardiac defects
- **T**racheal defects
- **E**sophageal defects
- **R**enal defects
- **L**imb defects

vacuole Space in the protoplasm of a cell.

vagal Related to the vagus nerve.

vagina Any tubular anatomical structure. Special reference is made to Vaginal which is the genital canal in female (vulva to cervix) This is the organ to receive male organ during intercourse.

vaginal That which is related with vagina.

vaginismus Owing to psychological and organic cause involuntary contraction of vaginal musculature contracts to produce severe pain. Hence painful intercourse is named as vaginismus.

vaginitis Infection and inflammation of the vagina

vagolytic Impulse of vagus gets inrturrupted and the action is called Parasympatholytic.

vagotomy By cutting the vagus nerve it's impulse is interrupted.

vagovagal When both Afferent and Efferent impulses are transmitted through vagus nerve.

vagus This is 10th Cranial nerve called Vagus Nerve.

valence Represents the combining power of an element in a chemical compound,

Valentin's corpuscles Amyloid bodies found in nerve tissues.

Valentine's position This position is used in the irrigation of urethra. Patient lies in supsine position with hips flexed.

valgus legs bent outward

validity Extent of purporting a test, particularly in case of screening test.

valine an essential amino acid, This is chemically α-aminovaleric acid which is an essential amino acid. It is essential for growth and nitrogen equilibrium.

valine transaminase This enzyme acts on valine and is a branched chain amino acid transaminase.

vallum Wall like anatomical structure such as nail wall which is called vellum unguis.

valone An anticoagulant used as rodenticide.

Valsalva's maneuver With closed glottis forced expiration produce high intrathoracic pressure that brings about lowered venous return to the heart.

value Value suggests the efficiency of a substance such as buffer value, P value, reference value, Z value etc.,

valva This is a Valve such as Aortic valve, Mitral valve etc., which are membranous folds which prevent backward flow or influx.

valvula Small valve such as valvulae anales (anal), Valvula ileocolic (ileocaecal) etc.,

VAMP Cancer regimen with **V**incristine, Methotrex**a**te, 6-**M**ercaptopurine, and **P**rednisone in cancer chemotherapy.

vancomycin An antibiotic from soil bacteria used in the treatment of staphylococci infections.

van den Bergh's test This is a qualitative test for Bilirubin . Here a standard solution of diazotized bilirubin is compared with serum containing bilirubin or plasma bilirubin is compared which is diazotized.

van der Hoeve's syndrome Osteogenesis Imperfecta Type I described by Van Der Hoeve

Vane British Pharmacologist who won Nobel Prize for his discovery of Prostaglandins.

van Hook's operation Ureter and Ureter anastomosis devised by Van Hook.

van Hoorne's canal The Thoracic Duct described by Van Hoorne.

Vanilla Mexican and Bourbon type of fruits which are sources of favoring agents in Ice creams.

Van Slyke's formula The formula is used to find out urinary coefficient by considering output of urine in a day and body weight.

$$\text{Urinary Coefficient} = \frac{D}{B \times \text{square root of body weight} \times V}$$

Where, D = Daily output of solids in urine in grams
B = Same solids in Grams per liter of blood
Body weight is = wt of patient
V = total volume of urine in one day

vapor Refer to steam, gas, or an exhalation.

vaporization Without any chemical change a solid or a liquid is converted into vapor.

vaporizer This refers to a Nebuliser which is used by asthma patient for inhaling medicated aerosol.

Vaquez's disease Polycythemia Vera described by Vaquez.

variable That which is variable or changes from time to time. It can be a symbol for a set in mathematics.

variance This is the square of S.D. for given set of values and is represented by the symbol σ^2.

$$\text{Variance} = \frac{Ó\,(X - x)^2}{n} \text{ or } \frac{Ó\,(X - x)^2}{n-1}$$

varicella Latin word meaning chickenpox

varicocele Varicose condition of the veins of the pampiniform plexus

variola Latin word meaning small pox which is globally eradicated .

varix Enlarged and tortuous vein

Varolius' bridge Bridging connections like Pons and Ileocaecal valve described by Varolius.

. **arus** bent inward like talipes varus.

vas Refers to an anatomical canal which carry spermatozoa, lymph or blood . Common vas in anatomical terms are:
- Vasa vasorum
- Vasa praevia
- Vas deference
- Vas epididymitis
- Vasa lymphatica

vascular Related to vessels i.e., blood vessels.

vasculitis Inflammation of a blood or lymph vessel.

vasectomy Surgical removal of portion of the vas deferens to induce infertility.

vasoconstriction Constriction of arterioles leading to decreased blood flow

vasodilatation Dilatation of arterioles leading to increased blood flow.

vasomotor Affecting the caliber of a blood vessel.

vasopressin Nonapeptide hormone that is formed by neuronal cells of hypothalamic nuclei and stored in the neurohypophysis which stimulates contraction of muscles of capillaries and arterioles, raising blood pressure

VATER abbreviation for birth defects complex which is composed of the following:
- o **V**ertebral defects
- o Imperforated **A**nus
- o **T**racgei **E**sophageal fistula
- o **R**adial and **R**enal dysplasia

Vater's ampulla Hepatopancreatic Ampulla described by Vater.

vault Domelike anatomical structure such as cranial vault.

VC Abbreviation for **V**ital **C**apacity.

VD Abbreviation for **V**enereal **D**isease Which is also called S.T.D.(**S**exually **T**ransmitted **D**iseases)

VDRL Abbreviation for **V**enereal **D**isease **R**esearch **L**aboratories .

vection Infection is transmitted from diseased person to normal person by different route, that is common in infectious and communicable diseases.

vector Refers to a carrier which can be an animal, an insect which can transmit disease from one person to another. Arthropods like mosquito, Flies, Ticks, Mites and Cyclops are common vectors in the transmission of infectious diseases. Different types of vectors known are:

Mechanical vector
Biological vector

vector-borne Refers to infectious diseases which spread one host to another by a vector

vecuronium bromide Neuromuscular blocking agent which is used (I.V.) as an adjunct to general anesthesia to induce relaxation of skeletal muscle and to facilitate endotracheal intubation and mechanical ventilation

vegetable Food from plant origin which are classified into a) Leafy vegetable b) Roots and Tubers and c) Other vegetables.

vegetative Related to asexual reproduction like budding and fission.

vein Venous or impure blood passes through these vessels and goes back to the heart for purification.

Vel blood group It was described in 1952 by taking into account of erythrocytic antigens and are grouped under two groups namely a) Vel 1 and b) Vel 2.

velar Related to Velum oa palate from where the sounds like G and K are produced.

Vella's fistula Term used in animal experiments in Physiology where in an artificial opening into an isolated segment of intestine is allowed with both ends opened and sutured to abdominal wall.

velocity This denotes the rate of movement of a body in a given direction. In Physics it is symbolically represented as V. Air velocity, Nerve conduction velocity etc.,

venation It tells how the veins are distributed.

venepuncture Cut open of a vein for the purpose of infusion which is commonly done when there is collapse of veins. It is also called Venesection.

venereal Related to sex related diseases and referable to S.T.D.

venereology This is the branch of medicine that deals with sexually transmitted diseases.

venom Poisonous substance secreted by snake, scorpion, spider, which can kill animals and human beings.

venous That which is related with veins.

ventilation This involves taking in of air (inspiration) and breathing out of air (expiration), both together constitute respiration .

ventilator Device or an instrument which is used to assist artificial respiration. It is also called Mechanical ventilator. Common types of Ventilators that are used in Intensive care unit are:

- Tank or Drinker Ventilator
- Cuirass negative pressure ventilator

ventral In man it is front portion or anterior surface of the body. In animals, it is lower portion or inferior surface of the body.

ventricular Related with ventricle.

Venturi mask This is device mask by Venturi which deliver a controlled mixture of oxygen and air. This is popularly called Face mask for Oxygen therapy.

VEP Abbreviation for **V**isual **E**voked **P**otential.

verapamil hydrochloride Drug used in Angina Pectoris (chest pain) that helps in the dilatation of coronary artery of the heart. This is a calcium channel blocker that dilates coronary arteries.

verbal That which is related with speech.

Veress needle This needle contains sharp trocar with slanted end that is surrounded by an inner cylinder with blunt end. This is used in case of insufflation of body cavity without injuring internal organs.

Verner-Morrison syndrome This is also called Diarrheagenic Syndrome which is characterized by ;

- Profuse watery diarrhea
- Hypokalaemia
- Achlorhydria
- High level of intestinal polypeptides

Vernet's syndrome This is Jugular foramen syndrome associated with the paralysis of 9th, 10th and 11th Cranial nerves. Clinical manifestations include Difficulty in swallowing, Loss of taste, Dysfunction of vocal cord.

verruca They are epidermal proliferations called Wart.

versicolor That which is changing it's color.

version This means tilting of uterus, This also means manual conversion of polarity of foetus in the uterus with reference to the mother.

vertebra Backbone which is made of 33 vertebrae which are named after their positions in the body such as Cervical, Thoracic, Lumbar, Sacral and Coccygeal vertebrae.

vertex Anatomical description for the top portion of an organ or of a structure. For example Vertex of cranium

vertical That which is perpendicular to the place of the body.

vertigo Dizziness due to ear problem or nervous system. Types of vertigo are:

- Labyrinthine vertigo
- Toxic vertigo
- Vestibular vertigo
- Angiopathic vertigo
- Cerebral vertigo
- Pilot's vertigo
- Arteriosclerotic vertigo
- Epileptic vertigo
- Postural vertigo
- Organic vertigo

Vesalius Vesalius lived during 1514–1564. He dissected and observed anatomical structure and wrote human body, which was the root for modern anatomy. He detailed osteology and Myology. Vesalius made naming of anatomical structures.

Vesalius' ligament Inguinal ligament described by Vesalius.

vesica Any receptacle such as gall bladder, Urinary bladder

vesicle a sac containing liquid such as auditory vesicle, brain vesicle, germinal vesicle, Occular vesicle, ophthalmic vesicle, seminal vesicle, optic vesicle

vesicovaginal Communicating with the urinary bladder and vagina.

vessel Channel for carrying blood.

vestibule Cavity at the entrance to a canal

vestibulocochlear Related to the vestibule of the ear and the cochlea.

vestibulum A space at the entrance to a canal or a depression or an invagination.

vestigium Remains of any structure which has undergone degeneration.

veterinary Related with diseases of domestic animals.

viable Foetus which is capable of living outside the uterus. Gestational age of 20 weeks and weight of more than 0.5 Kg especially said of a fetus that has reached such a stage of development that it can live outside of the uterus.

Viagra The ingredient is Sildenafil Citrate which is sex stimulator.

vial This refers to a small bottle that contains medicaments for parental administration.

Vibrio Gram-negative, facultative anaerobic, rod-shaped bacteria that are actively motile. They cause Cholera.

vicarious Any structure found in abnormal site other that it's normal position.

vigilance Actively watching over the disease occurrence in a community so that one is ready to respond to it's epidemic.

villikinin Duodenal hormone that stimulates villus movement. Villikinin is produced when HCl acts on gastric mucosa.

vinblastine sulfate Vinca alkaloids drug used intravenously in the treatment of cancers like Ca. breast, Choriocarcinoma, Neuroblastoma, Lymphosarcoma and Hodgkin's disease.

Vincent's angina Very painful condition of acute necrotizing ulcerative gingivitis.

vincristine sulfate Vinca alkaloids drug used intravenously in the treatment of Wilms's tumor, Sarcoma, Leukemia and brain tumors.

vindesine sulfate Vinca alkaloid drug used in the treatment of Lymphoid leukemia as anti cancer drug.

Vineberg operation By Pass heart surgery by implanting internal mammary artery into myocardium for a good collateral circulation.

vinegar Diluted acetic acid obtained by fermentation of cider and wine.

Vinson's syndrome Hypochromic anaemia in women with angular stomatitis, painful tongue and dysphagia. It is also called Plummer Vinson Syndrome.

viomycin sulfate Intramuscular preparation of antibiotic used in the treatment of Pulmonary tuberculosis.

viraginity Manly woman

Virchow was a pathologist from whom modern pathology started. He has described medical history, public health and anatomical pathology. According to him a cell is one citizen of human body and illness is a civil war in the body. He did not agree on Virchow's, Darwin's and Semmelweis's postulations.

virgin Unmarried which imply that the person not had sexual intercourse. It may also mean to keep away from intercourse.

virginity the condition of being a virgin.

viricidal That which kills virus i.e., virucidal agent.

virile Copulating power of male or Masculine.

virilism Female showing Masculine characters like developing hair on the body and beard, no breast development and more masculine

virion Viral particle which survives in living tissues.

virologist Person who is an expert in the study of virus and it's characteristics including it's diagnosis and management.

virology Science under microbiology which studies viruses and viral diseases.

virulence Severity with which a pathogen produce pathogenicity which is measured by Median lethal dose (LD_{50}) or Median infective dose (ID_{50}).

virus They are Ultra Microscopic organisms which can survive only in living tissues. There are many types of viruses that cause many viral infections in man. According to host specificity they are grouped under a) Bacterial viruses b) Animal viruses and Plant viruses. Other classifications include according to their origin, their mode of transmission, on clinical manifestations and on the name of place where they were detected first.

viscera This refers to body organs.

viscerotomy This is Forensic science word denoting incision of organ in Post Mortem examinations.

viscosity Physical property of a liquid which allow the resistance to it's flow.

viscous That which is sticky in it's physical property.

vision Special sense of vision which is by visual stimuli at retina of the eye.

visual That which is related to vision.

vital That which is related with life.

vitamin One of the requirement for the body growth and physiological functions of man which may be Fat soluble or Water soluble. Major Vitamins of public health importance are:

- Vitamin A
- Vitamin D
- Vitamin E
- Vitamin K
- Vitamin B complex
- Vitamin C

vitiligo Depigmented white patches with hyperpigmented border which is called Leucoderma that is attributed to an autoimmune disorders.

vitrectomy Extraction of contents of vitreous chamber of the eye

vitreous Vitreous body of the eye which is glasslike or hyaline

vivi Relationship to life.

vividialysis Peritoneal dialysis or Peritoneal lavage done in case of peritonitis .

viviparous Child bearing or offspring bearing in the womb from where the growing child or offspring gets nourishment.

vivisection Animal experiment for the purpose of research.

Vladimiroff's operation Removal of sternomastoid muscle in wry neck. (in torticollis) Orthopedic operation where the foot is brought into line with the leg in which heel, calcaneus are removed.

vocal Voice related.

Voges-Proskauer test It is a test to differentiate enterobacteriaceae. This is popularly called V P reaction. Development of red colour when a culture is treated with a solution of KOH and creatine, it indicates VP positive.

Vogt's syndrome This is attributed to disturbance of corpus stratum due to birth trauma which is characterized by the following clinical manifestations:

- Walking difficulties
- Spasmodic outbursts of laughing and crying,
- Speech disorder
- Bilateral athetosis

Vohwinkel's syndrome Mutilating Keratoma which is hereditary in nature described by Vohwinkel.

voice Sound produced by the larynx and modified by the vocal cords and other structures in the pharynx and oral cavity. Types are Whispering voice, Cavernous voice, double voice, woman voice.

void Excretion of urine or stool.

volar Related to palm or related to sole.

volatile Substance which has the tendency to evaporate.

Volkmann's canal Passage for the blood vessels in the bone.

Volkmann's contracture Severe contracture of fingers and wrist due to injury, tight pressure use like tourniquet that leads to ischaemic muscular atrophy.

volt This is the unit of E M F (Electro Motive Force) that is equal to 1 joule per coulomb.

voltmeter Instrument for measuring E M F

volume Quantity of a substance. E.g., Circulatory volume, blood volume etc.,

voluntary According to will (when a thing is accomplished)

volvulus Twisting that gives rise to Intestinal obstruction that constitute surgical emergency.

vomer Bone of the nasal septum.

vomit Content of stomach is casted out such as blood vomit, bilious vomit,

vomiting Emesisi or forcible expulsion of stomach contents

vomitus Content that is vomited.

Vossius' ring Because of contusion injury a ring is formed in papillary margin.

voyeurism Real involvement or fantasy observation of sexual activity that is repeatedly done. Intense sex urge.

VPC Abbreviation for **V**entricular **P**remature **C**omplex

VR Abbreviation for **V**ocal **R**esonance.

Vrolik's disease Osteogenesis Imperfecta Type II described by Vrolik.

VT Abbreviation for **V**entricular **T**achycardia.

vulcanize Process of producing flexible and hard rubber from raw Rubber. In rubber industry use of Sulphur, heat and high steam pressure are used.

vulgaris Refers to common condition such as Acne vulgaris.

vulnerability Susceptible to infection or disease.

vulsella Forceps with claw like hooks at the end.

vulva Female pudendum or external genital organs of the female

vulvorectal Related with vulva and rectum such as vulvorectal fistula.

VZIG Abbreviation for Varicella Zoster Immuno Globulin.

W

W Abbreviation for Watt in electricity science.

waist The body portion between hips and the thorax where waist belt is put.

wakefulness This refers to the state of consciousness.

Waksman Russian-born American microbiologist, 1888–1973 who discovered Streptomycin wonder drug for Tuberculosis Won Nobel prize in 1952 for Medicine and Physiology.

Waldenström's disease This refers to Osteochondrosis described by Waldenstrom.

walk The locomotor movement of man on the ground which is called Gait.

walker Physical support to the handicapped to move about with the help of crutch or a cane.

wall Harder surface of a structure or of a space or of a mass. E.g., Anterior wall of vagina, Cell wall etc.,

Wallenberg's syndrome This is anatomically called as Posterior Inferior Cerebellar Artery Syndrome as described by Dr. Wallenberg. Artery occlusion leads to

— Loss of pain and temperature on the face which Ipsilateral

— Loss of pain and temperature on the Trunk and extremities which is Contralateral

wallerian degeneration This is Secondary Degeneration commonly called Fatty degeneration of nerve fibers.

wandering Loosely attached anatomical part is referred to as wandering structure.

ward Hospital accommodation for In patient treatment which may be conservative or surgical in nature.

warfarin The word is coined from **W**isconsin **A**lumni **R**esearch **F**oundation Coum**arin** anticoagulant. This is a known Rodenticide used to kill rats.

Waring's method Sanitary method of disposal of sewage by Waring. This is called Sub Surface Irrigation method which allow Aerobic digestion.

Warren's incision see under Surgical cut is done through Thoracomammary fold which will allow access to all parts of the breast in surgery.

Warthin's tumor Adenolymphoma described by Warthiun.

wash In medical field the term used are Irrigation and Lavage for the cleansing done such as Mouth wash, eye wash Perineal wash etc.,

wasp Refers to insect stings that produce pain on prick. Multiple wasp sting need medical emergency treatment.

Wassermann test This test was described by Wassermann in 1906. This is Non Treponemal Antigen Serologic Test for Syphilis.

wasting General term for depletion of body store which is called Emaciation. Many illness produce wasting and major ones known are Tuberculosis, Cancer and AIDS

water This is Universal Solvent with the formula H_2O_n

water-borne Diseases that are transmitted through or water is vehicle for the transmission. They are:

- Bacterial — Typhoid, Paratyphoid, Dysentery, Infantile diarrhea, Cholera.
- Viral – Hepatitis A, Polio, Infantile Rota virus infection
- Protozoal – Amoebiasis, Giardiasis
- Helminthic – Roundworm, threadworm
- Leptospiral – Weil's disease
- Others – Schistosomiasis, Guinea worm infection, Fish tape worm.

water brash In hyperacidity or gastritis regurgitation of sour fluid and discomfort in epigastric region.

Waterhouse-Friderichsen syndrome This is manifested with Epidemic Cerebro spinal Meningitis and Bilateral Adrenal gland haemorrhage which is fulminating form of disease which ends with death due to coma and collapse.

Watson American biochemist who discovered the molecular structure of Nucleic acid in living tissues.

watt This is represented by "W" and is the unit of electric power at 1 joule per second or one ampere under a pressure of 1 volt.

wave Wave pattern in laboratory findings such as P wave, T wave in ECG or disturbances recorded like Brain waves.

wavelength Distance between the top of one wave to the other which is represented by λ.

wax They are esters of fatty acids and alcohols and is available in Yellow form and White form. Organisms like insects produce natural was. In human development of ear wax needs intervention to overcome hard of hearing.

WBC Abbreviation for **W**hite **B**lood **C**orpuscle.

wean To discontinue

weanling Infant is gradually allowed to artificial milk by discontinuation of breast milk by the mother.

web Meaning a membrane.

webbed That which is connected by a membrane.

Weber's corpuscle The Prostate Utriculus described by Weber.

Weber's disease This is clinically is called Encephalo Facial trigeminal angiomatosis where Port Wine stain is seen over the Trigeminal nerve area and on underlying meninges.

Weber's paradox This paradox described by Weber states 'Fully stretched muscle cannot contract'

Weber's syndrome This is clinically called as Alternating Oculomotor Hemiplegia wherein paralysis of the oculomotor nerve on the same side as the lesion producing ptosis, strabismus and loss of light reflex and spastic hemiplegia on the opposite side.

Weber's test When vibrating tuning fork is held on forehead and sound is heard well in affected ear it is conductive deafness. If the sound is heard well in normal ear it is sensorineural deafness.

Webster's operation Surgical correction by fixing the retro displaced uterus through round ligaments and broad ligaments.

Wechsler Adult Intelligence Scale This is abbreviated as W.A.I.S. a group of tests for assessment of intellectual functioning in adults.

Wechsler Intelligence scale for Children This is abbreviated as W.I.S.C. a group of tests for assessment of I Q in children between the age of 5 years and 15 years.

WEE Abbreviation for **W**estern **E**quine **E**ncephalomyelitis.

Wegner's disease In case of Hereditary Syphilis osteochondritis separation of the epiphyses is seen.

weight Importance given to a Mathematical Factor. The heaviness of an object which is due to gravitation force on that object.

Weil's syndrome This is a spirochetal infection causing Jaundice and is called LIH (leptospirosis ictero-hemorrhagica) always manifested in severe form of jaundice.

Weil-Felix test A test for the diagnosis of Typhus. The blood serum of patient suffering from typhus is tested against strains of Proteus vulgaris and is of three types. They are:

1. OX – 2
2. OX – 19
3. OX – K

Welch's bacillus The bacteria Clostridium perfringens discovered by Welch.

Wenckebach's phenomenon This is Second Degree Heart Block where one or more dropped beats occur periodically after a series of steadily increasing P – R intervals.

Werlhof's disease The Idiopathic Thrombocytopenic purpura described by Werlhof.

Werner's syndrome An Autosomal Recessive Trait characterized by Premature aging of the adult

Werner-His disease Trench Fever described by Werner and His.

Werner Schultz disease Werner syndrome (WS) or Werner's syndrome, also known as "adult progeria", is a rare, autosomal recessive disorder which is characterized by the appearance of premature aging.

Wernicke's encephalopathy This was described in 1981 by Wernicke now known as Thiamine deficiency disease which are common among alcoholics. This is manifested by neurological manifestations like confusion, drowsiness, altered gait, nystagmus and ophthalmoplegia.

Wertheim's operation This is a radical surgery for uterine cancer where the parts removed are Uterus, Fallopian Tubes, Parametrium, Tissues surrounding the upper vagina and Pelvic Lymphatics.

Westergren method This is the method of finding out E.S.R. (**E**rythrocyte **S**edimentation **R**ate)

Western blot technique It is a Technique for analysis and identification of a protein antigen. Electrophoresis is done to separate the proteins. Then is blotted or separated onto a membrane where they are binded for demonstration. Common Confirmatory test for ELISA done for HIV.

West Nile encephalitis It is a viral infection causing Encephalitis and was discovered in 1937 in Uganda.

wet-nurse A lactating women who give her breast milk to another's infant for nursing purpose.

Wharton's duct Submandibular Duct described by Wharton.

wheal A common manifestation of Allergy and is called Urticaria. Very common among sensitive people who can be provoked by mechanical irritation of skin.

wheeze Whistling noise of High pitch whistling noise generated from narrow airway. A common manifestation among asthma patients.

whey When the fat is removed from the milk the remaining proteins called lactalbumin and lactoglobulin are whey proteins.

Whipple's disease Intestinal Lipo Dystrophy described by Whipple.

whipworm A Nematode under Helminth Trichuris trichiura which cause intestinal parasitism.

whisper A soft, low, sibilant breathing sound which is soft and low that is air passing through glottis.

White Earlier work on prevention of Puerperal fever with the help of cleaning hand before delivery acclaimed as document in 1773 that was antedated the work of Ignaz Semmelweis in the crude discovery of sepsis during delivery which used to cause deaths among delivering women.

Whitfield's ointment Combined Benzoid acid and Salicylic acid ointment for skin lesions described by Whitfield.

WHO Abbreviation for **W**orld **H**ealth **O**rganisation under United Nation Organisation.

whoop In the phase of difficult inspiration of whooping cough the sonorous whoop is experience by the patient.

whooping cough One of the paediatric preventable infectious disease cause by a bacteria which has vaccine for proper prevention.

Wickham's striae Lines observed in Lichen Planus which are pale gray in colour.

Wigand's version In case of Transvers lie of foetus, Wigand's version is carried out by pushing the foetal head down with one hand and pushing buttocks up with the other hand to allow head presentation for normal delivery.

Wiggers diagram All events of a cardiac cycle are represented in a diagram which will give substantiate information on cardiac function. The events that are represented in the diagram are:

- ✓ ECG
- ✓ Pressure in Ventricle
- ✓ Pressure in atrium
- ✓ Pressure in the Aorta
- ✓ The ventricular volume
- ✓ Heart sounds Aortic Flow Rate
- ✓ Venous Pulse

Wilcoxon rank sum test This is a Non parametric statistical test to find out the significance of difference between matched pairs in two populations by using rank statistic.

wild Refers to the virulence of a pathogen

Williams' exercises To overcome Back Pain, this exercise is advocated wherein flexion of neck, trunk, pelvis, and lower limbs are done along with stretching extensor muscles in lower back and strengthening rectus abdominis muscle and gluteus maximum muscle.

Williams syndrome Also called Williams Beuren Syndrome after Willams and Beuren which has the following manifestations:

- ❖ Supra valvar aortic stenosis
- ❖ Mental retardation
- ❖ Hypercalcemia

This is also referred to as elfin facies syndrome by it's manifestation of elfin facies.

Wilms' tumor Malignant Tumor of the Kidney which grow rapidly. Nephroma as it is called is common in children below 5 years.

Wilson's disease An autosomal recessive trait with defective copper metabolism which allows the deposition of copper in liver, cornea and other organs giving rise to varied clinical manifestations.

Wilson's muscle Urethral sphincter muscle described by Wilson.

window An opening of an organ called fenestra.

windpipe This refers to the Trachea.

winking Closing and opening of the eyelids in quick succession.

Wintrobe hematocrit tube Used in the calculating haematocrit values.

Wirsung's canal, duct Pancreatic duct described by Wirsung.

withdrawal Patient suffering from schizophrenia and depression retreat from social contact and keep themselves aloof.

WMA Abbreviation for **W**orld **M**edical **A**ssociation.

wobble Unsteady movement of a person.

Wolfe's graft This is Full Thickness skin graft described by Wolfe

Wolff's duct Mesonephric duct described by Wolff.

womb Female reproductive major organ the Uterus.

World Health Organization (WHO) The agency of the U N in Geneva, Switzerland.

wound Tissue injury which cause altered structure and function. Types of wound are:

- Incised wound
- aseptic would
- Lacerated wound
- Opened wound
- Septic wound

W -plasty Technique in plastic surgery wherein lines of excision are put, triangular flaps are removed and segments are opposed. The surgery is ended with required sutures.

wrapping To put the cover around a structure.

Wright blood group Two group consisting of erythrocyte antigens a and b which are represented as under;-

- Wr^a
- Wr^b

wrist Joint which is articulated with radium bone and carpal bones at the junction of hand and forearm.

wristdrop Wrist not found functioning due to paralysis of the extensor muscles of the hand and fingers that is common in Leprosy and among painters with lead poisons

wryneck Tilted head due to torticollis or contracture of sternocleidomastoid muscle

wt Abbreviation for Weight.

Wuchereria Filaria worm is named after this physician who discovered it. W. bancrofti and W. malayi or Brugia malayi are two common filarial worms.

w/v This denote weight by per volume

Wynn method Reconstructive surgery method in Cleft lip. Repair by means of a long, narrow triangular flap.

X

x This represents the symbol for Abscissa in a graph.

ξ (xi) One of the Greek alphabet.

xanthelasma Eye lids showing xanthoma which is called xanthoma palpebrarum.

xanthematin When Haematin is mixed with Nitric acid a yellow substance is produced which is called xanthematin.

xanthene Xanthene (9H-xanthene, 10H-9-oxaanthracene) is the **organic compound with the formula $CH_2[C_6H_4]_2O$**. It is a yellow solid that is soluble in common organic solvents. Xanthene itself is an obscure compound, but many of its derivatives are useful dyes.

xanthin They are Carotenoids which are yellow pigments obtained from yellow flowers and other plants

xanthine In tissues it is in the form of Purine base that is produced by the degradation of Adenosine Mono Phosphate to Uric Acid.

xanthinuria Xanthine excretion in urine which is an Autosomal Recessive disorder where there is defect is there in Purine metabolism.

xanthism Albinism affecting skin and eye which is an autosomal recessive disorder.

xanthochromia Yellowish discoloration of the skin

xanthoma This is a tumor composed of lipid-laden foam cells

xanthosarcoma This is a tumor of malignant fibrous histiocytoma.

xanthosis Refers to yellowish discoloration

xeno That which is foreign or strange

xenoantigen More than one antigen detected in a person such as A and B antigens of the ABO blood group.

xenodiagnosis Animals are used in the diagnosis of pathological lesion in man. Animal inoculation followed by dissection of animals, Feeding insects and later entomological dissection of insects etc., are used in xenodiagnosis. In early century diagnosis of Chagas' disease and Trichinella spiralis infections were done through Xenodiagnosis.

xenograft Grafting or tissue transplanting is done between animals of different species.

xenology The science that deals with the relations of parasites to their hosts.

xenon Inert gas present in the atmosphere.

xenoparasite Organism becomes pathogenic because of weakening or reduced immunity of the host.

Xenopsylla They are wingless insects under the genus of fleas which are responsible in the transmission of Plague. Common Xenopsylla or Rat Flea are –

- X. astia
- X. brasiliensis
- X. cheopis

xero The word denotes Dryness.

xeroderma Dry, Rough and discolored skin which sometimes show desquamation.

xeroma Dry condition of conjunctiva which is called Xerophthalmia.

xeromenia All symptoms of menses is present but there will not be any blood flow.

xerophthalmia Symptom of vitamin A deficiency manifested by dryness of conjunctiva and of cornea.. Xerophthalmia is preceded by night blindness and conjunctival xerosis and it is succeeded by corneal xerosis and keratomalacia.

xeroradiography Dry recording of X-rays by using selenium and by photoelectric process.

xerosis Pathological dryness of eye, skin and mouth.

xerostomia Salivary gland dysfunction giving rise to dry mouth. Clinically it is present in Sjogren's Syndrome.

xerotic Characterized by or dryness.

xerotomography Dry tomography in which the images are recorded by xeroradiography.

xiphisternum Xiphoid process of sternum.

xiphoid Anatomical organ which is sword shaped. e.g., Xiphisternum.

xiphoomphaloischiopagus Condition where conjoined twins united from the level of the xiphoid process to the ischia.

xiphopagus Condition where symmetrical conjoined twins fused in the region of the xiphoid process.

X-linked Referred to Sex linked in genetics.

XO Denotes that one chromosome is present and the other either X or Y chromosome is absent.

X-ray Called Roentgen rays which are electromagnetic vibrations of short wavelengths Their penetrating property has helped in radiography for radiological diagnosis.

xylene It is Dimethyl Benzene that is used as solvent , as cleansing agent in microscopy.

xylitol A sugar alcohol used as sweetener in diabetes patients.

Xylocaine Local anesthetic containing Lidocaine.

xylol Chemically it is Xylene.

xylometazoline hydrochloride Drug used in Nasal congestion since it is a vasoconstrictor.

xylose Chemically it is an aldopentose with ribose from plants. Used as diagnostic agent in intestinal function.

xysma In stool of diarrhea bits of membrane is seen.

Y

y symbol for Vertical axis called Ordinate or y axis.

Y Upsilon the Greek letter.

yaw This refers to the lesions caused by Non Venereal or Non STD infection caused by a spirochete. Yaw is well differentiated from Syphilis by following manifestations:
It is not seen to produce CNS manifestations
It is not transmitted through placenta
Mother yaw is common skin lesions seen with the disease. Other types of lesions are a) Maize corn type of lesions b) ring like circular type of lesions

yawning Involuntary inspiration with the mouth open accompanied by body stretching.

yaws A non sexually transmitted disease caused by Treponema pertenue (a spirochete) in the tropics including India that is controllable or even eradicable with just Penicillin therapy.

yd Abbreviation for the measurement 'yard'.

yeast Single celled round fungi that belong to either Moniliaceae or to Endomycetales. Only a few yeasts are pathogenic.

yellow One of the primary colors in nature.

Yersinia Plague bacilli which cause bubonic plague which Gram negative and Facultatively anaerobic.

yohimbine This alkaloid is from Corynanthe or from Rauwolfia plants which has the Adrenergic blocking property . It is commonly used in Angina pectoris and as mydriatic. Yohimbine is known to have aphrodisiac property.

yolk It is the nutrient of the ovum. Egg yolk is a known nutrient.

Young's operation Surgical correction to form a new urethral tube in cases of epispadias.

Z

ζ One of the Greek alphabet zeta.

Zahn's infarct Hepatocellular atrophy gives rise to reddish blue discoloration in liver which is not a real infarct.

zeiosis Bubbling seen in a cell culture in artificial media.

Zeis' glands The name of Palpebral sebaceous gland.

zeisian stye Stye of palpebral sebaceous gland on the surface of the skin at the edge of the lid.

Zellweger syndrome The Cerebro Hepato Renal Syndrome described by Zellweger.

Zenker's degeneration Necrosis and hyaline degeneration of striated muscle, described by Zenker.

zidovudine Thymidine analog that inhibits replication of retroviruses and hence used in the treatment of AIDS.

Ziegler's operation This is undertaken to form an artificial pupil by **V** shaped iridectomy.

Ziehl-Neelsen stain Z N stain is done to identify Acid Fast Bacilli (AFB) They appear red against a blue background.

ZIFT Abbreviation for **Z**ygote **I**ntra **F**allopian **T**ransfer which is one of the treatments for infertility.

zigzagplasty To reduce the chance of long linear scars in surgery, short segments at right angles and alcute angles are done.

zoacanthosis Dermatitis caused by bristle, sting, hair, from animal origin.

Zollinger-Ellison syndrome This clinical condition is found to have the following triad:

1. Fulminating peptic ulcer
2. Severe gastric hyperacidity
3. Islet cell tumor of pancreas

zolmitriptan Drug used in Migraine

zona This is represented encircling area such as Zona ciliaris, Zona pellucida etc.,

zonula This is depicted by a small zonule such as Zonula ciliaris.

zonular That which is pertaining to a zonule.

zonule It is a small zone which is anatomically called as Zonula.

zonulitis Infection and inflammation of the zonula ciliaris.

zonulolysis When Chymotrypsin enzyme acts on Zonula ciliarus it dissolves and hence the name.

Zoogloea They are gram-negative, aerobic, rod-shaped bacteria of the family Pseudomonadaceae, present in water and sewage.

zoografting Graft tissue from different species taken for grafting to man.

zoology The scientific study of morphology, life cycle and habits of animals called zoobiology.

zoonosis They are mainly diseases of animals and man may get the disease from them. Common zoonotic diseases are;-

- Bacterial — Anthrax, Brucellosis, Leptospirosis, Plague
- Viral — Yellow fever, Japanese Encephalitis, Rabies
- Protozoal – Leishmaniasis, Trypanosomiasis
- Helminthic – Schistosomiasis, Echinococcosis,
- Taeniasis, Trichinellosis

zoonotic The related diseases of Zoonosis. Transmissible from animals to humans under natural conditions

zooparasite These are referred to animal parasites.

zoopathology This refers to Veterinary medicine.

zoophilia Fondness for animals in an unnatural way to the extent of sex with animals.

zoophilic Referred to mosquitoes which prefer to bite animals than man.

zooplankton Minute animal organisms called phytoplankton present in natural waters.

zooprophylaxis Preventive steps applied to animals so that the zoonotic diseases do not transmitted to man. Common example is to give rabies vaccine to dogs to prevent Rabies in man.

zoopsia Hallucination in which the patient thinks he sees animals.

zoopsychology Refers to animal psychology.

zoosperm This denote Spermatozoon.

zoospermia Live spermatozoa in the ejaculated semen.

zorubicin hydrochloride an antineoplastic chemically denoted - $\mathbf{C_{34}H_{35}N_3O_{10}\cdot HCl}$.

zoster Refers to Herpes Zoster.

Zovirax Preparations of Acyclovir the drug used in the treatment of AIDS

Z –plasty Plastic surgery for the release of contractures. With the help of Z shaped incision skin tensions is relaxed, brought to the desired position and two flaps are juxtaposed so that their apices cross the line of contracture.

Zumbusch's psoriasis Generalised Pustular Psoriasis described by Dr. Zumbusch.

zygal Any anatomical structure which looks like a yoke is suffixed with this word.

zygion A landmark at laterally situated point on either Zygomatic Arch. This is used in Craniometric analysis.

zygoma This is Zygomatic process of Temporal Bone and also called as Os Zygomaticum.

zygomatic That which is related with Zygoma.

zygomaticofacial Related to Zygomatic arch Zygomatic process Zygomatic bone and the face.

zygomaticofrontal Related to Zygomatic Arch, Zygomatic Process, Zygomatic Bone and the Frontal bone.

zygomatico-orbital Related to Zygomatic arch, Zygomatic process, Zygomatic bone and the orbit.

zygon The stem connecting the two branches of a zygal fissure.

zygosis conjugation of two unicellular organisms.

zygosity The condition relating to conjugation

zygospore Spore formed by the conjugation of two isogametes that are identical to each other

zygostyle This refers to the last coccygeal vertebra.

zygote This refers to the fertilized ovum. A male and a female gamete (sperm and ovum) unite to form Zygote.

zygotene The stage of the first meiotic prophase in which the two leptotene chromosomes undergo pairing

zymogen This is a proteolytic enzyme.